Textbook of Veterinary Medical Nursing

Edited by

Carole Bowden DipAVN(Surgical) VN
Head Nurse, Clifton Villa Veterinary Surgery, Truro; Trustee to RCVS; Senior BVNA Vice President;
Chief Examiner, RCVS VN UK

Jo Masters VN
VN Course Manager, Vetlink School of Veterinary Nursing, Somerset; BVNA Honorary Secretary; BVNA Pre-VN Chief
Examiner

Foreword by

Sharon Chandler VN DipAVN(Surgical)
Senior Nurse, Small Animal Wing, Queen's Veterinary School Hospital, Cambridge, UK

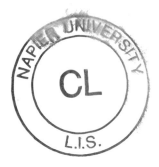

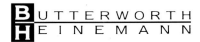
BUTTERWORTH
HEINEMANN

Edinburgh London New York Oxford Philadelphia St Louis Sydney Toronto 2003

Butterworth-Heinemann
An imprint of Elsevier Science Limited

ISBN 0 7506 5171 7

British Library Cataloguing in Publication Data
A catalogue record for this book is available from the British Library

Library of Congress Cataloging in Publication Data
A catalog record for this book is available from the Library of
Congress

Notice
Veterinary knowledge is constantly changing. Standard safety
precautions must be followed, but as new research and clinical
experience broaden our knowledge, changes in treatment and drug
therapy may become necessary or appropriate. Readers are advised to
check the most current product information provided by the
manufacturer of each drug to be administered to verify the
recommended dose, the method and duration of administration, and
contraindications. It is the responsibility of the practitioner, relying on
experience and knowledge of the patient, to determine dosages and
the best treatment for each individual patient. Neither the Publisher
nor the authors assume any liability for any injury and/or damage to
persons or property arising from this publication.

Where illustrations have been borrowed from other sources, every
effort has been made to contact the copyright owners to get their
permission. However, should any copyright owners come forward
and claim that permission was not granted for the use of their
material, we will arrange for acknowledgement to be made.

ELSEVIER SCIENCE your source for books,
journals and multimedia
in the health sciences
www.elsevierhealth.com

The
publisher's
policy is to use
**paper manufactured
from sustainable forests**

Printed in China by RDC Group Limited

Contents

Contributors

Victoria Aspinall BVSc MRCVS
Principal, Abbeydale Veterinary Training,
Gloucester, UK

Stephen J Baines MA VetMB PhD CertVR CertSAS
DipECVS MRCVS
Department of Veterinary Medicine, Queen's
Veterinary School Hospital, University of
Cambridge, Cambridge, UK

Joan Duncan BVMS PhD DipRCPath CertVR MRCVS
Clinical Pathologist, IDEXX Laboratories Ltd,
Wetherby, UK

Katie Dunn MA VetMB CVR CSAM MRCVS
Veterinary Editor, Vetstream, Cambridge, UK

Edward J Hall MA VetMB PhD DipECVIM-CA MRCVS
Senior Lecturer, Small Animal Internal Medicine,
Department of Clinical Veterinary Science,
University of Bristol, Bristol, UK

Alasdair Hotston Moore MA VetMB CertSAC CertVR
CertSAS MRCVS
Lecturer, Department of Clinical Veterinary
Science, University of Bristol, Bristol, UK

Karen Scott BSc AIBMS
Client Services Manager, IDEXX Laboratories
Ltd, Wetherby, UK

Melanie Simmonds DipAVN(Surgical) VN
Head Veterinary Nurse, The Veterinary Hospital
Group, Plymouth, UK

Jonathan Wray BVSc CertSAM MRCVS
Small Animal Hospital,
Department of Clinical Veterinary Science,
University of Bristol, Bristol, UK

Foreword

At last the arrival of a book that fills a niche in the veterinary nursing textbook market! To date all dedicated medical texts useful to the veterinary nurse have either been imported (usually from the American veterinary technician's market) or have required extrapolation from textbooks aimed at the veterinary surgeon.

Having read this textbook in its entirety I would recommend it to both students and qualified nurses alike. It is scientific in nature but nonetheless easy to read. The breadth and depth of the information presented is ample and well expressed, encouraging a practical approach to veterinary nursing.

The *Textbook of Veterinary Medical Nursing* is split into five chapters: *Fluid Management; Infectious Diseases; Common Medical Diseases; Medical Diagnostics; Laboratory Diagnostics*. This minimal split facilitates the speedy location of any particular subject area. At the beginning of each chapter there is a list of contents with the corresponding page numbers: this makes finding specific areas of interest extremely easy. Also within the text itself, bold sub-headings make navigation very straightforward.

The authors and editors have successfully maintained an easy-to-read style throughout, interspersing the text with much practical advice that not only brings medical nursing to life but also ensures that the book is enjoyable and interesting to read. Student nurses studying for their basic qualification will find the book a useful addition to the standard veterinary nursing text. It expands many theoretical aspects of medical nursing, whilst managing to keep information relevant to day-to-day nursing practice.

The medical nursing information supplied successfully covers much of the Advanced Medical Nursing Diploma's elective syllabus, and it does so to an appropriate level and in a manner that encourages nurses to assess patients more thoroughly, and have a more productive and informed input into patient care. For qualified veterinary nurses who wish to expand their medical nursing knowledge whilst studying for the Advanced Medical Diploma, or for others who simply want to improve their nursing skills, this book will undoubtedly be an essential acquisition. Much to the editors' and contributors' credit, the depth of scientific knowledge is of an advanced level, but easy to understand and well explained throughout. The use of well-annotated diagrams, clear illustrations and photography contributes effectively to the comprehension of the text. The inclusion of tabulated information makes the subject matter more accessible to the student.

The editors are both active veterinary nurses, who hold much knowledge of the requirements of the veterinary nurse in clinical practice. They are to be congratulated in their selection of contributors, all of whom have an active interest in the veterinary nursing profession and its advancement. They have skilfully managed to gather, both concisely and successfully, into a single textbook a large selection of theoretical and scientific knowledge, in addition to practical examples of medical nursing.

The *Textbook of Veterinary Medical Nursing* offers students and qualified nurses alike further knowledge and helpful practical advice to equip and enable them to implement improved patient care.

I feel sure that *The Textbook of Veterinary Medical Nursing* is set to become a core text for those studying for the Advanced Diploma in Veterinary Nursing (Medical).

Sharon Chandler

Preface

Medical nursing is a very well recognised and important role of the veterinary nurse. With the launch of the Diploma in Advanced Veterinary Nursing (Medical) in 2000, veterinary nurses are now able to further their knowledge and specialise in the medical nursing area. This in turn undoubtedly helps to improve job satisfaction and, most importantly, patient care.

Many books are available currently to address the demanding areas of veterinary nursing. We hope, however, that this book concentrating purely on the medical element will be able to offer something more dedicated and specialised.

We have included the medical nursing sections of the Royal College of Veterinary Surgeons (RCVS) Veterinary Nursing syllabus while providing full coverage of the syllabus for the Diploma in Advanced Veterinary Nursing (Medical). While it is difficult to cover every area in minute detail, we hope that this book will form the basis of reference and study materials both for those nurses embarking on the Diploma course and for those who have a vested interest in medical nursing. All contributors are well recognised within their chosen field, providing an invaluable source of knowledge and expertise, and we would like to take this opportunity to thank them for their continued support of the veterinary nursing profession and its development.

Carole Bowden
Truro and Langport 2003   Jo Masters

1

Fluid management

Melanie Simmonds

WATER IN THE BODY

COMPOSITION AND DISTRIBUTION OF BODY FLUIDS

Total body water in normal healthy animals represents approximately 60% of bodyweight although this varies considerably with age, sex and the proportion of body fat to lean tissues. In animals less than 6 months of age, water content may be as high as 70–80% of bodyweight but only 50–55% in those that are older or obese. This must be borne in mind when drawing up fluid therapy plans to ensure obese patients are not overhydrated nor young animals underhydrated.

Two thirds of total body water is contained within the intracellular compartment and the remaining one third is located extracellularly. Extracellular fluid (ECF) is further distributed between the water in the circulatory system but not including that contained within blood cells (i.e. plasma water), in the space between the cells of the tissues (i.e. interstitial fluid), and in the specialised transcellular fluids such as cerebrospinal and synovial joint fluids (see Fig. 1.1).

Sodium (Na^+), potassium (K^+), magnesium (Mg^{2+}) and chloride (Cl^{+-}) are the main ions contained within the body and together with calcium (Ca^{2+}), they are responsible for maintaining normal cellular function. Potassium and magnesium are the main cations contained within the intracellular fluid (ICF) together with phosphate anions (PO_4^{2-}), protein and smaller amounts of sodium. The ECF contains large volumes of sodium cations with chloride and

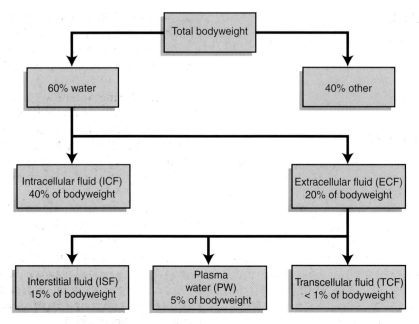

Figure 1.1 Distribution of water in the body. (Reproduced with permission from Cooper and Lane 1999.)

Table 1.1 Ionic composition of fluids in the body (reproduced with permission from Mathews 1996a)

	Plasma water	Interstitial fluid	Intracellular fluid
Cations (in mmol/l)			
Sodium	142.0	145.1	12.0
Potassium	4.3	4.4	150.0
Calcium	2.5	2.4	4.0
Magnesium	1.1	1.1	34.0
Total	**149.9**	**153.0**	**200.0**
Anions (in mmol/l)			
Chloride	104.0	117.4	4.0
Bicarbonate	24.0	27.1	12.0
Phosphate	2.0	2.3	40.0
Proteins	14.0	0.0	54.0
Other	5.9	6.2	90.0
Total	**149.9**	**153.0**	**200.0**

bicarbonate (HCO_3^-) as its neutralising anions (see Table 1.1).

HOMEOSTASIS OF EXTRACELLULAR FLUID

Two homeostatic mechanisms maintain the osmolality (concentration) and volume of the ECF (Hughes 1999):

1. Osmoreceptors in the hypothalamus detect the increase in plasma osmolality that occurs when water loss from the body exceeds water gain. This stimulates thirst and also the release of antidiuretic hormone (ADH), the latter of which acts upon the distal convoluted tubules (DCT) of the kidneys, promoting the reabsorption of water and concentration of the urine. When osmolality of the plasma reduces due to an excess of water gain over water loss, less ADH is produced resulting in reduced water reabsorption from the DCT and the production of more dilute urine.
2. Renal hypoperfusion stimulates the release of renin from the juxtaglomerular cells. Renin acts on angiotensinogen in the plasma to convert it to angiotensin I which is then converted to angiotensin II. Angiotensin II has a dual action acting on the proximal renal tubule to promote reabsorption of sodium and water, but also stimulating the release of aldosterone from the adrenal cortex which in turn promotes sodium reabsorption from the DCT.

WATER INTAKE

The normal healthy animal obtains water from two primary sources:

- ingestion of water
- metabolic water.

Ingestion of water

Ingested water, through the consumption of food and the drinking of fluids, provides the bulk of an animal's total water intake. The percentage of water in pet foods varies depending on the texture. Consequently, the volume of water that individual animals voluntarily drink will also vary depending on the composition and quantity of their diet. As tinned foods contain, on average, more than 70% water and dried foods less than 10%, animals fed only tinned food will obtain most, if not all, of their ingested water through diet alone and may need to drink voluntarily very little compared with those that are fed dried diets exclusively.

Metabolic water

Produced in the body as a result of nutrient oxidation, between 10% and 15% of an animal's total water intake is comprised of metabolic water. The actual volume produced will be dependent on the animal's diet as nutrients vary in the amount of metabolic water yielded. When metabolised, carbohydrates and fats are the greatest water-yielding nutrients, producing approximately 0.1 g of water per kilocalorie of energy released.

NORMAL WATER OUTPUT

The normal healthy animal loses water through:

- urinary losses
- faecal losses
- respiratory and cutaneous losses.

Urinary losses

Daily urinary water loss may be subdivided into *obligatory* water loss and *free* water loss (Kohn and DiBartola 1992). Obligatory water loss occurs even during periods of water deprivation and is necessary to excrete the daily renal solute comprised of dietary metabolites and by-products. The volume of free water loss varies and is increased during excessive water intake but decreased during periods of water deprivation to protect the animal from overhydration or dehydration, respectively. ADH controls the volume of free water loss from the kidneys and its secretion will be either stimulated or inhibited in response to water intake.

Normal urine output in the dog and cat is 1–2 ml/kg bodyweight/hour (i.e. 24–48 ml/kg bodyweight/24 hours). A urine output of less than 0.5 ml/kg bodyweight/hour is defined as oliguria and is indicative of renal hypoperfusion. If oliguria fails to improve with fluid therapy, the possibility of acute renal failure should be considered (Welsh 1994).

Normal urine specific gravity reference ranges in the dog and cat are:

- dog = 1.015–1.045
- cat = 1.020–1.060.

Faecal losses

Small obligatory water losses also exist to facilitate excretion of the faecal solute. Faecal water losses are elevated when the faecal solute increases or when gastrointestinal transit time decreases (e.g. with diarrhoea).

Respiratory and cutaneous losses

Together, these are described as *insensible* or *inevitable* losses as they cannot be regulated, even during periods of significant water deprivation. They may, however, be increased in response to elevations in ambient temperature or decreases in humidity.

Respiratory losses are particularly significant in dogs as they play an important role in thermoregulation, with panting increasing respiratory fluid losses. Cats' respiratory rates are raised to a lesser degree than dogs' in response to increases in ambient temperature and consequently respiratory losses are less significant. Cutaneous losses are less substantial in cats and dogs than other species because sweat glands are contained within the pedal pads only and do not play a significant role in thermoregulation. There have been reports however of cats in hot environments vigorously licking themselves with saliva to promote evaporative cooling (Chew 1965).

REQUIREMENTS FOR WATER INTAKE

It can be seen that each individual animal's specific water requirements vary and can only be quantified exactly when detailed and complex investigations and analyses of their ingested water intake, metabolic water gain and urinary, faecal and respiratory losses are undertaken.

As this specific information will not be routinely available on an animal's admission to the veterinary centre, a standard formula that best represents average water requirements is used to calculate maintenance needs and adjustments are then made to compensate for abnormal or ongoing losses. The formula used to calculate normal canine and feline maintenance water requirements is 50 ml/kg bodyweight/24 hours which represents:

- 20 ml/kg bodyweight/24 hours of normal urinary water loss
- 20 ml/kg bodyweight/24 hours of normal respiratory and cutaneous water loss

- 10 ml/kg bodyweight/24 hours of normal faecal water loss.

DEHYDRATION, FLUID AND ELECTROLYTE IMBALANCES

PATHOPHYSIOLOGY OF FLUID AND ELECTROLYTE IMBALANCES

Fluid imbalances can arise during periods of food and water restriction, whenever the usual sensible and insensible losses are exaggerated and/or when disease states cause other abnormal losses to occur. In some instances the losses will consist solely of primary water depletion although more commonly they will be accompanied by electrolyte imbalances. The possible causes of disturbances to water, electrolyte and acid–base balance are shown in Table 1.2.

Dehydration

Dehydration is the net reduction in the free water content of the body (Hughes 1999). It occurs when fluid losses from the body exceed the fluid intake and can be categorised according to the type of fluid lost and the effect this has on the tonicity of the remaining body fluids (DiBartola 1992b):

- Hypertonic dehydration. Losses of pure water and hypotonic fluid result in

Table 1.2 Common causes of the disturbances to water, electrolyte and acid–base balance (reproduced with permission from DiBartola 1992c)

Abnormality	Type of dehydration	Electrolyte balance	Acid–base status
Simple dehydration	Hypertonic	–	–
Heat stroke	Hypertonic	K+ variable Na+ variable	Metabolic acidosis
Anorexia/starvation	Isotonic	K+ loss	Mild metabolic acidosis
Vomiting	Isotonic or hypertonic	Na+, K+ and Cl− loss	Metabolic alkalosis
Diarrhoea	Isotonic or hypertonic	Na+ loss (K+ loss if chronic)	Metabolic acidosis
Diabetes mellitus	Hypertonic	K+ loss	Metabolic acidosis
Urethral obstruction or acute renal failure	Isotonic or hypertonic	K+ retention Na+ and Cl− variable	Metabolic acidosis
Hyperadrenocorticism	Isotonic	K+ loss	Mild metabolic alkalosis
Hypoadrenocorticism	Isotonic or hypertonic	Na+ loss, K+ retention	Metabolic acidosis
Haemorrhagic or endotoxic shock	Isotonic		Metabolic acidosis

Table 1.3 Clinical signs associated with dehydration

Estimated dehydration (% of bodyweight)	Clinical signs
<5%	Normal physical findings despite a history of fluid loss
5%	Dry oral mucous membranes
6–8%	Mild decrease in skin turgor. Dry oral mucous membranes. Slight tachycardia but normal pulse character. Slightly sunken eyes
8–10%	Moderate decrease in skin turgor. Dry oral mucous membranes. Tachycardia but normal pulse character. Eyes sunken within orbit. Slightly prolonged capillary refill time
10–12%	Marked decrease in skin turgor. Dry oral mucous membranes. Sunken eyes. Weak pulses. Prolonged capillary refill time (>2 s). Early signs of shock
12–15%	Marked decrease of skin turgor. Dry oral mucous membranes. Sunken eyes. Muscle weakness and collapse. Depression. Shock. Moribund

hypertonicity of the ECF relative to the ICF, causing the movement of water out of the cells and into the extracellular compartment.

- Hypotonic dehydration. Loss of hypertonic fluid results in hypotonicity of the ECF relative to the ICF, causing the movement of water out of the extracellular space and into the cells, thus exacerbating ECF deficits.
- Isotonic dehydration. No water movement occurs with the loss of fluid that has the same osmolality as ECF because, although the ECF volume is reduced, the tonicity is unaltered.

Degrees of dehydration are expressed as percentages of bodyweight. For each 1% of dehydration, a water deficit of 10 ml/kg bodyweight exists. Clinical signs associated with dehydration are outlined in Table 1.3.

Electrolyte imbalances

The causes of the principal electrolyte imbalances are described in Table 1.2. It can be useful to estimate the degree of any imbalance prior to commencing treatment by assessing plasma electrolyte levels. However, in the absence of such testing, diagnosis will be based solely upon history and clinical signs. The regular, ongoing assessment of plasma electrolytes can be useful in the monitoring of the effectiveness of fluid therapy.

Disturbances to acid–base status

The pH of a substance is defined as the negative logarithm of the hydrogen (H^+) ion concentration; i.e. the lower the pH the greater the concentration of hydrogen ions. The pH scale ranges from 1 to 14 with 7 being regarded as neutral, less than 7 as acidic and greater than 7 as alkaline.

The normal pH range of the extracellular fluid is 7.35–7.45, i.e. slightly alkaline. *Acidaemia* and *alkalaemia* describe serious states where the pH levels of the ECF are abnormal, i.e in acidaemia the pH has fallen below 7.35, rising to in excess of 7.45 in states of alkalaemia.

Acidosis and *alkalosis* describe pathophysiological processes that cause accumulation of either acid or alkali within the body. In acidosis and alkalosis, the pH of the blood remains normal because the body's secondary compensatory mechanisms act as lines of defence and prevent acidaemia or alkalaemia from occurring. These secondary compensatory mechanisms begin with a buffer response, which in turn stimulates a respiratory response and finally a renal response:

- Buffer response. Buffers are compounds that interact with acids and bases, preventing them from causing drastic changes in blood pH by trapping hydrogen ions until they can be delivered to the kidneys and excreted. Bicarbonate is the primary extracellular buffer with proteins and phosphates being the main intracellular buffers.
- Respiratory response. Respiration rate and tidal volume are controlled by chemoreceptors that detect changes in the H^+ ion concentration of the blood. Carbon dioxide (CO_2) when dissolved in water (H_2O) forms carbonic acid (H_2CO_3). In alkalosis,

respiration is decreased as this retains carbon dioxide (CO_2) which in turn increases the carbonic acid concentration in the blood. Increases in respiration are stimulated during acidosis to remove CO_2 from the body and lower carbonic acid concentration.
- Renal response: The kidneys regulate acid–base balance by controlling the levels of acid and base that are excreted in the urine. Plasma bicarbonate concentrations will dictate whether bicarbonate is either generated and reabsorbed by the kidneys or alternatively excreted. The kidneys are also capable of acid excretion.

Acidosis and alkalosis

These can each have metabolic or respiratory origins (see Table 1.2). Each of the primary metabolic disturbances will be accompanied by a secondary, adaptive response as the body attempts to overcome the initial insult (DiBartola 1992a):

- Metabolic acidosis. Characterised by a decreased plasma bicarbonate concentration. Secondary, adaptive response = respiratory alkalosis.
- Metabolic alkalosis. Characterised by an increased plasma bicarbonate concentration. Secondary, adaptive response = respiratory acidosis.
- Respiratory acidosis. Characterised by hypercapnia caused by alveolar hypoventilation. Secondary, adaptive response = metabolic alkalosis.
- Respiratory alkalosis. Characterised by hypocapnia caused by alveolar hyperventilation. Secondary, adaptive response = metabolic acidosis.

Simple acid–base disorders describe those where the disturbance is limited to the primary disorder and the secondary, adaptive response. Mixed acid–base disorders are said to occur whenever two primary disorders exist or when the secondary, adaptive response exceeds that expected.

ASSESSMENT OF FLUID, ELECTROLYTE AND ACID–BASE IMBALANCES

History

The route(s) of fluid losses, the length of time over which they have occurred and their approximate quantity need to be ascertained as accurately as possible. Owners should be asked open questions (i.e. those requiring descriptive responses) regarding the animal's food and water intake (e.g. anorexia, polydipsia, starvation), gastrointestinal losses (e.g. vomiting and diarrhoea), increased or decreased sensible or insensible losses (e.g. polyuria, oliguria, excessive panting, fever) and other traumatic/non-traumatic losses (e.g. haemorrhage, vulval discharges).

Physical examination

The degree of dehydration can be estimated by assessing the colour and moistness of the oral mucous membranes and corneas, heart rate and peripheral pulse character, capillary refill time, and the position of the eyes within the orbits. Skin turgor can also be assessed but is relatively subjective, being dependent not only on interstitial fluid volume but also on the subcutaneous fat content and skin elasticity of the animal. Bodyweight measurement can be useful as an acute loss of 1 kg implies a 1000 ml fluid deficit. Unfortunately, an accurate weight of the animal prior to the onset of illness is rarely available, making bodyweight comparisons difficult. Additionally, third space losses as seen with intestinal obstruction and peritonitis can cause dehydration due to a loss of circulating volume but as the fluid lost from the ECF remains within the body, weight loss will not be a factor in these particular animals.

Laboratory analyses

It is important to run basic laboratory tests prior to commencing fluid therapy to provide a base level against which follow-up tests can be compared. Such tests should include the following as a minimum:

- packed cell volume (PCV)
- haemoglobin (Hg)
- total plasma protein (TPP)
- urine specific gravity (USG).

Blood urea, creatinine and plasma electrolytes are also useful.

PCV, Hg and TPP will increase with all fluid losses except acute haemorrhage, although care must be taken when interpreting the results of either Hg in anaemic animals or TPP when there is a pre-existing hypoproteinaemia.

USG will be expected to increase in the dehydrated animal as the urine should become more concentrated. Failure of the urine to concentrate may indicate the existence of diabetes insipidus. A refractometer should be used to measure USG accurately. Dipsticks are calibrated for human urine and are not reliable for use with veterinary patients.

FLUID THERAPY

INTRODUCTION

Fluid therapy is a supportive treatment, the aims being to restore the volume and composition of body fluids to normal by correcting water and electrolyte imbalances, to improve and maintain renal function, and to provide the necessary water and electrolytes required for maintenance and replacement of ongoing losses. Fluids may also be used to provide parenteral nutrition. When drawing up a fluid therapy plan it is important to consider the following (DiBartola 1992c):

1. Is fluid therapy indicated?
2. What type of fluid is indicated?
3. What route should be used to administer the fluid?
4. What rate should the fluid be administered at?
5. What volume of fluid is required?
6. When should fluid therapy be stopped?

ROUTES OF ADMINISTRATION OF FLUID THERAPY

Intravenous

This is the chosen route to replace severe and acute losses in shocked, dehydrated and hypotensive patients. As fluids can be administered quickly and directly into the vascular space, rapid improvements in the animal's condition may be achieved. The most frequently used veins in the cat or dog are the cephalic and jugular, although the lateral and medial saphenous veins are also available. Intravenous fluid therapy in rabbits is best achieved using the marginal ear vein. A range of different fluids can be administered by this route including hypertonic, hypotonic and isotonic electrolyte solutions, as well as blood products. However, hand-in-hand with these advantages are a number of disadvantages including the need for specialised, sterile equipment, and the increased risk of side effects such as thrombophlebitis, embolism and overinfusion.

Subcutaneous

In dogs and cats, the subcutaneous space is relatively large allowing the administration of approximately 10 ml/kg bodyweight of isotonic or hypotonic fluids per site although the actual volume that can be administered is also dependent on skin elasticity. Volume overload is unlikely to occur. However, it is unsuitable for the correction of severe or acute losses and is inadequate in hypothermia or moderate to extreme dehydration as the peripheral vasoconstriction that occurs reduces the absorption and dispersion of the fluid. Care is necessary with repeated administration as it is associated with pain, infection and in the worst cases, skin sloughing.

Oral

Physiologically, this is the ideal route for the administration of water, electrolytes and nutrients as the intestine acts as a selective barrier absorbing only substances that are needed. Its use is limited to animals that are willing to eat and drink, are only mildly dehydrated and not suffering from any form of gastrointestinal dysfunction. It is relatively inexpensive, associated with minimal side effects and simple to undertake, so much so that it can be performed by owners as part of a home nursing programme. This route is unsuitable for severely dehydrated patients as the rate of absorption is not sufficiently rapid.

A number of different feeding techniques enable this route to be used in anorexic animals. Short-term therapy can be administered by stomach tube or per os syringe. Longer-term therapy is better performed via nasogastric, pharyngostomy or gastrostomy feeding tubes.

Intraperitoneal

The peritoneum has a large surface area that allows the rapid and efficient absorption of relatively large volumes of fluid. To prevent the osmotic movement of fluid from the ECF and into the abdomen, the use of hypertonic solutions is contraindicated and only isotonic or hypotonic solutions should be administered. Aseptic technique is essential to prevent infection which can lead to peritonitis. The risk of damage to the internal abdominal organs is minimised by ensuring the animal is adequately restrained and the procedure is performed by experienced personnel. This route is useful in neonates and rodents.

Intraosseous (intramedullary) (Fig. 1.2)

The intraosseous route is useful in very young or small animals where venous access is difficult to achieve. Unlike an animal's veins, the bone mar-

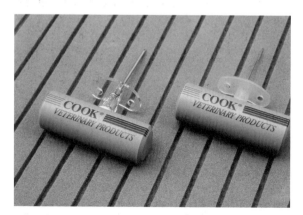

Figure 1.2 Intraosseous needle. (Reproduced with permission from Cook Veterinary Products.)

row does not collapse during periods of hypovolaemia and so access to the bone marrow is more rapidly achieved and with greater success than a venous cutdown. The most suitable sites include the intertrochanteric fossa of the femur, the tibial tuberosity, the wing of the ileum and the greater tubercle of the humerus. Initial placement of the intraosseous needle is painful although ongoing administration of the fluid is generally well tolerated. Aseptic technique is vital to avoid infection and osteomyelitis. Damage to the growth plates is a potential complication when used in young animals.

Rectal

This is employed fairly infrequently as fluid selection is limited to isotonic or hypotonic solutions and it cannot be used in the presence of diarrhoea. Fluid is easily administered although it must be instilled into the colon where water absorption is efficient. Administering into the rectum rather than the colon will simply produce an evacuant enema.

RANGE AND COMPOSITION OF FLUIDS AVAILABLE FOR PARENTERAL ADMINISTRATION

Table 1.4 shows the ionic composition of the commonest fluids available.

Crystalloids

These are sodium-based, non-colloidal, electrolyte solutions most of which are similar in composition and tonicity to plasma water. They enter the ECF and temporarily increase blood volume before passing through cell membranes and equilibrating with the ICF. If renal function is normal, they are rapidly excreted in the urine. Examples of crystalloids are:

1. Normal saline (0.9% NaCl). This contains mainly water with sodium and chloride but no potassium. It is indicated in acute secondary dehydration or to replace fluid and electrolyte losses where the nature of the clinical disorder is associated with hyperkalaemia.

Table 1.4 Ionic composition of the common replacement fluids (adapted with permission from Hughes 1999)

Solution	Electrolyte concentration (in mmol/l)					Osmolality (mOsm/l)
	Na$^+$	K$^+$	Ca^{2+}	Cl$^-$	HCO$_3^-$ precursor	
NaCl 0.9%	150			150		308
Dextrose 5%						252
NaCl 0.18% + 4% dextrose	30			30		
Hartmann's	131	5	2	111	29 (lactate)	272
Ringer's	147	4	2	155		310
Gelofusine	77			62.5		279
Haemaccel	145	5.1	6.25	145		

2. Dextrose 5% (or glucose 5%). This consists of water with dextrose (or glucose) added at a concentration of 50 mg/ml. As the solution contains no electrolytes, it is indicated in situations of primary water loss such as simple dehydration, or to treat hypoglycaemia.

3. Dextrose saline (4% dextrose + 0.18% NaCl). This consists of water with small amounts of sodium and chloride added, and also dextrose at a concentration of 40 mg/ml. It is used in primary water loss or as a maintenance fluid as it contains the correct amount of sodium per unit volume necessary for maintenance. If used for long-term maintenance, hypokalaemia is prevented by adding potassium to the drip bag and administering at a maximum rate of 0.5 mmol/kg bodyweight/hour.

4. Hartmann's solution (also called lactated Ringer's or compound sodium lactate). The electrolyte concentration of Hartmann's is similar to that of ECF. It contains potassium, calcium and relatively high levels of sodium and chloride. It also contains lactate as a precursor of bicarbonate, the bicarbonate being produced when lactate is metabolised by the body. Indicated in the treatment and correction of metabolic acidosis.

5. Darrow's solution. This has a similar composition to Hartmann's solution but contains increased amounts of potassium and lactate. Its primary indication is in the correction of metabolic acidosis where there is also a potassium deficiency, e.g. chronic diarrhoea.

6. Ringer's solution. This has a similar composition to Hartmann's solution except that it contains no lactate. It is used mainly to treat cases of metabolic alkalosis where there is also a potassium deficiency, e.g. persistent vomiting.

7. Sodium bicarbonate (2.74% or 5.0% or 8.4%). Used as an alternative to lactate in the treatment of acidosis. When acidosis is suspected but cannot be measured, sodium bicarbonate is administered at a rate of 1–2 mmol/kg i.v. (An 8.4% solution of sodium bicarbonate contains 1 mmol/ml of bicarbonate.)

Colloids

These contain large molecules that remain in the intravascular space for up to 24 hours before being excreted. They increase the effective osmotic pressure of plasma, expand plasma volume and are indicated during severe hypovolaemia where a rapid improvement in cardiovascular function is required. It is important to remember that following severe haemorrhage, although plasma expanders will increase the circulatory volume they will not replace lost red cells. Therefore, following colloid administration, although the effective circulatory volume will be restored, the blood's oxygen-carrying capabilities will remain reduced. Consequently, in instances of severe haemorrhage when whole blood is unavailable, colloids should be administered whilst simultaneously providing oxygen supplementation. Examples of colloids are:

1. 'Haemaccel'/'Gelofusine'. These isotonic gelatin-based fluids are used as plasma expanders, remaining in the circulation for approximately 5 hours and being almost fully excreted within 24 hours. Occasional sensitivity

reactions have been reported. Otherwise these are very safe and useful agents. They are stored at room temperature and administered through standard fluid-giving sets. Their administration will not interfere with blood cross-matching tests.

2. Dextrans. Dextran 40 and Dextran 70 are hypertonic solutions that contain high-molecular-weight glucose polymers in either 5% dextrose or 0.9% sodium chloride. Care is needed as the administration of large volumes may interfere with blood clotting mechanisms, causing either haemolysis or the clumping together of red cells. Their administration also interferes with the interpretation of blood cross-matching tests. The hypertonicity of these solutions can result in intravascular cellular dehydration which is prevented by simultaneously administering crystalloids. Depending on the molecular weight, these solutions will remain within the circulation for between 2 and 24 hours.

3. Mannitol. This hypertonic solution must not be used as a plasma expander. Instead, it is used to promote osmotic diuresis in poisonings, cerebral oedema, and also to re-establish renal function.

Blood products

1. Whole blood. Administration is species specific. It is indicated in haemorrhage, hypovolaemia or circulatory deficiency where there is effectively >30% loss of blood volume. Dependent on the anticoagulant, blood can be refrigerated for up to 4 weeks.

2. Plasma. Administration is species specific. It contains all of the clotting factors except platelets and is indicated in multiple clotting factor defects and hypoproteinaemia. It is also used in the correction of hypovolaemia whenever whole blood is unavailable. Plasma can be stored safely for up to 6 months at −70°C.

3. Packed red cells. Indicated in the treatment of anaemia. Prior to administration, packed red cells are resuspended in 0.9% NaCl to reduce viscosity. Solutions such as Hartmann's and Ringer's are unsuitable for resuspension as the calcium they contain can react with the citrate used to collect the blood resulting in

coagulation. After collection and separation, packed red cells can be refrigerated for up to 3 weeks.

Donor selection

When selecting a donor certain criteria must apply:

- Donors must be fit, healthy, free of disease and fully vaccinated.
- Donor PCV measurements must be >40% in dogs and >30% in cats.
- Feline donors must test negative for feline leukaemia virus (FeLV), feline immuno-deficiency virus (FIV), feline infectious anaemia (FIA) and feline infectious peritonitis (FIP).
- Canine donors must weigh at least 25 kg; feline donors must weigh at least 4 kg.
- No donor is to be obese.
- Donors must have a suitable temperament to permit the collection of the blood.
- No donor should be bled more frequently than at 3–4 weekly intervals.
- There should be no history of a donor having previously received a blood transfusion.

Eight different blood groups have been identified in dogs and one in cats (see Box 1.1). Of the canine blood groups, DEA 1.1, 1.2 and 7 will produce antibodies if incompatibly transfused, thus increasing the incidence of incompatibility reactions when the recipient receives second and subsequent transfusions. Incompatibility reactions are unlikely in dogs receiving first transfusions as naturally occurring antibodies to these blood groups are rare. Ideally, canine donors should be

---

Box 1.1   Canine blood groups and feline blood types

Canine blood groups
DEA = dog erythrocyte antigen
Eight canine blood groups exist:

DEA 1.1	DEA 1.2
DEA 3	DEA 4
DEA 5	DEA 6
DEA 7	DEA 8

Feline blood types
One blood group with three blood types exists:
  Blood type A
  Blood type B
  Blood type AB (rare)

negative for DEA 1.1, 1.2 and 7 (Knottenbelt and Mackin 1997a).

Unlike dogs, naturally occurring antibodies to red cells of other blood types exist fairly commonly in cats. Reactions to first transfusions are not uncommon. Type A cats given type B blood will usually show signs of only a mild transfusion reaction. However, type B cats that receive type A or AB blood show very acute and severe signs with the incompatibility reaction often proving fatal. For this reason, feline donors and recipients should be blood typed or cross-matched prior to transfusion (Knottenbelt and Mackin 1997b).

Collection of blood

In the UK, the Royal College of Veterinary Surgeons (RCVS) ethically approves the collection of blood for immediate transfusion but not the storage of blood or blood products for future needs (Hughes 1999). Donated blood should ideally be transfused immediately after collection and if plasma or packed red cells are required instead, these should be promptly separated by centrifugation. When blood is to be transfused immediately after collection, either heparin or ethylenediaminetetraacetic acid (EDTA) anticoagulants can be used. If however, there is to be a delay in transfusion, anticoagulants with preservative properties such as Citrate Phosphate Dextrose (CPD) or Acid Citrate Dextrose (ACD) are necessary. With CPD the blood can be refrigerated for 4 weeks and up to 3 weeks with ACD.

In dogs, blood is usually collected into commercially prepared blood bags that contain a specific volume of anticoagulant for one unit (450 ml) of blood. If less than 450 ml of blood is to be donated, a proportion of the anticoagulant should be removed from the bag prior to collection as there is a risk of hypocalcaemia in the recipient when too great a concentration of citrate anticoagulant is present in the transfusion. In cats, blood is best collected into a 60 ml syringe that contains 1.4 ml of ACD or CPD anticoagulant (withdrawn from a standard blood collection bag) for every 10 ml of blood that is to be donated.

The total blood volume in ml of canine and feline donors can be calculated as follows:

- canine = 90 × lean bodyweight in kg
- feline = 66 × lean bodyweight in kg.

Generally, 10% of a donor's blood volume can be collected without causing the donor any adverse effects. Up to 20% of the donor's blood volume can be collected if intravenous crystalloid fluids are administered simultaneously during the donation and for 45 minutes afterwards. The volume administered should be 2–3 times the amount of blood collected – this compensates for the rapid movement of 75% of the fluid out of the circulation shortly after administration (Knottenbelt and Mackin 1997a).

Blood for transfusion is usually collected from the jugular vein. The cephalic vein is not recommended as its lower pressure can increase the risk of clots forming during collection due to the slow movement of the blood. The patient is restrained in a sitting position or in lateral recumbency and the skin then surgically prepared before applying sterile Xylocaine gel to minimise discomfort during venepuncture.

Collection requires a minimum of three personnel. At least one person (and possibly two) will need to restrain the patient. Collection of one unit takes several minutes and full cooperation of the patient is maximised with good restraint and by providing praise and reassurance. Another person will perform the jugular venepuncture keeping the needle in position and maintaining the raised pressure of the vein throughout collection. Finally, another assistant gently rotates the bag to ensure the blood evenly mixes with the anticoagulant. It is advisable to weigh the bag at regular intervals to determine when the correct volume of blood has been collected. As 1 ml of blood weighs approximately 1 g, one whole unit will weigh 450 g (plus the weight of the bag and anticoagulant). The blood bag must be fully labelled with the date of collection, the donor name and blood group (if known), and the expiry date.

EQUIPMENT AVAILABLE FOR INTRAVENOUS FLUID THERAPY

Intravenous access

A range of needles and catheters are available (Fig. 1.3). Selection will usually depend on

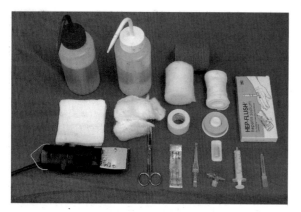

Figure 1.3 Intravenous catheter equipment. (Courtesy of Adam Coulson, Veterinary Hospital Group.)

availability, personal preference, patient requirements and cost:

- Over-the-needle catheters. Well suited for placement into peripheral veins, their soft construction minimises trauma or the risk of displacement outside of the vein.
- Through-the-needle catheters. Their length makes this type well suited for central venous access from peripheral sites.
- Winged (butterfly) needle catheters. More suitable for single use rather than indwelling purposes as the needle can easily traumatise the vein when left in situ.

Giving sets

A wide range is available. Standard fluid giving sets are simple in construction delivering either 15 or 20 drops per ml and can be used to administer crystalloids or colloids. Variations of the standard giving set include the addition of a burette to enable measured volumes of fluid to be delivered at a time, coiled tubing to prevent twisting and kinking of the giving set in restless animals, multiple port flow connectors to permit simultaneous infusion of compatible solutions, and paediatric sets that deliver 60 drops per ml enabling more accurate administration of fluid in small animals.

Also available are blood giving sets that incorporate an in-line filter to remove clots and debris.

Infusion pumps and syringe drivers

Two types of fluid pump are available – the rate consistent pump and the volumetric pump (Fig. 1.4). Syringe drivers are a type of rate consistent pump used to deliver drugs or fluids at a constant rate (Fig. 1.5). In practical fluid therapy, volumetric pumps are more useful as they enable a prescribed volume of fluid to be delivered over a period of time. In each case, these pumps

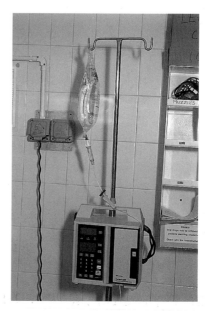

Figure 1.4 Infusion pump. (Courtesy of Alasdair Hotston Moore, University of Bristol.)

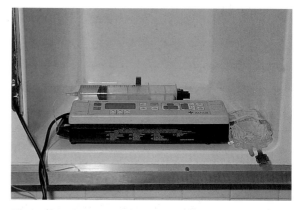

Figure 1.5 Syringe driver. (Courtesy of Alasdair Hotston Moore, University of Bristol.)

deliver fluid at the desired rate and under sufficient pressure to overcome resistance caused by viscous solutions, filters and kinks in the giving set. Many pumps will stop delivery of fluid when air bubbles are detected in the tubing. Usually, an alarm sounds to alert personnel to this and to any other problems such as emptying of the fluid bag or catheter blockage.

PRACTICAL FLUID THERAPY

Over-the-needle catheter placement is a procedure that qualified veterinary nurses should be competent and confident in performing. The placement of through-the-needle catheters is less commonly performed in small animal practice and only veterinary nurses working in intensive care units may actually be inserting these on a regular basis. Intraosseous needle placement is most likely to be performed by a veterinary surgeon. Veterinary nurses who have a familiarity with and understanding of each of these procedures will be more effective when preparing the equipment and assisting during placement (see Appendices 1, 2 and 3).

The general equipment that should be prepared for intravenous catheter and intraosseous needle placement is described in Box 1.2.

BLOOD TRANSFUSION THERAPY

Donor/recipient matching

There are two methods available to determine compatibility of canine and feline donors and recipients: *cross-matching* and *blood typing*.

Cross-matching

Two tests are performed (see Box 1.3):

• Major cross-match: performed with recipient serum and donor cells, this is necessary prior to the transfusion of whole blood and packed red cells but not plasma.
• Minor cross-match: performed with donor serum and recipient cells, this is necessary prior to the transfusion of whole blood and plasma but not packed red cells.

Box 1.2 Equipment required for the placement of intraosseous needles or vascular catheters

• Suitable needle or cannula depending on the procedure, e.g. intraosseous needle, over-the-needle cannula, or through-the-needle cannula
• Clean latex examination gloves
• Clippers with a number 40 blade or blunt, curved scissors
• Gauze swabs
• Skin preparation agents, e.g. chlorhexidine gluconate or povidone–iodine skin scrub, 70% isopropyl alcohol, skin antiseptic
• 1 ml syringe filled with lidocaine (lignocaine) hydrochloride (for intraosseous catheter placement) and a 23G/25G hypodermic needle
• No. 11 scalpel blade
• 2 ml syringe filled with heparinised saline (1–2 IU heparin/ml)
• Bung, three-way tap and/or giving set
• Tape to secure cannula in place
• Suture material, needle and needle holders for securing in place intraosseous catheters or cannulae inserted into the medial saphenous or femoral veins
• Padding material and cohesive bandage

Box 1.3 Blood cross-matching method (reproduced with permission from Knottenbelt and Mackin 1997a)

Major cross-matching method
Apparatus should be maintained at 38°C.

1. Donor blood is collected into ethylenediaminetetraacetic acid (EDTA) anticoagulant and centrifuged at 3000 rpm for 10 min.
2. The supernatant (plasma and buffy coat) is drawn off and discarded. The red cells are washed by resuspending in warm saline (at 38°C).
3. Centrifugation is repeated and the saline supernatant removed.
4. The red cells are resuspended in a measured volume of warm saline to produce a 3–5% solution.
5. Two drops of the donor erythrocyte suspension are added to 1–2 drops of heparinised recipient plasma in a test tube or well plate (slides can be used if necessary but produce less reliable results).
6. The mixture of cells and plasma is examined for evidence of haemolysis (seen as reddening of the solution that fails to separate out) or agglutination (seen as irregular buttons or clumping).
7. Compatibility is demonstrated by the absence of haemolysis, and the lack of agglutination which is shown by sedimentation into a smooth button at the bottom of the tube.

Minor cross-matching is performed using the same steps but with donor plasma and recipient cells.

Blood typing

Commercial desktop kits are available to identify canine donors that are DEA 1.1 and 1.2 negative, and also to determine the blood typing of feline donors and recipients.

Administration of blood products

Collected blood must be inspected prior to use for clots, deterioration and any damage to the packaging that may affect sterility. The expiry date must also be checked. Refrigerated blood and fresh or frozen plasma should be steadily warmed in a water bath to 37°C and the bag should be gently rocked to mix the contents.

Blood giving sets must be used as they contain an in-line filter to remove small clots and debris that might otherwise embolise within the recipient. Blood that has been collected from a feline donor into a syringe should be transferred aseptically into a blood bag (from which all anticoagulant has been removed) to enable administration through a blood giving set.

For the first 15 minutes, blood should be administered slowly at a rate of 0.25 ml/kg bodyweight to allow for the observation of reactions. Baseline levels for temperature, pulse, respiratory rate, mucous membrane colour and PCV should be recorded prior to administration with continued monitoring of these parameters throughout transfusion. After 15 minutes, the transfusion rate is increased to a maximum of 22 ml/kg/24 hours although in severely hypovolaemic animals, this rate can be increased temporarily to 22 ml/kg/hour. ECG monitoring is recommended with the latter, as cardiac arrhythmias can occur with rapid transfusion rates (Mathews 1996b).

Complications of blood transfusion therapy

These should rarely occur if blood typing, cross-matching, collection and administration are performed correctly. The animal should be closely monitored for signs of complications which include:

- Immunologic transfusion reaction. When seen in dogs at first transfusions, these are not usually life threatening and signs are limited to pyrexia, facial oedema, urticaria and vomiting. More severe reactions may be seen during second transfusions or when type B cats receive type A blood and include haemoglobinuria due to the intravascular destruction of red blood cells, tachycardia, weakness, disseminated intravascular coagulation (DIC) and renal failure.
- Hypocalcaemia. A result of citrate toxicity, it can occur when blood products anticoagulated with ACD or CPD are administered too rapidly, or when the anticoagulant is too concentrated within the transfusion (Hughes 1999). It is also seen in hypothermic animals or those with liver disease due to an altered metabolism of citrate (Authement 1992). Signs include restlessness, muscle tremors, cardiac arrhythmias and vomiting. The transfusion should be slowed and calcium gluconate may be administered if necessary, although through a different intravenous line to avoid coagulation of the blood product being transfused.
- Circulatory overload. This is most likely to occur when packed red cells or plasma are administered to normovolaemic patients to correct anaemia or hypoproteinaemia. Pulmonary oedema and restlessness will be evident. The transfusion should be stopped. Diuretic therapy may be indicated.
- Sepsis. Bacterial contamination of the blood can occur if aseptic technique is breached during collection or if the product is inappropriately stored.

CALCULATION OF FLUID THERAPY REQUIREMENTS

The golden rule of 'replacing like with like' in fluid therapy applies not only to the type of fluid used but also the rate of replacement. Depletions that occur over a long period of time require slow, steady replacement whereas very sudden losses need to be replaced rapidly. Fluid therapy can therefore be categorised as *acute* or *chronic* (Hughes 1999).

Acute fluid therapy

The degree of hypoperfusion dictates the rate of administration. Provided there are no contraindications to rapid fluid therapy (e.g. the presence of cardiorespiratory disease or renal failure), the maximum rates of infusion are as follows (Hughes 1999):

- mild hypoperfusion: 20–40 ml/kg bodyweight for the first hour
- moderate hypoperfusion: 40–60 ml/kg bodyweight for the first hour
- severe hypoperfusion: 60–90 ml/kg bodyweight for the first hour.

Chronic fluid therapy

Chronic rather than acute losses occur in animals that are dehydrated but not seriously hypo-volaemic. These losses should be replaced over 12–24 hours. In calculating the volume required, the following need to be evaluated:

- Pre-existing deficits. Presenting clinical signs indicate the percentage of dehydration which enables the approximate fluid deficit to be calculated. (For every 1% of dehydration, an approximate deficit of 10 ml/kg bodyweight exists.) Generally, half of this volume should be delivered during the first 6–8 hours of fluid therapy.
- Maintenance requirements. A formula of 50 ml/kg bodyweight/24 hours is used. Maintenance requirements are calculated from the point when fluid therapy is commenced until food and water intake is resumed.
- Ongoing losses. Occasionally, it will be possible to measure ongoing losses accurately

---

Box 1.4   An example of a fluid therapy plan

Patient
A 3-year-old, female neutered German Shepherd weighing 34 kg. Normal ratio of body fat to lean tissue. No pre-existing disorders.

History
Fully vaccinated. Anorexia of 3 days' duration. Eight episodes of diarrhoea over the past 48 hours.

Clinical examination
Tachycardia (130 beats/min). Moderate pulse strength. CRT of 2s and slight pallor of oral mucous membranes. Moderate decrease in skin turgor observed when skin between the shoulder blades is raised. Dry oral mucous membranes. Eyes sunken within orbits. Depressed. Elevated PCV and Hg.

FLUID REQUIREMENT

Replacement
Each 1% of dehydration represents a fluid deficit of 10 ml/kg bodyweight. Clinical signs indicate a dehydration of 10%
= 10 (ml) × 34 (kg) × 10%
= 3400 ml   *Use Darrow's solution*

Maintenance
Maintenance fluid requirement = 50 ml/kg bodyweight/day
= 50 (ml) × 34 (kg)
= 1700 ml   *Use 4% dextrose + 0.18% NaCl*

Ongoing losses
Use formula 4 ml/kg bodyweight/diarrhoea and readjust fluid plan accordingly. In this patient, the approximate fluid lost with each motion of diarrhoea
= 4 (ml) × 34 (kg)
= 136 ml

Daily fluid requirement
Replacement and maintenance requirements to be delivered over 24 hours, with half the replacement requirements being delivered over the first 6 hours. Giving set delivers 20 drops per ml.
First 6 hours: = half of replacement losses
                = 1700 ml of Darrow's solution
                = 283 ml/h
                  (i.e. 1700 ml divided by 6 h)
                = 4.7 ml/min
                  (i.e. 283 ml divided by 60 min)
                = 94 drops per minute
                  (i.e. 4.7 ml × 20 drops/ml)
Next 18 hours: = remaining 1700 ml of Darrow's
                solution + 1700 ml of dextrose saline
                = 188 ml/h
                  (i.e. 3400 ml divided by 18 h)
                = 3.1 ml/min
                  (i.e. 188 ml divided by 60 min)
                = 62 drops per minute
                  (i.e. 3.1 ml × 20 drops/ml)
The infusion of Darrow's solution will end after the fifteenth hour of fluid administration. Dextrose saline will be administered for the last 9 hours.
Fluid requirements will be re-evaluated after 24 hours or as and when ongoing losses occur.

although normally they can only be estimated. Fluid lost from diarrhoea and vomiting is estimated using the formula of 4 ml/kg bodyweight for each motion of vomit or diarrhoea.

An example of a fluid therapy plan is given in Box 1.4.

MONITORING DURING FLUID THERAPY

Regular monitoring of the patient and the equipment is vital (see Box 1.5). Fluid therapy is a dynamic process and should be reviewed at frequent intervals and adjusted according to the animal's progress and ongoing needs. Parameters such as peripheral pulse rate and quality, capillary refill time (CRT), mucous membrane colour and the temperature of the extremities give a good indication of the adequacy of peripheral perfusion. In hypovolaemic or shocked patients with hypotension, blood flow to the peripheral tissues is reduced in an attempt to maintain normal perfusion of the vital organs. A weak pulse, prolonged CRT and pale mucous membranes will be evident but should improve with fluid therapy as the blood pressure is restored. Chest auscultation allows the detection of abnormalities such as pulmonary oedema and cardiac arrhythmias.

Central venous pressure (CVP) is a measurement of the pressure in the cranial vena cava immediately proximal to the right atrium and is used to assess intravascular fluid requirements and monitor the effectiveness of fluid therapy (Fig. 1.6). The normal CVP range in small animals is 0–5 cm of water (Mathews 1996a). However, as CVP varies considerably between individual animals, one-off measurements have little value except to indicate an abnormally high or low circulating volume. Repeated measurements will demonstrate changing trends and so are far more useful in the monitoring of fluid therapy (see Appendix 4).

Box 1.5 Monitoring patients receiving fluid therapy (reproduced with permission from Cooper and Lane 1999)

Temperature
- Core body
- Limb (extremities)

Cardiovascular system
- Peripheral pulse rate, rhythm and strength
- Heart rate, rhythm and character
- Capillary refill time
- Mucous membrane colour
- Jugular distension
- Central venous pressure
- Mean arterial blood pressure
- Thoracic auscultation (to detect cardiac arrhythmias and pulmonary oedema)

Respiratory system
- Respiratory rate, depth and pattern
- Thoracic auscultation (to detect pulmonary oedema)
- Venous and arterial blood gases

Other observations
- Urine output (to assess renal function)
- Peripheral oedema
- Bodyweight
- Skin turgor
- Demeanour

Equipment checks
- All connections and the patency of tubing and catheters
- Fluid administration rates
- Catheter insertion site for evidence of phlebitis or extravasation

---

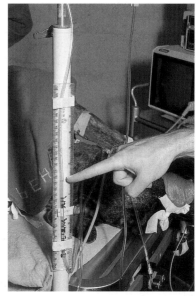

Figure 1.6 Central venous pressure measurement. (Courtesy of Alasdair Hotston Moore, University of Bristol.)

A number of complications can occur, particularly with intravenous fluid therapy. These can be due to equipment faults or problems with the patient. Regular monitoring enables complications to be detected and treated at an early stage. Detailed and accurate record keeping is vital.

COMPLICATIONS OF INTRAVENOUS FLUID THERAPY

There are a number of possible complications of intravenous fluid therapy although most are avoidable if catheters are inserted correctly, maintained aseptically and cared for appropriately.

Thrombophlebitis

A combination of localised endothelial inflammation and thrombus formation, thrombophlebitis can be initiated by many different factors including:

- mechanical, e.g. placement of the catheter in close proximity to a joint
- chemical, e.g. following administration of irritant drugs
- infectious, e.g. poor aseptic technique during catheter insertion.

Localised signs of inflammation will be seen such as pain and erythema of the skin overlying the catheter, which will progress to hardening of the vein and ultimately, complete occlusion of the blood vessel. Systemic signs of thrombophlebitis such as pyrexia may also be evident (Hansen 1992).

Thrombosis

Intravenous catheters left in situ for more than 3–4 hours will become enclosed in a sheath comprised of fibrin and platelets. As the catheter is removed, the sheath detaches from the surface and a thrombus forms that either becomes incorporated within the wall of the vein, or enters the circulation as an embolus. Usually, such thrombi or emboli are so small in size and number they remain insignificant although very occasionally they will combine or increase in size causing a blockage. Mechanical factors are most likely to cause thrombi formation including the use of stiff or damaged catheters and veins that overlie joints (Hansen 1992).

Infection

Risks of localised and systemic infection are significantly reduced if the catheter is placed and maintained aseptically. Incidence of infection is likely to be increased with patients that contaminate the insertion site or the giving set tubing with urine, faeces or saliva. Localised and systemic signs will be similar to those of thrombophlebitis. When infection is suspected, the skin is given a full surgical preparation and the catheter then removed.

Perivascular administration (extravasation)

The infiltration of fluid into the perivascular tissues is most likely to occur when the catheter is displaced outside of the vein. The use of butterfly needles or stiff catheters is most likely to cause this as they can easily penetrate the vein wall. Signs of peripheral vein extravasation include localised swelling and tenderness at the site of the catheter tip. If irritant fluids or drugs are administered, the signs will be more severe and possibly accompanied by localised necrosis and sloughing of the skin. Central venous extravasation may not become apparent until much larger volumes of fluid have been delivered. Dyspnoea as a result of fluid build-up in the mediastinum or pleura will be evident.

Extravasation is avoided by using the smallest and softest catheters available and selecting a large vein, ideally positioned away from a joint. If the catheter must be inserted close to a joint, limiting movement by immobilising the limb with a splint is advisable. All catheters should be flushed with saline prior to injecting irritant drugs to confirm patency and positioning (Hansen 1992).

Catheter embolism

This occurs when a section of the catheter becomes detached inside the vein and carried around the circulation until it lodges in the heart or pulmonary artery. Rarely, it will be due to a faulty catheter where the shaft becomes disconnected from the hub. More commonly it is a result of accidental severing of the catheter due to poor insertion, carelessness when cutting the tapes securing the catheter in place, or following patient interference.

If severing of the catheter is seen to occur, action needs to be swift if there is to be any hope of successfully retrieving the fragment. A tourniquet is applied proximally to the site of insertion with the aim of impeding further movement of the embolus. The location of a section of a radiopaque catheter can be identified by radiographing the animal. If possible, the fragment should then be removed surgically (Hansen 1992).

Air embolism

This is potentially a very serious complication as it may, in some cases, result in respiratory or cardiac arrest. Very small air bubbles will usually go unnoticed although larger emboli will cause respiratory distress, pulmonary oedema and cardiovascular collapse (Hansen 1992).

Although it can occur whenever an intravenous catheter is in place, the risk is greatest during catheter insertion. Proper bleeding of giving sets to remove all air is vital. If someone else has set the equipment up ready for use, it is imperative to check this has been carried out. Never assume this is the case as removing air from the vascular space once it has been administered necessitates central venous catheterisation and aspiration of the air from the right atrium and ventricle, which is both invasive and not guaranteed to be successful.

Exsanguination

This is a complication that can arise whenever the giving set tubing becomes detached from the catheter, but the catheter remains securely in place. Usually this occurs because the patient has bitten through the giving set or has moved in such a way as to cause disconnection. If the animal is not being observed closely and such disconnection occurs, a significant volume of blood will continually ooze from the vein with disastrous consequences (Hansen 1992).

Overinfusion

Circulatory overload can occur whenever an animal is receiving intravenous fluid therapy although it is particularly likely with the following (Welsh 1994):

- when cardiac output is reduced, e.g. if fluids are being administered to support an animal with congestive heart failure
- when renal function or urine output is reduced, e.g. if fluids are being administered in acute renal failure or to a patient with a blocked urethra
- when fluids are being administered to normovolaemic patients, e.g. if blood is being used to treat chronic anaemia.

Signs of volume overload include restlessness, tachypnoea, serous nasal discharge, chemosis, weight gain, vomiting, subcutaneous oedema and pulmonary oedema.

Recommendations for the prevention of complications of intravenous fluid therapy

1. Use the smallest and softest catheter that is adequate.
2. Use the largest appropriate vein.
3. Avoid placing catheters close to the site of a joint, and when this is unavoidable, immobilise the limb with a splint.
4. Ensure that aseptic technique is not broken during the placement of the catheter and that the catheter is maintained aseptically and managed properly.
5. Ensure that all equipment is functional, correctly assembled, in date and sterile.
6. Unwrap bandages or tapes when removing catheters rather than using scissors. If

scissors must be used, cut at a site that is distant from the catheter.

7. Apply Elizabethan collars to animals that are biting or nibbling at the catheter or giving set.

8. Never attempt to withdraw or reinsert misplaced catheters with the needle positioned below the surface of the skin. Instead, the misplaced catheter and needle should be fully withdrawn as a whole unit and reinserted only if they are undamaged.

9. Reinforce attachments between catheters and giving set tubing with tape to prevent disconnection.

10. Remove catheters after 48 hours or before if there is evidence of localised or systemic infection.

11. Calculate accurately the volume of fluid required and ensure this is delivered at the correct rate.

12. Perform regular checks of the patient and the equipment to ensure complications and faults are detected early on.

URINARY CATHETERISATION

Monitoring urine output is essential with all patients receiving fluid therapy to confirm that renal function is adequate. During fluid therapy, urine should be produced at a minimum rate of 1 ml/kg bodyweight/hour.

Aseptic technique, atraumatic insertion and proper patient monitoring are vital to ensure that complications such as trauma, cystitis and catheter blockage are prevented.

Equipment (Fig. 1.7)

Catheters

Dog catheters Available in sizes 6FG, 8FG and 10FG, these catheters are constructed from polyamide and consist of a rounded tip and two small drainage holes proximally, and a Luer hub distally. They are designed for single use only but can be adapted for indwelling use by applying zinc oxide butterfly tapes to the catheter and then suturing to the preputial or perivulval skin. Their

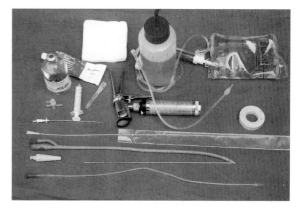

Figure 1.7   Equipment for urinary catheterisation. (Courtesy of Adam Coulson, Veterinary Hospital Group.)

main disadvantage is their length (50–60 cm) which can be excessive in smaller breeds.

Bitch catheters There are three types of catheter:

• Foley. Available in sizes 8FG to 16FG, these are made from latex rubber. The catheter comprises an inflatable balloon situated just distally to the drainage holes at the catheter tip. Inflation of this balloon with air or sterile water/saline after correct insertion into the bladder makes the catheter indwelling. Balloon deflation allows catheter removal. The volume of air or water required to inflate the balloon is stated on the port at the distal end of the catheter. Foley catheters are soft and flexible and so non-traumatic during insertion. However, this lack of rigidity can also mean that placement into the urethral orifice is difficult, although it is made easier by inserting the tip of a metal stylet into one of the drainage holes.

• Tieman's. Although originally designed for use in the human male, these have since found favour in veterinary practice as the curved tip can assist insertion. Available in sizes 8FG to 12FG, its excessive length (43 cm) is disadvantageous except in very large breeds.

• Metal. Although the rigidity of these catheters can make insertion of the tip into the urethral orifice easier, there is also the significant risk of causing urethral trauma during placement. The use of these catheters is no longer recommended.

Dog catheters have also been used with great success in the bitch as a result of their extra rigidity over the Tieman's and Foley types.

Cat catheters Two types of catheter are available, both in sizes 3 FG and 4FG:

- Jackson. These are made from flexible nylon and comprise a thin metal stylet that extends along the length of the catheter lumen. This stylet provides rigidity to the catheter and greater control during insertion. The stylet is removed once the catheter has been placed. The catheter flange comprises a number of small holes that can be used to secure it in place by suturing to the preputial or perivulval skin.
- Conventional. These are a smaller version of the dog catheter. They are unsuitable for indwelling use as they are excessively long (30 cm) and also the catheter hub does not contain holes to allow it to be secured in place.

Urinary catheters are designed for single use only. When a decision is taken to clean and re-sterilise catheters, this is often false economy as the time and resources necessary are often more costly than the catheters themselves. Additionally, after repeated use, the catheters can become damaged, which increases the risk of trauma during insertion. Foley catheters must never be reused as the balloon weakens after each inflation, with the risk of bursting on subsequent insertions.

Lubricants

Three types of lubricant are available:

- petroleum-based, e.g. 'Vaseline'
- water-based, e.g. 'KY Jelly'
- water-based with local anaesthetic added, e.g. 'Xylocaine Gel'.

It is important to check the contents of lubricants prior to use as they may not be compatible with all catheters. Petroleum-based lubricants must not be used with latex catheters such as Foley types as the rubber will deteriorate. The lubricants used should be sterile and applied sparingly – normally it is necessary to lubricate just the tip to ensure non-traumatic passage along the urethra. The advantage of using lubricants that contain local anaesthetics is they desensitise the urethral opening during insertion.

Specula/light sources

These aid catheter placement by retracting the vaginal tissues thereby allowing good visualisation of the urethral orifice. Some specula have built-in light sources. If not, a pen torch can be held in place by an assistant to illuminate the vaginal tissues. Speculum blades should be sterile. Various varieties of speculum can be used to aid urinary catheterisation including nasal specula, rectal specula and auriscopes.

Miscellaneous

Other equipment will also need to be available when preparing for urinary catheterisation including gloves, antiseptic solution and swabs to clean the urogenital area, and a spigot (necessary with Foley catheters to create a Luer connection).

Procedures for urinary catheterisation

Equipment is prepared in advance and laid up on a clean, draped surface where it is easily accessible. The urogenital area is cleansed with a mild antiseptic and then rinsed with saline. This removes discharges, surface dirt and debris and is important to avoid introducing infection into the bladder. With long-haired animals, it can be useful to clip the hair around the prepuce and vulva although permission must first be sought from the owner.

Once the tip of the catheter enters the bladder, urine should start to flow down the lumen. At this point there should be no further advancement of the catheter as there is a risk of it knotting if too much length is positioned inside the bladder. The knotted catheter would need surgical removal.

It is sensible to fit Elizabethan collars to patients with indwelling catheters to prevent self-removal.

Dog

Most dogs can be catheterised without the need for chemical restraint. With the dog in either a standing or laterally recumbent position, one hand is used to grasp the caudal os penis and retract the prepuce caudally, whilst the other inserts the catheter.

The lubricated tip of the catheter is aseptically inserted, usually by feeding the catheter through its protective sleeve, although alternatively, a sterile glove could be worn. Once inserted into the urethral opening, the catheter is gently and steadily advanced into the bladder. Resistance to the passage of the catheter may be experienced at the caudal point of the os penis where the urethra narrows slightly. Steady, gentle pressure should be applied to overcome this resistance. It may be necessary to re-catheterise with a smaller-gauge catheter.

Bitch

Although catheterisation can be performed without chemical restraint, mild sedation is useful to aid positioning, particularly if dorsal recumbency is to be used. Alternatively, the bitch may be restrained in a standing position or in lateral recumbency.

The blades of a vaginal speculum are passed through the vulval lips and into the vestibule, taking care to avoid the clitoral fossa, which is located ventrally. The lubricated catheter tip is inserted into the external urethral orifice, which can be visualised on the floor of the vestibule, and advanced into the bladder. If difficulty is experienced locating the urethral opening, caudal retraction of the vulva by an assistant can sometimes aid visualisation (White 1999).

Tom

If the patient's health permits it, sedation or light anaesthesia can be useful to avoid causing undue stress.

The tom is restrained in dorsal or lateral recumbency with the hindlimbs pulled cranially. The penis is extruded by pushing the prepuce cranially and the tip of the lubricated catheter is inserted into the urethral opening and advanced into the bladder. Once inserted into the urethra, gentle retraction of the prepuce caudally can assist further advancement if resistance is experienced.

Queen

Chemical restraint is usually necessary. Lateral recumbency is preferred.

The vulval lips are grasped gently and retracted caudally. The catheter tip is inserted along the floor of the vestibule and blindly into the urethral opening, a small depression located on the vestibular floor. If the urethral opening cannot be located blindly, a small auroscope head may be used as a vaginoscope to allow visualisation.

Urine collection systems

Indwelling catheters should be connected to sterile closed urine collection systems. Commercial systems are available although an empty and aseptically assembled intravenous fluid giving set and bag will suffice (Fig. 1.8). With the latter, care must be taken to ensure that the giving set control is not accidentally turned off as this will prevent urine from flowing out of the bladder.

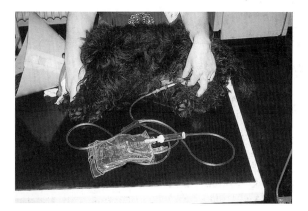

Figure 1.8   Urine collection bag connected to patient. (Courtesy of Alasdair Hotston Moore, University of Bristol.)

Urine scalding and an ascending bacterial infection resulting in cystitis are potential complications of indwelling urinary catheters that are not attached to closed collection systems. Both of these complications will cause unnecessary suffering to the patient and may prolong recovery.

SHOCK

INTRODUCTION

Many textbook definitions of shock exist. The earliest are fairly vague and non-specific. It is only during recent years that definitions have become more specific to describe the manifestations of shock with particular emphasis on the deranged tissue perfusion and disrupted cellular oxygen utilisation that occurs.

A definition by Tobias and Schertel (1992) states 'Shock is the clinical state resulting from an inadequate supply of oxygen to the tissues or an inability of the tissues to properly utilise oxygen'. Note there is deliberately no mention of hypovolaemia as a derangement in tissue perfusion can also occur in the presence of normovolaemia and hypervolaemia. Additionally, the term 'clinical state' cannot be qualified more specifically as the presenting clinical signs vary considerably depending on the aetiology of the condition and the individual case.

CLASSIFICATION OF SHOCK

Various types of shock exist. Classification is based on pathophysiology, i.e.:

- hypovolaemic
- traumatic
- cardiogenic
- distributive.

Hypovolaemic shock

This occurs when a loss of circulating volume causes severe tissue hypoperfusion. The physiological response to hypovolaemia is vasoconstriction as this raises blood pressure, improves venous return and redistributes blood from non-essential tissues to the coronary and cerebral circulation. Hypovolaemic shock can develop as a result of mixed water and electrolyte losses or severe haemorrhage. Healthy animals will normally be able to tolerate acute losses of up to 10% of the circulating volume before signs of shock start to develop.

Traumatic shock

Shock due to trauma is relatively common and is often complicated by haemorrhage or sepsis. An initial increase in cardiac output, heart rate and contractility occurs after an intense vasoconstrictive response. However, tissue damage following the initial insult stimulates the release of inflammatory mediators from traumatised cells which in turn causes further cellular damage.

Cardiogenic shock

This results from impaired cardiac systolic or diastolic function. Causes include myocardial, pericardial or valvular diseases that impair contractility and ventricular filling. Hypotension is a common factor of this type of shock as cardiac output is reduced even though blood volume remains normal or may even be increased. Increased intra-atrial pressures develop due to the reduced cardiac output and this leads to congestion and oedema in the dependent tissues (i.e. the lung and liver).

Distributive shock

Septic shock and anaphylactic shock both fall into this class. Vasoactive inflammatory mediators interfere with normal physiological mechanisms that regulate blood pressure. This leads to hypotension, maldistribution of blood flow and vasodilation causing clinical signs that are unlike those seen with other forms of shock. Hyperaemic mucous membranes, a rapid CRT, a bounding pulse quality and warm extremities are all characteristics of this type of shock.

Sepsis results when bacteria or their toxins are present in the circulation of a patient. Septic shock exists when signs of shock accompany clinical signs of sepsis. Anaphylactic shock occurs following an allergic reaction to an antigen to which the patient has been sensitised and signs of shock may be accompanied by urticaria, bronchospasm and laryngeal oedema.

Failure to reverse shock

Failure to correct the state of shock will result in irreversible cell damage as a consequence of the following (Aldrich 1999):

- Vasoconstrictive compensatory measures affect vital organs causing ischaemia, hypoperfusion and tissue hypoxia.
- A prolonged reduction in coronary blood flow damages the myocardium resulting in decreased cardiac output and further compromised coronary perfusion.
- Reduced cerebral perfusion impairs the vasoconstrictive response causing further decreases in cerebral and coronary blood flow.
- Cells damaged during shock release inflammatory mediators which in turn cause further cellular damage.

THE SHOCKED PATIENT

Patient evaluation

Evaluation of the patient should incorporate:

- history taking
- physical examination
- laboratory tests.

This is vital to ensure that shock is correctly diagnosed and the cause identified, thereby enabling an appropriate plan of treatment to be drawn up.

History

Depending on the circumstances under which the animal is presented, the quantity or quality of the history will vary considerably. There will be times when there is limited history available as the animal is brought in as an injured stray. On other occasions, the owner will be able to provide a detailed history. Open questions should be used ensuring that leading questions are avoided if an accurate and detailed history is to be obtained.

Physical examination

As shock is a dynamic and progressive condition, a thorough and accurate examination of the patient at an early stage is vital not only to achieve an initial diagnosis but also to provide a baseline against which a subsequent improvement or deterioration can be measured. The following clinical signs are associated with abnormalities of intravascular and/or interstitial volume.

Mental state

The brain has a high metabolic rate, requiring constant supplies of oxygen and glucose to function normally (Aldrich 1999). Hypoperfusion of the brain and the subsequent reduction in availability of oxygen and glucose result in altered behaviour and a reduced level of consciousness.

Colour and moistness of mucous membranes

Pallor of the mucous membranes is indicative of either anaemia or vasoconstriction of the peripheral blood vessels. Red, injected, hyperaemic mucous membranes due to peripheral vasodilation are common in cases of distributive shock. Dryness of the mucous membranes is associated with reduced interstitial fluid volume although this is a difficult parameter to assess, particularly in the presence of hypersalivation, for example due to nausea or periodontal disease (Aldrich 1999).

Capillary refill time

This is usually evaluated using the oral mucous membranes and should be less than 2 seconds in a normal healthy animal but may be prolonged in states of vasoconstriction or lessened in the presence of vasodilation. It is important to remember that the CRT provides an indication of peripheral vasomotor tone only and not cardiac output (Aldrich 1999).

Heart rate

Heart rate during shock becomes elevated in an attempt to increase cardiac output. Tachycardia is commonly seen but will usually respond to any treatment that restores circulating volume. In severe shock, tachycardia can be so pronounced that there is insufficient time for ventricular filling to occur adequately, resulting in a decreased stroke volume and consequently cardiac output will be reduced rather than increased.

Pulse quality

Peripheral pulses should be palpated to assess their quality. The pressure of the pulse represents the difference between systolic and diastolic blood pressure and gives an indication of stroke volume and vasomotor tone. Vasoconstriction and small stroke volume are common reasons for a poor pulse quality.

Temperature (core body and extremities)

Comparing core temperature with that of the extremities provides useful information about the degree of peripheral perfusion. Normally, a 4°C difference will exist between the two (the core temperature being the highest). When peripheral vasoconstriction occurs, the extremities will feel cool as the blood flow to the area is reduced and a greater difference between the two measurements will be recorded.

Laboratory tests

Blood samples should be obtained at the earliest possible opportunity and prior to commencing treatment. As a minimum, PCV, haemoglobin and total plasma proteins should be assessed.

TREATMENT OF THE SHOCKED PATIENT

Any treatment plan needs to focus on addressing the underlying cause as well as correcting each of the signs and symptoms. Many shocked patients will be exhibiting a number of different problems and so prioritising their treatment is vital. Triage assessment is often undertaken by veterinary nurses who must be able to identify accurately and prioritise the needs of shocked patients if treatment is to be swift and effective. The role of the triage veterinary nurse may involve:

- initial assessment of the animal as it arrives at the veterinary centre
- alerting the veterinary surgeon, advising of the animal's condition
- providing first aid in the absence of a veterinary surgeon
- preparing equipment to enable diagnosis and treatment to be undertaken by the veterinary surgeon
- liaising with the client, as necessary, to ensure he/she is kept informed.

The plan of treatment will include first aid to correct any life-threatening aspects of the syndrome followed by circulatory volume restoration to improve tissue perfusion and then drug therapy as necessary to treat acidosis, provide antibiosis and guard against any complications. Importantly, each patient must be treated as an individual as the causes of shock, the manifestations and the response of different patients to certain types of treatment can be so variable.

First aid treatment

The rules of A, B, C (airway, breathing, circulation) must be observed.

Compromised ventilatory effort must be supported with the provision of oxygen therapy. Masks will usually be tolerated by animals that have a reduced level of consciousness, although for other patients this may only heighten any fear or distress. Nasal catheters and oxygen tents are useful and less distressing alternatives, with endotracheal intubation being suitable for unconscious patients. Control of haemorrhage and the dressing of burns is vital in animals presented with hypovolaemic shock.

Resuscitation in the event of cardiac or respiratory arrest will be necessary in some instances and this is a procedure with which all veterinary nurses must be able to assist efficiently.

Fluid therapy

Fluid therapy has been discussed extensively in the previous section. The choice of fluid used will depend upon the cause of shock and the degree of hypoperfusion.

Drug therapy

There are various indications for drug therapy:

- to treat metabolic acidosis
- to treat anaphylaxis
- to provide antibiosis
- to suppress the inflammatory response.

Metabolic acidosis is common in shocked patients as decreased tissue perfusion and anaerobic metabolism cause an increase in blood lactate levels. Lactate accumulates intracellularly and then diffuses into the extracellular space where it causes a decrease in bicarbonate and a resulting acidosis. As perfusion improves and oxygen delivery to the tissues is restored, the liver becomes more capable of metabolising lactate and the acidosis is resolved. Therefore, acidosis is best treated with fluid therapy and oxygen delivery although administration of bicarbonate may also be indicated.

Intravenous adrenaline (epinephrine) is indicated to treat life-threatening anaphylactic shock.

Broad-spectrum antibiotics are indicated in cases of severe shock and particularly where sepsis is suspected or when there is a likelihood of intestinal tract trauma/ischaemia, as the latter can lead to the development of bacteraemia and endotoxaemia.

The use of corticosteroids to suppress the inflammatory response is questionable. There is no doubt that their use is associated with many potential benefits including stabilisation of lysosomal membranes and improved oxygen transport in peripheral tissues. Concern exists over their potential for causing gastrointestinal and renal injury and increased susceptibility to infection.

Nutrition

Hypermetabolism may be a factor of septic or traumatic shock, with the basal metabolic rate being increased by 50–100... little or no caloric intake... develop. High-quality nu... be provided at the earliest op... enteral route cannot be used it will ... to address caloric needs using intraven... fluids. However, it is unlikely that the full calorie requirements of these patients can be provided parenterally and enteral nutrition should therefore be instituted as early as possible.

MONITORING OF THE SHOCKED PATIENT

The standard of nursing of shocked animals can contribute significantly to either the recovery or deterioration of the patient. Nursing includes supportive care but also close monitoring to detect subtle changes in the condition of the animal.

Monitoring of the patient will include many of those parameters that are assessed in patients receiving fluid therapy (as outlined in Box 1.5). Urine output is important as it provides a fairly reliable indication of tissue perfusion. A urine output of less than 0.5–1.0 ml/kg bodyweight/hour in an otherwise healthy patient without pre-existing renal disease indicates hypoperfusion of the kidneys, and from this it can be assumed that hypoperfusion of other tissues exists simultaneously. CVP and mean arterial blood pressure are also useful with sequential readings to demonstrate trends, being preferable to single one-off measurements. In many veterinary practices, CVP and arterial blood pressure monitoring may not be readily available. However, good-quality monitoring can still be performed by simply using the senses of sight, hearing and touch as well as basic tools such as a thermometer and stethoscope.

Detailed record keeping is vital. This enables other personnel to see at a glance what treatments have been given, the animal's current state and also its response to therapy. It also demonstrates the degree of monitoring that has been performed, which is vital should an owner question the standard of care that the pet has received – an important consideration as we now work within a very litigious society and our

er records must back up the high standards
care we are providing.

APPENDIX ONE

Procedure for the placement of an over-the-needle intravenous catheter

The full equipment required should be selected beforehand. Aseptic technique is essential. If aseptic technique is broken due to contamination of the insertion site or the catheter shaft, the procedure must be started again with fresh equipment. Proceed as follows:

1. A wide margin of hair is clipped from the skin at the intended site of venepuncture. Ideally, electrical clippers and a no. 40 blade are used as these clip much closer to the skin. However, with fractious patients scissors may be less frightening.
2. The operator washes the hands and dons a pair of clean examination gloves.
3. The skin is prepared in the same way as for surgery. Gauze swabs soaked in a surgical scrub solution are used to clean surface debris from the skin, a process that will normally take 2 minutes or more. The swabs should be changed frequently, with each one being inspected before discarding. This process should continue until used swabs appear clean. Isopropyl alcohol (70%) is applied and the skin preparation finished by painting with an iodine or povidone–iodine solution.
4. The operator changes the gloves. An assistant restrains the animal and raises the vein. Once the operator has visualised the position of the raised vein, the assistant releases pressure to enable the operator to make a small stab incision in the skin at the correct site but without the vein raised at the time – damage to the raised vein could occur if the animal were to move unexpectedly.
5. The assistant re-raises the vein. The operator grasps the combined catheter and stylet unit between the thumb and forefinger of the dominant hand and the limb is grasped in the palm of the other. The catheter unit is inserted

bevel edge upwards through the stab incision and into the vein. Once blood is visualised in the hub of the stylet, the whole unit is inserted a further 2–3 mm to ensure that both the stylet and also the catheter shaft have penetrated the wall of the vein.

6. The less dominant hand is adjusted to grasp the hub of the stylet between the thumb and either the second or third finger. At this point, it is important for the operator not to release grasp of the leg as the animal may pick up on this sudden change in restraint and react by withdrawing the leg. With the stylet held in position, the dominant hand is used to advance the catheter into the vein. The catheter should advance freely without resistance or kinking and blood should continue to flow into the hub of the stylet. If kinking or resistance is noted, both the catheter and stylet should be removed and pressure placed over the insertion site to minimise haematoma formation. Under no circumstances should blind attempts be made to advance the stylet into the catheter whilst either unit is positioned under the animal's skin as this could result in damage to the vein or catheter embolus.
7. Once the catheter has been successfully advanced, the assistant releases the pressure and the stylet is removed and discarded. A three-way tap or bung (or giving set) is attached and the whole unit flushed with 1–2 ml of heparinised saline to clear any blood from the catheter lumen and to confirm correct positioning. If not, signs of perivascular administration or 'blowing' will be seen at the site overlying the catheter tip as the heparinised saline is administered.
8. The whole unit must be secured in place. With cephalic and lateral saphenous veins, this is best achieved by anchoring tape around the catheter hub and then around the leg. Catheters inserted into the medial saphenous or femoral veins can be successfully anchored in place by suturing.
9. Finally, a sterile gauze swab covered with sterile antiseptic ointment is placed over the insertion site before bandaging, firstly with a padding material followed by a self-adhesive

conforming bandage. This protects the catheter from damage and contamination.

APPENDIX TWO

Procedure for the placement of a through-the-needle intravenous cannula

As for over-the-needle catheter placement, equipment must be prepared beforehand. A full surgical scrub of the insertion site is performed with aseptic technique being maintained throughout the following procedure:

1. When cannulating the external jugular vein, proper positioning is vital to maximise accessibility and minimise patient movement. Lateral recumbency, if tolerated, is ideal for large dogs with thin skin and easily visible veins. Animals that resist lateral recumbency or have thick skin or poorly visible veins are better restrained in a sternally recumbent or sitting position with the hind limbs positioned away from the side that is to be used for venepuncture, as this reduces the depth of the jugular groove and maximises accessibility of the vein (Hansen 1992).

2. The assistant holds the animal's head with the nose in a horizontal position, directed 35–45° away from the site of venepuncture. Further elevation of the nose may assist visualisation of the vein in animals with very loose skin.

3. The operator uses the thumb of the less dominant hand to occlude the vein at the point of the thoracic inlet and the forefinger of this hand to palpate the vein. The pressure is then released to allow a stab incision to be made approximately 1–2 cm laterally to the site of the vein.

4. The catheter and needle are held with the catheter tip lying inside the needle. Inserted bevel edge upwards, the needle should pass subcutaneously for 2 cm before introduction into the vein to create a tunnel that acts as a barrier, preventing bacterial migration from the skin surface and into the vein. The catheter is advanced once blood is seen within the hub of the needle.

5. Occasionally, flashback of blood will not occur despite successful venepuncture (Hansen 1992). In this case, an attempt should be made to advance the catheter. If there is resistance, the whole unit is removed.

6. Haemorrhage at the site of insertion is sometimes seen as the insertion site hole is larger than the catheter diameter. Positioning the animal in such a way that the insertion site is raised above the level of the heart minimises localised haemorrhage by reducing venous pressure (Hansen 1992).

7. Depending on the style of catheter, the needle is either split away or, alternatively, enclosed within a plastic sheath.

8. The bung or three-way tap is attached. Air is aspirated from the catheter using a sterile syringe followed by the aspiration of blood which confirms it has been successfully placed. The whole unit is flushed with heparinised saline.

9. The catheter is withdrawn a sufficient distance (not more than 1–2 cm) and dried with a sterile gauze swab to allow a small piece of waterproof tape to be attached, thus creating two wings that enable the catheter to be secured in place.

10. The point of insertion is covered with a gauze swab or sponge treated with a sterile antiseptic solution.

11. Further tape is applied to the base of the needle guard and taken dorsally to anchor the whole unit before carefully applying layers of bandaging material.

APPENDIX THREE

Procedure for the placement of an intraosseous needle (Fig. 1.9)

The equipment required is prepared in advance and arranged ready for use on a clean trolley. Procedure is as follows:

1. The site is clipped of hair and prepared surgically as for intravenous catheter placement.

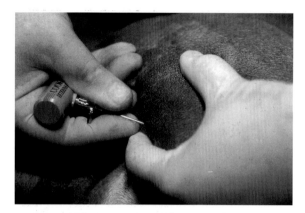

Figure 1.9 Placement of intraosseous needle. (Reproduced with permission from Cook Veterinary Products.)

When the procedure is performed in conscious animals, it is important to anaesthetise the skin and periosteum with lidocaine (lignocaine) hydrochloride, as insertion of the needle is associated with pain.

2. An assistant stabilises the limb. A stab incision is made in the skin and the needle introduced through the wound and advanced to the periosteum. Positioning of the needle into the cortex is achieved using a rotating action whilst simultaneously applying gentle pressure to push the needle forward.

3. Further rotation and pressure are then applied to force the needle through the cortex so that the tip is lying within the bone marrow.

4. Suction is applied to the hub of the needle using a 12 ml syringe. If the needle is correctly placed, a small amount of bone marrow matter will be aspirated and the needle is then flushed with a small volume of heparinised saline. If no aspiration of bone marrow contents occurs or if resistance to flushing is experienced, the needle should be rotated as the bevel may be lying against the inner cortex (Hansen 1992).

5. Once the needle is correctly positioned the infusion is started. Localised tissues should be palpated for evidence of fluid leakage from the bone.

6. A suture passed through the periosteum is used to anchor the needle in place. Antiseptic ointment is used to treat the insertion site and the needle is then bandaged in place.

APPENDIX FOUR

Central venous pressure monitoring technique

1. A through-the-needle catheter is placed aseptically into the intrathoracic cranial vena cava via the jugular vein.

2. Extension tubing is attached to the catheter and a three-way tap connected to the other end of the extension tubing.

3. A crystalloid infusion and giving set are attached to one of the ports on the three-way tap.

4. The third port on the three-way tap is connected to a fluid-filled manometer measured in centimetres. The zero point of the manometer scale is positioned so that it is level with the right atrium.

5. A CVP measurement is taken prior to infusing fluid. To do this, the three-way tap is turned off at the giving set port so that there is a direct connection between the jugular catheter and the manometer. If the catheter is patent and correctly positioned, the fluid meniscus in the manometer will fluctuate slightly with each heart beart and rise and fall more significantly with each ventilation due to changes in intrathoracic pressure. If there is any doubt as to whether the catheter is correctly positioned, radiography can be used to confirm.

6. To administer fluids to the patient, the three-way tap is turned off at the point of the manometer to create a direct connection between the jugular catheter and the infusion.

Elevated CVP measurements are seen with volume overload and primary right-sided myocardial failure. A low CVP measurement indicates a low circulating volume. Administration of fluid in hypovolaemia rapidly results in a temporary increase in CVP which then quickly declines. Fluid that is administered to an animal with circulatory overload or congestive heart failure will also cause a rise in CVP, but instead of declining rapidly the elevation will be sustained or it will very slowly decrease back to the baseline measurement.

REFERENCES

Aldrich J 1999 Shock. Manual of canine and feline emergency and critical care. BSAVA, Cheltenham, pp 23–35

Authement J 1992 Blood transfusion therapy. Fluid therapy in small animal practice. WB Saunders, Philadelphia, pp 371–383

Chew RM 1965 Water metabolism of mammals. In: Mayer WW, VanGelder RD (eds) Physiologic mammalogy: Vol II Mammalian reaction to stressful environments. Academic Press, New York, pp 43–177

DiBartola SP 1992a Introduction to acid–base disorders. Fluid therapy in small animal practice. WB Saunders, Philadelphia, pp 193–215

DiBartola SP 1992b Disorders of sodium and water. Fluid therapy in small animal practice. WB Saunders, Philadelphia, pp 57–88

DiBartola SP 1992c An introduction to fluid therapy. Fluid therapy in small animal practice. WB Saunders, Philadelphia, pp 321–340

Hansen B 1992 Technical aspects of fluid therapy. Fluid therapy in small animal practice. WB Saunders, Philadelphia, pp 341–370

Hughes D 1999 Fluid therapy. Manual of canine and feline emergency and critical care. BSAVA, Cheltenham, pp 7–22

Knottenbelt C, Mackin A 1997a Practical blood collection in the dog. Veterinary Practice Nurse. TBP, pp 27–30, Autumn

Knottenbelt C, Mackin A 1997b Practical blood collection in the cat. Veterinary Practice Nurse. TBP, pp 4–7, Winter

Kohn CW, DiBartola SP 1992 Composition and distribution of body fluids in dogs and cats. Fluid therapy in small animal practice. WB Saunders, Philadelphia, pp 1–29

Mathews KA 1996a Fluid therapy. Veterinary emergency and critical care. Lifelearn, Guelph, 12.1–12.21

Mathews KA 1996b Blood/plasma transfusion. Veterinary emergency and critical care. Lifelearn, Guelph, 28.1–28.22

Tobias TA, Schertel ER 1992 Shock – concepts and management. Fluid therapy in small animal practice. WB Saunders, Philadelphia, pp 436–470

Welsh E 1994 Fluid therapy and shock. Veterinary nursing. Pergamon, Oxford, pp 455–472

White R 1999 Emergency techniques. Manual of canine and feline emergency and critical care. BSAVA, Cheltenham, pp 307–340

2

Infectious diseases

Victoria Aspinall

INTRODUCTION

Much of the everyday work of a veterinary nurse is the nursing of animals with infectious diseases and the prevention of spread of the disease to other susceptible animals. So what are infectious diseases? What causes them and how are they transmitted between animals? Armed with an understanding of this, the veterinary nurse can develop strategies to prevent further infection within the practice. Helpful definitions are given below:

- An **infectious disease** is one that is caused by a micro-organism that is capable of invading and growing within the tissues of the host animal.
- A **non-infectious disease** is one that is not caused by a micro-organism and cannot be spread from one animal to another. Many non-infectious diseases are caused by an upset in the normal function of an organ, e.g. the kidneys, liver or endocrine glands.
- A **contagious disease** is one that can be transmitted from one animal to another by direct or indirect contact. This includes all the infectious diseases and all diseases caused by internal and external parasites.

Infected animals shed disease-causing micro-organisms from their bodies in significant quantities, and these can either be transmitted directly from one animal to another – direct contact – or they may contaminate the environment in which the animal is living – indirect contact (Fig. 2.1). The pathogen enters the body of a susceptible

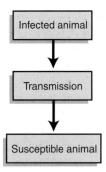

Figure 2.1 The way in which infectious diseases are transmitted.

animal and affects it in such a way that symptoms of the disease develop. Both the ability of the micro-organism to survive off the animal's body and the degree of contamination of the environment are important factors in the efficiency of spread of a disease and of its control.

INFECTIOUS DISEASES – OVERVIEW

CAUSAL ORGANISMS

Infectious diseases are caused by micro-organisms. These organisms are too small to be seen with the naked eye. The majority of micro-organisms are either harmless or play an important part in the balance of life. For example if there were no bacteria and fungi to break down dead material in the soil, dead bodies would soon overcome us. However, a small proportion of micro-organisms are able to cause disease in the host animal and are known as pathogens.

The most commonly occurring pathogens in small animal practice can be divided into four groups:

- bacteria
- viruses
- fungi
- protozoa.

Bacteria

Bacteria (sing. bacterium) are unicellular organisms whose size varies from 0.5 μm to 5 μm (1 μm or

1 micrometre = 1000th of a millimetre or 10^{-6} m). Inside the host animal they live in the intercellular spaces or in the blood. Outside the body, many are able to survive for varying amounts of time depending on the species.

Bacteria are differentiated by their shape (Fig. 2.2) and by their reaction to Gram stain. This is determined by the structure of the cell wall and enables bacteria to be divided into:

- Gram positive – stain purple, e.g. *Staphylococcus* spp., *Streptococcus* spp.
- Gram negative – stain red, e.g. *Escherichia coli*, *Campylobacter* spp.

When considering the ability of a pathogen to cause disease (virulence) and its ability to survive outside the body, certain structural factors are important:

1. Most bacteria are surrounded by a cell wall (Fig 2.3). This is a rigid structure of varying thickness which protects the cell from external damage.
2. Some species of bacteria have an outer slime coat (Fig 2.3). This reduces the risk of drying

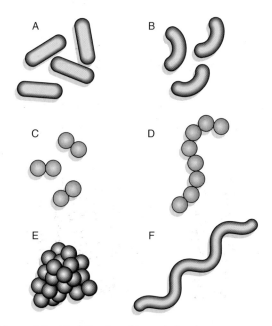

Figure 2.2 Classification of bacteria by shape. (Reproduced with permission from Cooper and Lane 1999.)

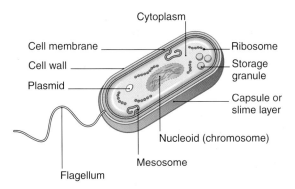

Figure 2.3 Cross section of a generalised bacterial cell. (From *Pre-Veterinary Nursing Textbook* by Masters and Bowden (2001). Reprinted by permission of Elsevier Science.)

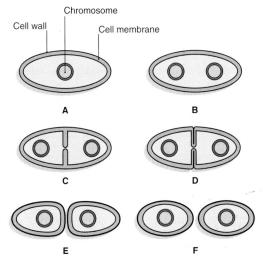

Figure 2.4 Sequence of events seen in bacterial sporulation. (From *Pre-Veterinary Nursing Textbook* by Masters and Bowden (2001). Reprinted by permission of Elsevier Science.)

out, helps the cell to adhere to the cells of the host animal and may prevent phagocytosis by the white blood cells of the host.

3. Some bacteria have appendages known as pili (sing. pilus) or fimbriae (sing. fimbria) which protrude and enable the bacterium to stick to the host cell.

4. Bacteria replicate asexually by binary fission – one cell divides into two, two into four, etc. The time between successive divisions is the generation time. Under optimal environmental conditions the generation time may be very rapid, e.g. *Escherichia coli* will divide every 20 minutes, but excess heat, lack of moisture or a change in pH may slow down the rate of division.

5. Certain species are able to survive in unfavourable conditions by forming spores or endospores – sporulation (Fig. 2.4), e.g. *Bacillus anthracis* – anthrax; *Clostridium tetani* – tetanus. These spores are very resistant and can survive extremes of heat, ultraviolet radiation, pH and some disinfectants. In order to kill *all* micro-organisms and their spores, sterilisation techniques have to be used.

Rickettsia and *Chlamydia* are a group of micro-organisms that have characteristics in common with both bacteria and viruses. They are small intracellular parasites and examples include *Haemobartonella felis* which causes feline infectious anaemia and *Chlamydia psittaci* which causes chlamydiosis in cats.

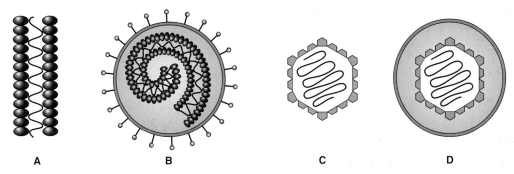

Figure 2.5 Four types of viral structure. (Reproduced with permission from Cooper and Lane 1999.)

Box 2.1 Replication of animal viruses (adapted with permission from Cooper and Lane 1999)

Part 1
Once the virus has reached a suitable host cell, it attaches to receptor sites on the host cell membrane.

Part 2
(A) The envelope of the virus may fuse with the cell wall and release the nucleocapsid into the cell or (B) the virus may be taken into the cell by endocytosis.

Part 3
The virus enters the host cell and the protein coat (capsid) breaks down to release the viral nucleic acid.

Part 4
The viral nucleic acid replicates (either in the host cell cytoplasm or nucleus) and directs the host cell metabolism to make new virus material.

Part 5
The new viruses are assembled.

Part 6
They leave the host cell either by rupture or the cell membrane or

Part 7
Through the cell membrane

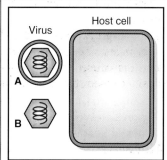

(1) Once the virus has reached a suitable host cell, it attaches to receptor sites on the host cell membrane.

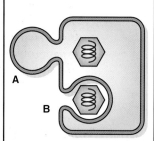

(2) (A) The envelope of the virus may fuse with the cell wall and release the nucleocapsid into the cell or
(B) the virus may be taken into the cell by endocytosis.

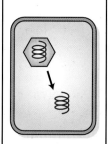

(3) The virus enters the host cell and the protein coat (capsid) breaks down to release the viral nucleic acid.

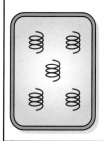

(4) The viral nucleic acid replicates (either in the host cell cytoplasm or nucleus) and directs the host cell metabolism to make new virus material.

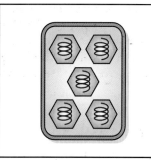

(5) The new viruses are assembled.

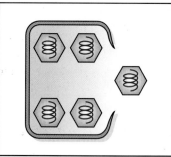

(6) They leave the host cell either by rupture of the cell membrane; or

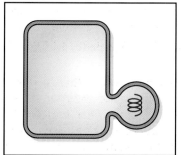

(7) through the cell membrane.

Viruses

Viruses are tiny obligate intracellular parasites, i.e. they have to live inside a host cell and cannot survive for long outside the body. Each virus particle or virion consists of a core of nucleic acid of either RNA or DNA surrounded by a protein coat – the capsid. Some viruses are also enclosed in an envelope which gives additional protection. The different shapes of virus particles (one of the ways used to classify them) are illustrated in Figure 2.5.

Viruses replicate by attaching to the host cell and penetrating the cell membrane. Once inside, the virus programs the cell to obey the instructions of the virus (Box 2.1). New virus particles are formed by the host cell and they are released. This process may damage the cell permanently or leave it intact depending on the type of virus involved.

As viruses are intracellular organisms and are protected by the host cells, they are difficult to overcome once inside the host. However, most viruses do not survive for long outside the body, so control of viral diseases is aimed at preventing transmission between animals by direct or indirect contact.

Fungi

Fungi are a large group of organisms and form a kingdom on their own. Their size ranges from giant mushrooms to microscopic moulds and yeasts. As with other micro-organisms, very few are pathogenic and those of veterinary importance include:

- **Dermatophytes** – these are the 'skin eaters' which have the ability to invade healthy tissue. *Trichophyton mentagrophytes* and *Microsporum canis* both cause ringworm in the dog, cat and rabbit. The spread of infection may be by direct contact between animals or by fungal spores on fomites. Prevention of spread by spores is relatively easy as they are killed by most disinfectants.
- **Yeasts** – unicellular organisms that reproduce by binary fission and spread by direct

contact. Examples include *Candida albicans* which causes 'thrush' in many different species and *Malassezia pachydermatis*, a common underlying cause of many skin diseases in the dog.

Protozoa

Protozoa are unicellular organisms with a definite nucleus and a cytoplasm containing structures such as mitochondria and ribosomes. Many are capable of independent movement and survive outside the body in films of moisture. Sources of infection include water, food and soil contaminated by infected faeces.

Protozoal diseases of significance in the dog and cat include giardiasis caused by *Giardia duodenalis,* toxoplasmosis caused by *Toxoplasma gondii* and coccidiosis caused by *Eimeria* and *Isospora* species.

INFECTIOUS AGENTS

Spread of infection from an infected animal to a susceptible animal may occur in two ways:

- direct contact
- indirect contact.

Direct contact

Direct contact is said to occur when the infected animal comes into physical contact with the susceptible animal. Animals may touch each other when lying together, or grooming, fighting, by sexual contact or when the dam is feeding her young.

Indirect contact

Indirect contact means that there is no physical contact, and spread between animals is achieved by some form of infectious agent.

Infectious agents may be:

- **Fomites** – inanimate objects that carry disease. Such objects may be anything with which the infected animal has come into contact, e.g. litter trays, kennel walls, grooming equipment, blankets, surgery floors, surgical instruments or even clothing or footwear. This is environmental contamination. Fomites may be contaminated by blood, faeces or saliva containing pathogens from the infected animal. Survival on the fomite depends on the structure and nature of the pathogens and of the material surrounding them. Prevention of spread by fomites is a vital part of the daily routine of the nurse.

- **Vectors** – animate or living organisms that carry disease. These include flies, fleas, ticks and mites but there are many others.

There are two types of vector:

1. **Biological vectors** – also called **intermediate hosts.** A certain amount of development of the organism occurs within the intermediate host and the infective stage of the organism cannot be reached without it.

   Examples are seen in the tapeworm family:

   a. The egg of the tapeworm *Dipyllidium caninum* develops into a larva inside the cat flea *Ctenocephalides felis*. The flea must be eaten by a dog or cat for the larval tapeworm to be released and to develop into the adult form in the small intestine. Dogs and cats must be treated for tapeworm infection at the same time as treating for fleas in order to break this lifecycle.

   b. The pork tapeworm *Taenia solium* uses the pig as an intermediate host or biological vector. The larval tapeworm develops in the muscle of the pig and may be ingested by a human eating raw or undercooked pork. Once in the gut, the larva is released, develops into the adult form and attaches to the wall of the intestine where it begins to produce segments which pass out in the faeces. Good standards of public sanitation and making sure that pork is always well cooked before eating will break the lifecycle.

2. **Mechanical vectors** – these transmit infection, but no development occurs in the vector. There are two types:

   a. A **transport** host keeps the pathogen viable and infective but is unaffected by it. The pathogen must be shed from the transport host before it can pass to the susceptible animal. The cat flea *Ctenocephalides felis* is thought to transmit viruses such as those causing feline leukaemia and feline infectious enteritis. The flea ingests blood from an infected cat and this is passed on by biting a susceptible cat.

   b. A **paratenic** host must be eaten by the susceptible host for the pathogen to be transmitted. If the paratenic host is not eaten the organism remains unchanged and causes no harm to the host. The protozoan, *Toxoplasma gondii*, encysts in the tissues of many vertebrates and they remain unaffected. Cats eating contaminated mice or raw meat may become infected and subsequently transmit the disease toxoplasmosis to humans and other vertebrates via their faeces.

MODES OF INFECTION

Infectious diseases pass from one animal to another in three stages (Fig. 2.1):

1. The pathogen leaves the infected animal.
2. The pathogen passes between the infected animal and the susceptible animal.
3. The pathogen enters the susceptible animal.

The time taken for this process to occur could be a few milliseconds or several weeks or years depending on the type of pathogen:

- Canine parvovirus may survive in the environment for up to 6 months – thus one infected dog may shed the virus in faeces, which could be ingested several months later by another dog that then develops the disease.
- Feline calicivirus, one of the causal agents of the cat 'flu syndrome, does not survive out of the host body for more than a few days – spread of infection by sneezing has to take place quickly.

- *Bacillus anthracis* causes anthrax and, although rare, this can affect most warm-blooded animals. The bacteria have been recorded surviving as spores in soil for up to 50 years – time taken for the spread of this disease is then almost immeasurable.

The pathogen leaves the infected animal

Pathogens leave the infected animal from any of the normal body orifices and are protected by body fluids or secretions.

Examples include:

1. Secretions:
   a. Saliva – rabies virus, feline leukaemia virus (FeLV).
   b. Nasal discharge – cat 'flu viruses, *Pasteurella multocida* in rabbits, canine distemper virus, kennel cough group including *Bordetella bronchiseptica*.
   c. Ocular discharge – *P. multocida* in rabbits, *Chlamydia psittaci*.
   d. Semen – *Brucella canis* (brucellosis in dogs in the USA).
   e. Vaginal discharge – *B. canis*.
   f. Vomit – canine parvovirus, feline infectious enteritis virus.
2. Excretions:
   a. Faeces – canine parvovirus, canine distemper virus, feline infectious enteritis, *Salmonella* spp., rabbit viral haemorrhagic disease.
   b. Urine – canine adenovirus-1 (infectious canine hepatitis), *Leptospira* spp.
3. Body fluids:
   a. Blood – *Haemobartonella felis* (feline infectious anaemia), FeLV.
   b. Foetal fluids – *B. canis*.
   c. Milk – FeLV, *Toxocara canis* larvae.
4. The skin may be a source of infection by ectoparasites such as lice and fleas.

The pathogen passes between the infected animal and the susceptible animal

Pathogens are protected from drying out by the fluids in which they leave the animal. This prolongs their survival and increases the chances of transmission from the infected animal to the susceptible animal. Methods of transmission from clinical cases include:

- Direct contact – physical contact between animals allows rapid spread of secretions or ectoparasites.
- Indirect contact – spread by vectors or fomites contaminated by fluids and secretions produced by the infected animal.
- Aerosol transmission – the act of coughing and sneezing releases large numbers of droplets containing pathogens from the nasal and oral cavities. These leave the body at high velocity and they can travel distances of up to 1.5–2 metres from a dog or cat. Prevention of spread includes separation of infected animals by distance or by solid barriers, good ventilation systems and reducing the number of animals in one air space.
- Contamination of food and water
  — Food – may contain pathogenic bacteria such as *Salmonella, Campylobacter* and *Staphylococcus*, all of which cause gastro-enteritis. *Toxoplasma gondii* and larval tapeworms may be present in meat.
  — Water – may contain the bacteria *Leptospira,* and protozoa such as *Cryptosporidium* and *Giardia*. Contamination of water courses by sewage and buried carcasses may be a source of infection.
- Carriers – defined as animals that harbour a pathogen but show no clinical signs of the disease or evidence that the pathogen is being excreted. They are of particular risk to other animals in close contact, such as in boarding kennels or veterinary practices, as they are unidentifiable until others show symptoms of infection. Carriers may be:
  — Convalescent carriers – the animal has had the disease and recovered. These cases are of less risk to other animals providing that their medical history is known and precautions are put in place. For example, dogs recovered from infectious canine

hepatitis or leptospirosis may secrete the
pathogen in urine for some time
afterwards. Cats that have had cat 'flu may
secrete the virus in nasal discharges for a
long time. This becomes more likely when
the cat is under stress, e.g. at the time of
neutering, in a cattery, or when affected by
another disease.
— Healthy carriers – the animal has never
shown any symptoms of infection despite
being exposed to the pathogen. These
animals are usually immune but
contaminate the environment with the
pathogen and are of high risk to any in-
contact animal. For example, some cats
may shed spores of *Microsporum canis*
without suffering from ringworm
themselves. The spores contaminate
fomites such as kennels, blankets and
grooming equipment.

Both convalescent and healthy carriers may
be either:

— Open carriers – shed the pathogen
continuously and will contaminate their
environment, or
— Closed carriers – harbour the pathogen but
do not shed it.

The pathogen enters the susceptible animal

Pathogens will enter the body through all the
normal routes. They may also penetrate the skin or
mucous membranes or be introduced congenitally:

• Ingestion – this is one of the more common
routes of entry and includes eating
contaminated food and water, faeces of other
animals, infected urine and other body
secretions, vectors such as fleas, mice and
birds, grooming other animals, licking and
chewing fomites.
• Inhalation – via the respiratory tract. Includes
droplets transmitted by the aerosol effect,
dust particles carrying pathogens and fungal
spores.
• Inoculation – penetration through the skin

which is normally an intact barrier. It can be
damaged by wounds which may become
infected; biting insects such as the flea
Ctenocephalides felis or the sucking louse
Linognathus setosus and the larvae of the
hookworm *Uncinaria stenocephala* may
penetrate the skin. Dirty needles or surgical
instruments may introduce infection and for
this reason it is essential to maintain sterile
procedures.
• Through the mucous membranes – the
membranes of the respiratory and digestive
tracts, conjunctiva, vagina, penis and prepuce
may all be penetrated by pathogens.
• Congenital route – pathogens infect the
developing embryo or foetus by
transplacental or transuterine infection. This
is known as **vertical transmission** and may
cause resorption, abortion, stillbirth or
congenital abnormalities in the neonate.
Pathogens that may cause this include FeLV,
feline infectious enteritis, *Toxoplasma gondii*,
canine parvovirus and *Toxocara canis* – canine
roundworm infection.

The major groups of pathogens generally use
one or two routes of transmission rather than
every route, e.g. viruses leave an infected animal
protected by the secretions of the body as they
cannot survive for long in the desiccating atmosphere of the environment. The most common
routes are summarised in Table 2.1.

PREVENTATIVE MEDICINE

The maintenance of health and the prevention of
the spread of disease within any collection of
animals are of prime importance. This is the aim
of preventative medicine and the intention is to
prevent animals developing the disease rather
than to treat them once they have become
dangerously ill. Animals within a veterinary
surgery are at a higher risk than most animals as
they may be in close contact with infectious
diseases and may be immunologically weakened
by concurrent disease, routine surgery, or just the
stress of being away from home.

Table 2.1 Examples of routes of transmission favoured by the major groups of pathogens

Pathogen	Route of transmission	Example of disease	Species affected
Bacteria	Faeces and vomit	Salmonellosis	Dog and cat
		Campylobacter	Dog and cat
	Urine	Leptospirosis	Dog
	Bites (saliva)	Pasteurellosis	Cat and rabbit
Viruses	Saliva	Rabies	All warmblooded species
		FeLV	Cat
		FIV	Cat
	Ocular discharge	Chlamydiosis	Cat
	Respiratory secretions	Calicivirus	Cat
	(aerosol effect)	Herpesvirus	Cat
		Kennel cough	Dog
	Faeces	Feline infectious enteritis	Cat
		Distemper	Dog
		Canine parvovirus	Dog
		Viral haemorrhagic disease	Rabbit
	Urine	Infectious canine hepatitis	Dog
	Blood	FeLV	Cat
		Myxomatosis	Rabbit
		Feline infectious anaemia	Cat
Fungi	Spores from skin	Ringworm	Dog, cat, rabbit
Protozoa	Faeces	Giardiasis	Dog
		Toxoplasmosis	Cat

FeLV, feline leukaemia virus; FIV, feline immunodeficiency virus.

Knowledge of how diseases are transmitted between susceptible animals is the basis of preventative medicine and this must be understood by veterinary surgeons, veterinary nurses and the owners of the animals. The range of methods used in the control of disease can be applied to the steps involved in transmission (Fig. 2.6).

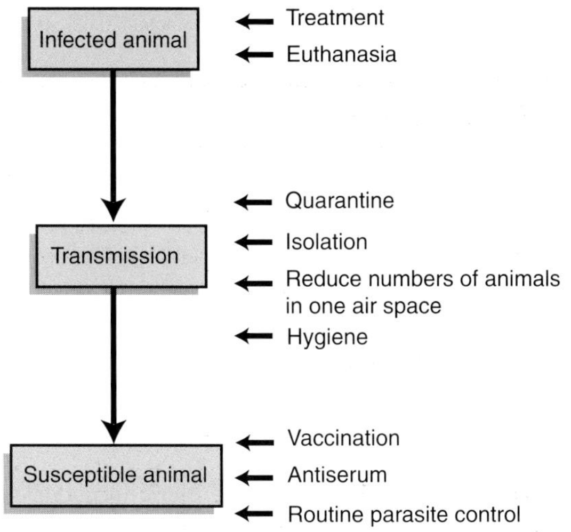

CONTROL METHODS APPLIED TO THE INFECTED ANIMAL (Fig. 2.6)

Treatment

A rapid diagnosis is essential to prevent:

- unnecessary suffering
- further spread of the disease
- deterioration of the animal's condition
- development of zoonoses.

Treatment of an animal with an infectious disease will kill the pathogens and prevent spread, but a treatment may not always be available. Many viruses cannot be effectively killed but the use of antibiotics will prevent secondary bacterial infection that could further weaken the animal. Treatment may not be economically viable, particularly when considering the cost against the value of farm animals or small rodents – this is a decision which must be taken by the owner.

Figure 2.6 Methods of disease control.

Euthanasia

Usually considered to be a means of preventing further suffering in a terminally ill animal, it is also used as a means of preventing further spread of an infectious disease. By euthanasing an infected animal, the pathogens are killed and cannot spread to other susceptible animals, e.g. in cases of feline leukaemia infection where there is no treatment and the cat may be a source of infection to other cats in the household or in the same neighbourhood.

After the death of the infected animal, the nurse must be able to explain to the owner that:

- The animal's body may be a further source of infection to other animals in the house, so cremation is recommended.
- Equipment used by the animal, e.g. feeding bowls and litter trays, may act as fomites and should be thrown away or thoroughly disinfected.
- The correct disinfectants must be used to kill pathogens in the house and on fomites.
- A new animal should not be brought into the house until a sensible period has elapsed. This depends on the type of disease involved. Any new animal must be fully vaccinated before it enters the house.

CONTROL METHODS THAT INTERFERE WITH ROUTES OF TRANSMISSION (Fig. 2.6)

Quarantine

This is the physical separation of an animal that is outwardly healthy but may be carrying or incubating an infectious disease. It may be used as follows:

- Classically this is taken to mean the compulsory quarantine period for animals being imported into the UK. The recent introduction of the PETS scheme means that fewer animals will have to undergo the 6 months' stay in quarantine kennels.
- When introducing new animals or groups of animals into an established colony. This may be applied to:

— breeding colonies
— zoos
— pet shops.

If an infectious disease is present, the clinical signs will manifest themselves during the quarantine period. As the animal is already separated from any susceptible animals, transmission is prevented.

Isolation

This is the physical separation of an animal that is exhibiting clinical signs to minimise the risk of spreading the disease by direct or indirect contact.

As soon as an animal shows signs of an infectious disease, it should be removed to the isolation unit in the practice and looked after by barrier nursing. The facilities should be designed in such a way as to prevent any possibility of transmission of the pathogens to other animals. The unit should:

- be a self contained room equipped with a range of kennels, with a separate entrance from that of the practice and a separate means of disposal of waste materials
- have its own water supply for cleaning and its own kitchen for the preparation of food
- have a separate supply of feeding, cleaning and nursing equipment and of cleaning and disinfectant chemicals
- have a separate treatment room stocked with its own supply of medicines and necessary equipment
- have a ventilation system of an appropriate design; it may be necessary to filter the incoming and outgoing air supplies.

One or two nurses should be designated to work in the unit and should not work in any other areas of the practice. This may be done on a weekly or monthly rota. No visitors are allowed into the unit. All nurses working in the unit should:

- Wear appropriate clothing which must be left in the unit at the end of the day. The clothing should not be taken into the main practice and should not be taken home. Disposable clothing is the most efficient method of preventing disease transmission by this route. A changing room used only by nurses working in the unit should be provided.

- Wear special footwear kept for use in the unit or shoes which may be covered by disposable overslippers. A disinfectant footbath at the entrance to the unit may also be used.
- Have hair tied back and covered by disposable caps.
- Wear surgical masks and gloves when dealing directly with the infected patients. This prevents transmission of disease and reduces the risks of infection with zoonotic diseases.
- Personal hygiene must be strictly observed.

In an owner's home or in smaller practices, isolation may have to be achieved in more difficult circumstances, but the aim is still the same:

- The infected animal must be separated from all others of the same species but a cat may be put in the dog kennels and vice versa as most infectious diseases do not cross the species barrier.
- Cages must be separated by solid walls and arranged in a straight line to prevent spread across a central corridor.
- If the animal cannot be put in a separate room, then prevent transmission by covering the cage with a towel or blanket.
- Provide a separate set of cleaning, feeding and medical equipment for use only on the infected animal. This should be thrown away or thoroughly disinfected after recovery or death.
- Wear protective clothing when dealing with the animal and do not wear it at any other time.
- Always wash your hands after handling the patient.
- If there are other susceptible animals in the house, they should be given booster vaccinations if appropriate.

Reduce the numbers of animals in one air space

The greater the numbers of animals in one air space, the greater the chances of spreading infectious diseases. Boarding and hospital kennel design should incorporate the idea of several smaller rooms rather than one large room containing the kennels.

Care must be taken to reduce the chances of pathogen survival and should ensure that:

1. Building design allows air to circulate freely through the kennels, but avoids draughts and air pockets.
2. Air is actively changed by the ventilation system: 6–12 air changes per hour will provide a healthy atmosphere.
3. The temperature and humidity of the kennels must not promote condensation and a damp unpleasant atmosphere.

Hygiene

This is the most vital method of disease prevention particularly where transmission of infection is indirect. None of the other methods discussed so far will be effective unless hygienic practices are strictly observed. There are three 'degrees' of hygiene:

1. cleaning
2. disinfection
3. sterilisation.

Cleaning

This is an important part of the daily routine. The aim is to reduce the number of microorganisms in the environment by physical actions such as wiping, scrubbing and flushing with large quantities of hot water. The chemicals used in cleaning are detergents whose action is to break down the surface tension between dirt, grease or organic matter and water. This results in the fragmentation and subsequent removal of all dirt particles. Cleaning must precede disinfection as organic matter inactivates disinfectants.

Disinfection

This is the removal or destruction of all micro-organisms except bacterial spores. These are highly resistant to the actions of most disinfectants, leaving an area or object as a potential source of infection by spores even after thorough disinfection.

Disinfectants are used in the environment, e.g. kennels, floors, litter trays, grooming equipment, surgical instruments, but not for disinfecting living tissue. Many disinfectants are harmful to skin and gloves should be worn when coming into direct contact with some of the more concentrated formulations.

Antiseptics are disinfectants designed for use on skin and other living tissues.

Disinfectants are classified according to their antibacterial activity as:

- **Bacteriostatic** – stop growth of bacteria but do not necessarily kill them. If the disinfectant is too diluted or used incorrectly, bacterial growth may begin again.
- **Bactericidal** – destroy or kill bacteria. These are the more efficient disinfectants.

There is a wide range of disinfectants available and all have different uses (see Table 2.2). General points that should be observed when using disinfectants are:

- Observe the Control of Substances Hazardous to Health Regulations 1988 (COSHH) as applied to the product.
- Select the correct disinfectant to use against the particular pathogen.
- If recommended wear protective clothing, e.g. gloves, goggles or overalls.
- Use the recommended dilution. Too strong a solution may be dangerous to you, to the animal or to the equipment; too weak a solution may be ineffective.
- Use hot water rather than cold unless otherwise recommended.
- Make fresh solutions when needed. Some disinfectants become ineffective if left around for long periods, e.g. hypochlorites are inactivated by sunlight.
- Never mix disinfectants – you may create a toxic mixture!

- Never mix disinfectants and detergents – leave this to the manufacturers who will take note of the chemical nature of the products.
- After use rinse thoroughly and dry the area or object.
- **Never use phenolic disinfectants for cleaning areas used by cats.**

General rules for cleaning and disinfection

1. All equipment, work surfaces, kennels, runs and areas where food is prepared must be cleaned thoroughly with a detergent to remove organic matter such as grease, faeces and fur every day. Any remaining organic matter will inactivate disinfectants used later.
2. After cleaning, rinse well and use a disinfectant to remove and/or kill pathogens.
3. Where possible use disposable equipment and bedding. Make sure that it is disposed of correctly as it can act as a fomite if left around.
4. Do not prepare food in the same areas as waste disposal or sterilisation of surgical equipment.
5. Store food for animals in a separate place to that used for humans.
6. Do not feed raw meat to animals.
7. Keep cooked food away from uncooked food.
8. Maintain a high standard of personal hygiene:
   a. Wash hands and nails after going to the toilet and after handling animals.
   b. Wash hands before eating and before smoking a cigarette.
   c. Never smoke or eat in the operating theatre, prep room or kennels.
   d. Wear clean protective clothing at all times.
   e. Tie your hair back, remove all rings and studs and remove nail polish.
9. Keep all vermin and flies under control – remember they may be vectors of disease.

Sterilisation

This is the destruction of all micro-organisms including bacterial spores. All equipment used

Table 2.2 The range of disinfectant groups and their uses

Disinfectant group	Use	Area of activity	Method of action	Examples of product	Comments
Alcohols	Skin disinfection Commonly used for swabbing injection sites	Bacteria. TB. Not viruses	Coagulates bacterial protein	Ethyl alcohol. Isopropyl alcohol. Methylated spirit. Surgical spirit	Organic compound. Evaporates quickly. Becomes contaminated once open to the air
Aldehydes 1. Formaldehydes	Environment. Sterilant for vaccines and for pathological specimens	Sporicidal. Highly irritant to skin	Fixes bacterial cell proteins making them useless	Parvocide. Formula H	Specimens are stored in 10% solution. Evaporates easily
Aldehydes 2. Glutaraldehydes	Environment. Cold sterilisation	Bacteria, viruses. Will kill spores if left in contact for long enough	Protein inactivation	Cidex	Less irritant to tissue than formaldehydes
Diguanides	Skin disinfection. Surgical scrub	Gram-positive bacteria, fungi	Unknown	Hibiscrub. Hibitane	Easily inactivated by organic matter. Make sure area is really clean and rinsed before use
Halogens 1. Iodines	Skin disinfection. Surgical scrub	Bacteria, fungi, protozoa, some viruses	Oxidises the cell of the micro-organism causing inactivation	Aqueous iodine solution	Used as a 2% tincture. Can be irritant. Stains area brown if left too long
Halogens 2. Iodophors	Skin disinfection. Surgical scrub. Environment if preparation includes a detergent	Bacteria, fungi, protozoa, some viruses	Oxidation	Pevidine. Wescodyne	Iodine molecule is bound to organic molecules which act as carriers. Makes them less toxic but more readily inactivated by inorganic matter
Halogens 3. Hypochlorite (Bleach)	Environment	All pathogens including bacterial spores	Oxidation	Domestos. Milton. Chloros	Irritant to tissue. Corrosive to metals. Inactivated by sunlight and organic material
Peroxide	Environment. Skin application	Bacteria, especially anaerobes	Oxidation	Virkon (environment only). Hydrogen peroxide	Can be used as a flush for abscesses or to cauterise bleeding
Phenols 1. Black/white/clear	Environment	Bacteria, TB, viruses, fungi	Denatures proteins	Jeyes fluid. Izal	Strong smelling, absorbed by rubber. **Toxic to cats**
Phenols 2. Chlorinated	Environment. Skin disinfection	Gram-positive bacteria	Denatures protein	Dettol. Ibcol	Less irritant. Inactivated by hard water and organic matter. **Toxic to cats**
Phenols 3. Hexochlorophane	Skin disinfection	Gram-positive bacteria	Denatures protein	Phisohex	Used in soaps and detergents
Quaternary ammonium compounds (QACs)	Environment. Skin disinfection	Gram-positive and -negative bacteria. Some viruses, fungi and bacterial spores	Dissolve lipids in the cell walls of the pathogen	Trigene, Vetaclean, Savlon, Zephiran	Non-toxic, Cheap. Colourless and odourless. Inactivated by hard water, organic matter and soap

during surgery and for any procedure that involves breaching the primary defence system of the body – mainly the skin – such as injections and implants must be free of pathogens – they must be sterile. The methods of sterilisation are classified according to the agents used:

- heat
- cold chemicals
- gas
- irradiation.

The choice depends on the size and type of equipment to be sterilised, the cost and in some cases the size of the room available. In most practices, several methods may be used.

Heat sterilisation

This is the most common method used in practice. It can be subdivided into:

- **Wet heat** – this is a simple but old-fashioned method of sterilisation. To kill all pathogens and spores, the water must be boiling for a minimum of 5 minutes. This is difficult to achieve and absolute sterility cannot be guaranteed. With the development of more modern and efficient methods it is not recommended.
- **Wet heat under pressure** – this method uses the autoclave and is considered to be the easiest way of achieving sterility in current practice. The steam, introduced under pressure, drives air out of the autoclave chamber. When it meets the cooler surfaces of the instruments in the chamber, the steam condenses. The latent heat released coagulates the proteins in the micro-organisms, so killing them. Efficient sterilisation relies on correct packing of the equipment and instruments and in putting them into the autoclave itself. If the steam is unable to circulate freely, there may be pockets where there is inadequate sterilisation. There are various types of autoclave on the market and care must be taken to read the instructions and observe the recommended timings.

- **Dry heat** – this method is incorporated into small hot-air ovens heated by electrical elements. Dry heat kills micro-organisms and spores by oxidation but they are more resistant to the effect in the absence of moisture so operating times have to be increased to achieve sterility. Destruction of bacterial spores cannot be guaranteed at temperatures below 140°C for less than 4–5 hours. At the end of the period, a long cooling time is essential before the instruments can be handled. For these reasons and for reasons of safety, dry heat is less often used nowadays.

Cold chemical sterilisation

This involves immersion in a chemical solution for a prolonged period. It does not produce a reliable level of disinfection unless the instruments are submerged for at least 24 hours.

This method is used for:

- equipment that may be damaged by heat, e.g. plastics which would melt or sharp-pointed instruments which may become blunt
- sterilisation of endoscopes and arthroscopes
- suture materials – supplied in cassettes containing chemical sterilants or prepacked with swaged needles
- needles ready for emergency use – kept in glass trays or bowls covered in sterilising solution.

Chemicals used include isopropyl alcohol, ethyl alcohol, glutaraldehyde (COSHH regulations prevent use of this in veterinary practice) and many commercially produced solutions. Solutions must be disposed of appropriately after use.

Gas sterilisation

This uses ethylene oxide which is a highly effective sterilant and a penetrative, but toxic, gas. Instruments are packed in polythene bags, placed in the steriliser and an ampoule containing liquid ethylene oxide is broken to release the gas. The steriliser is sealed for 12 hours and the room temperature must be at least 20°C. At the end of the cycle, the door must remain closed for 2 hours and the packs must then be left for a further 24 hours in a well ventilated room to allow the gas to dissipate.

Use of this method of sterilisation is limited by the size of the container, the time taken and the toxicity of the gas. COSHH regulations may eventually preclude its use in veterinary practice.

Irradiation

Many prepackaged items including needles, syringes, gloves and catheters are sterilised using gamma rays under commercial conditions.

CONTROL METHODS APPLIED TO THE SUSCEPTIBLE ANIMAL (Fig. 2.6)

- **Vaccination** – this provides a susceptible animal with immunity against a range of specific infectious diseases, e.g. distemper, feline infectious enteritis, myxomatosis. An animal should be vaccinated when it is young and levels of immunity must be maintained throughout the animal's life by annual boosters. In a disease outbreak, if other preventative measures fail, the vaccinated animal has the added protection of immunity. It is worth noting that we do not have vaccines for every infectious disease, so the safeguards created by other preventative measures must never be relinquished.
- **Antiserum** – or hyperimmune serum. This contains antibodies (see later) to a specific infectious disease and provides instant immunity to an animal at risk during an outbreak of the disease. Antiserum is of use to:
  — an unvaccinated animal
  — an animal that is too young to form antibodies – immunologically incompetent
  — an animal whose immune system is defective in some way – immunodeficient.
- **Routine parasite control** – treatment against ectoparasites and endoparasites does not protect against subsequent infection – it is not a form of vaccination, but it does ensure that

the animal is in optimum condition for a short time afterwards, enabling it to overcome any challenge from infectious diseases.

Any animal going into boarding kennels or entering a veterinary practice for elective surgery should have been recently treated for parasites and have up-to-date vaccinations in order to reduce the risk of contracting infectious diseases from its surroundings.

IMMUNITY AND VACCINATION

PROGRESS OF A DISEASE

When a pathogen enters the body of an animal by any of the routes previously described, it starts a chain of events that culminates in the clinical signs of the disease. The time between the entry of the pathogen into the animal and the development of the clinical signs is known as the **incubation period.** The incubation periods of the more common infectious diseases of the dog, cat and rabbit are shown in Table 2.3. During the incubation period, the infected animal may shed the pathogen in large quantities and is a source of infection to other animals – the disease is at its most infectious.

Incubation periods are expressed as a range of days, weeks or months. The period varies with:

1. The size of the dose of the pathogen – clinical signs develop as soon as the numbers of individual pathogens have increased to the optimum numbers to cause an effect. If the original numbers are small, the incubation period will be longer and vice versa.
2. Immune status of the infected animal – clinical signs are unlikely to develop in a vaccinated animal, if the levels of antibody reach significant levels within the incubation period. If the animal has no immunity to the disease, the pathogen will be able to replicate easily and quickly and the incubation period will be short.
3. Health status of the infected animal – an animal weakened by such things as parasites,

Table 2.3 Incubation periods of the major infectious diseases

Species	Disease	Incubation period	Causal organism
Dog	Distemper	7–10 days	Morbillivirus
	Infectious canine hepatitis	5–9 days	CAV-1
	Kennel cough	5–7 days	*Bordetella bronchiseptica* CAV-2, parainfluenza
	Leptospirosis	1–7 days	*Leptospira canicola* *L. icterohaemorrhagiae*
	Lyme disease	Variable	*Borrelia burgdorferi*
	Parvovirus	4–7 days	Parvovirus-2
Dog and cat	Rabies	Up to 6 months	Lyssavirus
Cat	Chlamydiosis	3–10 days	*Chlamydia psittaci*
	Leukaemia	Few weeks to months	Retrovirus (FeLV)
	Infectious anaemia	Unknown	*Haemobartonella felis*
	Infectious enteritis	2–10 days	Parvovirus
	Infectious peritonitis	Variable	Coronavirus
	Immunodeficiency virus	Variable	Retrovirus (FIV)
	Calicivirus – upper resp. tract disease	2–10 days	Calicivirus
	Herpesvirus – upper resp. tract disease	2–10 days	Herpesvirus
	Toxoplasmosis	2–5 weeks	*Toxoplasma gondii*
Rabbit	Myxomatosis	Unknown	Poxvirus
	Viral haemorrhagic disease	1–2 days	Calicivirus

FeLV, feline leukaemia virus; FIV, feline infectious virus.

concurrent disease, starvation or poor management will be easily overcome by pathogens and the incubation period may be shorter than might be seen in a healthy animal.

4. Age – younger animals are more easily infected by infectious diseases than older ones who may have developed an immunity. This is reflected in the length of the incubation period.

5. Site of entry – many pathogens have a preferred target tissue in the body which they reach via the blood or the lymph. Once reached, clinical signs will then develop. It takes a finite amount of time to reach the tissue from the site of entry – the further away it is the longer will be the incubation period.

Once inside the host animal, the pathogen may remain at the site of entry or spread further into the body. It is carried around the body in the blood or in the lymphatic system and the infection is said to be **systemic**. The pathogen will then establish itself and begin to multiply within the tissues. Clinical signs of a disease may result from:

- direct damage to the cells resulting in a change in the physiology of the cells
- an inflammatory reaction which initiates many of the clinical signs
- release of toxins which may cause breakdown or lysis of the cells, or cell death
- antigen–antibody reactions causing tissue necrosis or allergic reactions
- damage to the immune system – immunodeficiency.

To prevent this invasion, the body has evolved many defence mechanisms and these make up the immune system of the body.

THE IMMUNE SYSTEM

The immune system is the body's means of fighting the invasion by foreign particles known as antigens. An **antigen** is anything that the body can recognise as foreign and which stimulates the production of a specific protein known as an **antibody**. It is usually protein molecules within the antigen that stimulate antibody production. Certain materials such as metal pins or plates do not stimulate antibodies and can be successfully introduced into the body without being rejected. The body is under constant attack by many types of antigen including dust particles, pollen, fur and house mites, but the most dangerous antigens are the disease-causing organisms – the pathogens.

There are two types of immunity:

- innate immunity
- acquired immunity.

Innate immunity

This is present from birth and does *not* depend on exposure to any particular antigens. It is described as being **non-specific.**

There are three components to this type of immunity:

1. genetically controlled factors
2. external defence mechanisms
3. inflammatory response.

Genetically controlled factors

These include:

- Species – myxomatosis will affect rabbits but not dogs; leptospirosis affects dogs and rats but not rabbits; this is due to an innate insusceptibility influenced by the genotype of the species.
- Strain – certain strains of animals are more susceptible to diseases than others, e.g. some strains of laboratory mice have been bred to develop tumours for oncology studies.
- Age – infectious diseases are more severe in very young animals, due to immature immune systems, and in very old ones due to physical abnormalities which cause increased susceptibility to infection.
- Sex – this is linked to hormonal influences, particularly the production of glucocorticoids. They have an anti-inflammatory action which leads to an increased susceptibility to infectious diseases. Fluctuating levels of oestrogen and progesterone in the female may predispose to certain conditions, e.g. diabetes mellitus often develops after oestrus.

External defence mechanisms

These provide an effective barrier against entry by non-pathogenic and pathogenic organisms, providing they remain intact and the animal is healthy:

- Skin
  - Provides an impermeable barrier which can only be breached by injury, biting insects, surgical equipment and hypodermic needles.
  - Sebaceous glands in the skin secrete sebum which acts as a source of nutrition for commensal bacteria living on the skin. These create an acid pH which deters growth of pathogenic bacteria on the skin surface.
  - Sweat from sweat glands contains lysozymes which have an antibacterial action.
- Digestive tract
  - Lined with mucous membrane which secretes sticky mucus to which particles adhere and these are either swallowed or are spat out.
  - Saliva contains lysozymes with antibacterial action.
  - pH of the stomach is acid. This will destroy any organisms that enter the stomach.
  - Proteolytic enzymes are secreted by gastric glands in the stomach wall. They act on protein within the antigens and digest them.
- Respiratory tract
  - Lined with ciliated mucous membrane. Particles collect in the mucus and are then swept up the trachea towards the larynx and pharynx by the cilia (Fig. 2.7).
  - The cough reflex is initiated by particles stuck in the area of the pharynx and larynx which are coughed out or swallowed.
- Urogenital tract
  - Lined by mucous membrane.
  - pH of the vagina is acid which destroys pathogens.
  - Urethra is regularly flushed by urine which removes any organisms in the tract.

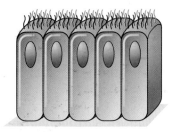

Figure 2.7 Ciliated mucous membrane. (From *Pre-Veterinary Nursing Textbook* by Masters and Bowden (2001). Reprinted by permission of Elsevier Science.)

The inflammatory response

If the external defences are breached, then the internal defence mechanisms begin to work. The inflammatory response is non-specific and is the same whether it is stimulated by bacteria entering a wound, a bruise, a burn or a biting insect inoculating a virus through the skin.

When tissue is damaged, mast cells in the tissue release a substance known as **histamine** which causes:

- local vasodilation of the capillaries in the area. This results in reddening of the affected area and local heat
- increased permeability of the blood capillaries which allows plasma proteins and fluid to leak out into the surrounding tissues. This causes swelling of the area.

Chemicals released into the area attract neutrophils and macrophages (mainly monocytes) – this is known as **chemotaxis.** They stick to the walls of the capillaries and squeeze between the endothelial cells into the tissues. Their function is phagocytosis of dead and damaged tissue and of bacteria (Fig. 2.8). Pus is formed from dead tissue, bacteria, neutrophils and macrophages. Clinical signs of inflammation include reddening, swelling, heat and pain and usually result in loss of function.

During the inflammatory reaction, a range of bactericidal proteins are released into the tissues. The most important are:

- complement
- interferon
- pyrogens.

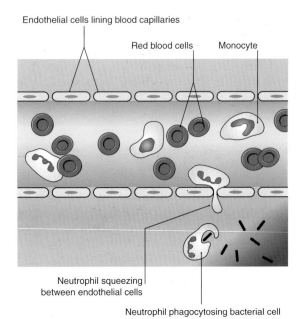

Endothelial cells lining blood capillaries

Red blood cells   Monocyte

Neutrophil squeezing between endothelial cells

Neutrophil phagocytosing bacterial cell

Figure 2.8 Movement of cells out of the blood capillaries during the inflammatory response.

Complement is a complex series of proteins normally present in serum. It helps the destruction of invading Gram negative bacteria by interacting with the antibody once it has attached to its specific bacterial cell. Phagocytosis and cell lysis are increased by the action of complement.

Interferon is released in response to virus attack. It is produced when a cell is penetrated by a virus and is a chemical belonging to a group known as the cytokines. Interferon interferes with virus replication and stimulates other uninfected cells to produce chemicals, which then protect them from attack. It is also important in the immune response to viruses.

Pyrogens are released from inflamed tissue and are responsible for causing **pyrexia** or a raised body temperature – one of the more common clinical signs of infection. Pyrogen enters the circulation and has two effects:

- It reaches the thermoregulatory centre in the hypothalamus of the brain and effectively resets the 'thermostat' of the body, which keeps the body temperature within the normal range – the body temperature rises. This higher temperature slows down bacterial growth: bacteria prefer to grow at around 38°C.

- It stimulates the liver cells to take iron out of the blood into storage in the liver. Reduced levels of iron in the blood slow down bacterial growth and increase the rate of recovery.

Acquired immunity

This develops during life as a result of exposure to particular antigens that have managed to by-pass the innate mechanisms. It is described as being **specific.**

There are two types of response, which usually develop in parallel:

1. Humoral immunity – antibody production by B cells
2. Cell-mediated immunity – T cells develop the ability to destroy specific antigens.

Antibodies, specific to a particular antigen, are produced by small rounded cells known as **lymphocytes.** These are the main cell type in the lymphatic system. During embryonic and foetal development, undifferentiated stem cells produced in the bone marrow, liver and spleen migrate to the primary lymphoid organs. These are:

- Bone marrow, Peyer's patches in the small intestine, and other unidentified sites. Stem cells become **B cells** or **B lymphocytes,** so-called as they resemble cells found in the Bursa of Fabricius of birds.
- Thymus gland – lies in the cranial thoracic inlet and anterior mediastinum of the foetus and young animal. The gland atrophies during the first year of life. Stem cells become **T cells** or **T lymphocytes.**

The differentiated lymphocytes then migrate to the secondary lymphoid organs, e.g. lymph nodes, spleen and bone marrow, where they await antigenic stimulation.

Humoral immunity

This is the production of specific antibodies or immunoglobulins by B cells in the lymph nodes, spleen and bone marrow.

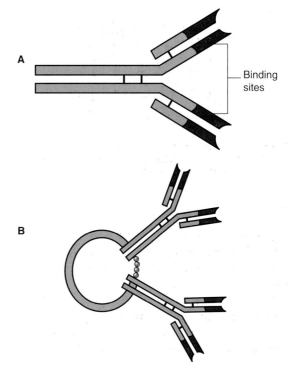

Figure 2.9 Diagrammatic representation of two common types of antibody.

Antibodies are proteins. They are typically Y-shaped with specific binding sites for the antigen at the tips of the Y (Fig. 2.9). The antibody binds with the antigen and this results in the destruction of the antigen. Each antibody is only able to bind to the specific antigen – thus distemper antibodies will only 'fit' distemper antigen; infectious canine hepatitis (ICH) antibody will only 'fit' ICH antigen.

When the antigen enters the body of the animal, it is carried in the blood or lymphatic system and will eventually pass through the secondary lymphoid organs, principally the lymph nodes. Here the B cells are stimulated by the presence of the antigen (primary response) and begin to divide rapidly, forming plasma cells. These secrete antibodies – rates of 2000 per second have been measured for several days before the cell dies. The blood carries the antibodies to the target antigens, which are then destroyed.

Certain B cells remain in the lymphoid organs and retain a memory of the type of antibody

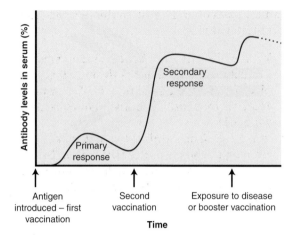

Figure 2.10 Graph to show antibody response to introduction of an antigen by natural exposure or vaccination.

produced. If the animal encounters the antigen again (secondary response), these cells are capable of producing the specific antibody very quickly and the antigen is overcome. The animal is described as being **immune.**

The antibody response (Fig. 2.10) can be detected by measuring levels of antibodies in the blood and is divided into:

1. **Primary response** – antibodies are produced within 7–10 days. Levels are relatively low, slowly reach a peak and fall as antigen–antibody reactions mop them up.
2. **Secondary response** – antibodies are produced within 12–24 hours. Levels are 10–50 times higher and remain high for several months. Subsequent exposure to the antigen will boost levels still higher.

Humoral immunity is the underlying principle of vaccination. A vaccine contains the antigen in a harmless form. The initial dose stimulates the primary response without causing the disease. The second dose stimulates the secondary response and the animal develops a life-long immunity. Booster vaccinations are recommended annually to 'top up' the levels of antibodies as the memory retained varies according to the type of antigen – some are more immunogenic, i.e. better at stimulating antibody production than others. If

an animal receives only the initial dose, it will retain the memory of the antigen, but the response to an antigenic challenge may be less effective.

Cell-mediated immunity

This involves the T cells in the lymph nodes, spleen and bone marrow. They are stimulated by the presence of certain types of antigen. These include those that enter cells such as viruses, tubercle bacilli that cause TB and certain chemicals including nickel and those found in sticking plaster.

The T cells divide to form plasma cells. These secrete antibodies which remain fixed to the surface of the cell and are known as killer T cells. They are carried by the bloodstream to the site of antigen attack where they release substances known as **lymphokines,** chemicals similar to cytokines. Lymphokines attract and activate other T cells and destroy the infected cell by perforating it, allowing the cell contents to leak out. This releases the pathogens inside, which are attacked and destroyed by the surface antibodies.

Antibody/antigen detection tests

Detection of a specific antibody can be used to identify whether an animal has been exposed to a specific antigen. This is an aid to diagnosis and is also useful in determining the degree of exposure of a population to the antigen. Tests involve the measurement of antibody–antigen reactions in the serum and are referred to as serology.

In small animal practice the most commonly used tests are based on the enzyme-linked immunosorbent assays or ELISA test (Fig. 2.11) for the diagnosis of infection with FeLV and feline immunodeficiency (FIV) viruses.

Types of immunisation (Table 2.4)

An animal may be protected against infectious diseases in two ways:

- Active immunisation – antibodies are formed by the susceptible animal and protection is lifelong.

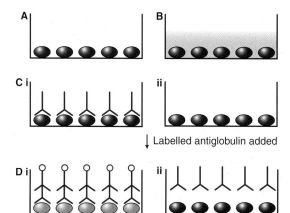

Figure 2.11 Diagrammatic representation of enzyme-linked immunosorbent assay (ELISA). (Reproduced with permission from Cooper and Lane 1999.)

↓ Labelled antiglobulin added

- Passive immunisation – preformed antibodies are taken from an immune animal and given to the susceptible animal. Protection is transient.

Maternal immunisation

Neonatal animals are protected from infectious diseases during the first few weeks of life by antibodies that are derived from the dam. This is natural passive immunity. Antibodies are transferred in two ways:

- Via the placenta – antibodies in the maternal circulation enter the foetus through the placenta and the umbilical cord. This only accounts for about 5% of the total maternal antibodies.
- In the colostrum – this is the first milk secreted by the dam after parturition. It contains 95% of the total maternal antibodies and is therefore essential for neonatal protection.

Colostrum is rich in antibodies to any antigen with which the dam has been in contact. This includes antibodies to diseases in the dam's immediate environment. Moving the young to a new area after parturition will expose them to different pathogens to which they have no maternal immunity. Ensuring that the dam has been recently vaccinated before she is mated will increase the levels of antibodies. Booster vaccinations may be given during pregnancy providing that care is taken to avoid the use of live vaccines, which may harm the developing foetuses.

Antibodies, ingested in the colostrum, pass undigested through the lining of the small intestine

Table 2.4 The types of immunisation

Type	Method		Comments
Active – animal forms its own antibodies	**Natural**	Animal becomes infected with the disease and survives	Antibodies take several days to develop. Protection lasts for life. In some diseases there is a risk of animal being left with residual damage, e.g. fits, paralysis, etc.
	Artificial	Vaccination – antigen inoculated in a harmless form	Antibodies take several days to develop. Protection lasts for life. Regular booster vaccinations are recommended
Passive – animal is given preformed antibodies	**Natural**	Maternal antibodies passed to the foetus via the placenta and the neonate via the colostrum	Provides instant protection to diseases with which the dam has been in contact. Lasts for approximately 12 weeks
	Artificial	Antiserum or hyperimmune serum	Provides instant protection. Used in cases of disease outbreak. Lasts for approximately 4 weeks

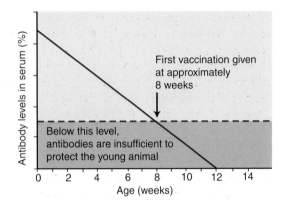

Figure 2.12 Graph to show levels of maternal antibody in the young animal.

for 24–48 hours post-partum. After this, the lining of the intestine 'closes' and the antibodies are digested along with all other proteins. This makes them useless in overcoming antigens so it is essential that neonates receive colostrum within the first 24 hours of life.

Maternal antibodies survive in the body of the young animal for approximately 12 weeks. During this period, the levels slowly fall and the animal's own immune system develops the ability to form antibodies. The timing of the vaccination (Fig. 2.12) has to be considered in relation to the levels of maternal antibody. High levels of maternal antibody actively interfere with formation of antibodies by the young animal. By approximately 8 weeks, the maternal antibodies have fallen to levels within which the animal may be at risk from disease and this is traditionally the time of the first vaccine.

VACCINATION

Vaccination is the means by which active immunity is stimulated artificially in a susceptible animal. It provides protection, which develops over a period of several days but lasts for a long time. Regular booster vaccinations are recommended to keep antibodies up to therapeutic levels.

A **vaccine** contains an antigen in a harmless form so that it loses its virulence (ability to cause disease), but is able to stimulate the production

of specific antibodies against it. If the vaccinated animal is challenged by the natural disease, a secondary response is produced and antibody levels rise to fight the antigen (Fig. 2.10) so preventing the onset of clinical signs. The antibodies resulting from vaccination are specific to the antigen, although some pathogens are so closely related that immunity to one will protect against infection by another, e.g. canine adenovirus (CAV-2), one of the causes of kennel cough, will also protect against CAV-1, the causal organism for infectious canine hepatitis.

Types of vaccine

Vaccines are produced by modifying the antigen in some way so that it cannot cause the disease. They may be:

- **Live and attenuated** – the antigen is live but the virulence of the antigen is reduced or lost. This is done by a process known as attenuation in which bacteria are cultured under abnormal conditions or viruses are grown on successive tissue cultures. Live vaccines undergo limited replication when injected, which may cause a mild infection, and there is a very slight risk of the antigen regaining its virulence and causing disease. For this reason they should never be given to pregnant females as they may affect the developing foetuses. Live vaccines stimulate a good level of immunity, require fewer boosters and are less likely to initiate an allergic reaction.
- **Killed** – the antigen is allowed to replicate in the laboratory and is then killed by the use of heat, ultraviolet or chemicals such as formaldehyde. The dead antigen is quickly removed by phagocytosis, so levels of antibodies must be raised by repeated doses. Killed vaccines are safe to use in pregnant animals.
- **Adjuvenated** – the addition of an insoluble adjuvant enhances the immune response elicited by a killed antigen. Common adjuvants include oil and aluminium hydroxide which form a depot and slow

down the release and removal of the killed antigen. The antigen leaks out of the granulomatous reaction to the adjuvant and may remain for several weeks. Without the adjuvant it may remain for only a few days. The use of an adjuvant means that only one dose of vaccine has to be used. The disadvantage of adjuvants is that they are associated with systemic reactions and aluminium in particular has been recently linked with fibrosarcomata in cats.

- **Toxoid** – in veterinary practice, the most common use of a toxoid is in vaccination against tetanus. *Clostridium tetani*, an anaerobic bacteria responsible for causing tetanus, secretes a toxin that damages the neurons. The body responds by producing antitoxins. To vaccinate against the disease tetanus toxoid or heat-killed toxin is given. Tetanus antitoxin (similar to antiserum) is given to provide instant protection in the case of a wound or bite.

The search for new and improved vaccines continues and has led to many different types including:

- **Genetically engineered** – the genetic makeup of the pathogen is altered so that it stimulates the formation of antibodies but cannot cause disease.

- **Sub-unit** – the pathogen is fragmented to release the part that stimulates the formation of antibodies which is used in the vaccine, leaving the parts responsible for causing disease. Feline leukaemia vaccine is a sub-unit vaccine based on the protein coat of the virus.
- **Autogenous vaccine** – derived from pathogenic bacteria or viruses taken from the individual animal. This is injected into the animal to form antibodies against the pathogen. It is used particularly in cases of intractable staphylococcal skin infections.

Diseases for which vaccines are available

See Table 2.5.

Vaccine administration

Vaccines are supplied as solutions or as freeze-dried pellets, which must be reconstituted with sterile water, supplied by the manufacturers. Different vaccines may be mixed to avoid giving multiple injections, but this must only be done following the manufacturer's instructions. Once the vaccine has been reconstituted, it must be stored in the fridge and used within a few hours.

The **route of administration** depends on the vaccine to be used:

Table 2.5 Range of vaccines available in the UK

Species	Vaccine/disease	Type of vaccine	Route of adminstration
Dog	Distemper	Mod live	Subcutaneous
	Canine parvovirus	Mod live or killed adj	Subcutaneous
	Infectious canine hepatitis/CAV-1	CAV-2 – mod live	Subcutaneous
	Leptospirosis	Killed adj	Subcutaneous
	Kennel cough	Mod live	Subcutaneous or intranasal
Dog and cat	Rabies	Killed adj	Subcutaneous
	Tetanus toxoid	Killed adj	Subcutaneous
Cat	Feline infectious enteritis of feline panleucopenia	Mod live or killed adj	Subcutaneous
	Cat 'flu – feline herpesvirus	Mod live or killed adj	Subcutaneous
	– feline calicivirus	Mod live or killed adj	Subcutaneous
	Feline leukaemia virus	Killed adj/GE/SU	Subcutaneous
	Chlamydiosis	Mod live or killed adj	Subcutaneous
Rabbit	Viral haemorrhagic disease	Killed adj	Subcutaneous
	Myxomatosis	Mod live	Subcutaneous/intradermal

GE, genetically engineered; SU, sub-unit.

1. **Subcutaneous injection** – this is the most common method and is given in the scruff of the neck. Normal sterile techniques must be observed in preparing the site and the equipment, but do not use a spirit swab to wipe the top of the vaccine bottle as spirit may inactivate live vaccines. If multiple injections are given, it is important to vary the site in order to avoid causing a local skin reaction.
2. **Intranasal** – used for kennel cough vaccination – canine parainfluenza/*Bordetella bronchiseptica*. A special applicator is used to squirt the vaccine into the nasal cavity. The antigen stimulates the formation of local antibody and cell-mediated immunity in the nasal mucosa which gives a greater degree of protection to this respiratory disease than that produced by a subcutaneous vaccine.
3. **Oral** – used to vaccinate wildlife in Europe against rabies. Vaccination against lungworm in cattle is achieved by oral administration of irradiated lungworm larvae.

After vaccination, owners should be warned that the animal may show a minor reaction such as:

• slight lethargy a few hours afterwards
• loss of appetite and depression within 24–48 hours
• small swelling at the injection site.

More severe reactions have been reported and seem to be particularly linked with vaccinations against rabies and feline leukaemia. These include allergic reactions such generalized itching, swelling of the face and 'blue eye' – a corneal reaction linked with the use of CAV-1 vaccine against infectious canine hepatitis. The vaccine has been changed so this is less common nowadays. If a severe reaction occurs, the owner should report it to the vet who may inform the vaccine manufacturer if appropriate.

Timing of vaccination

The timing of vaccination depends on individual practice protocols and the choice of vaccine:

• Most vaccination programmes begin when the puppy or kitten is 8–9 weeks old. At this time the maternal antibodies have fallen to levels that no longer interfere with the vaccination (Fig. 2.12).
• Recent research has led to the development of vaccines that are able to overcome higher levels of maternal antibody and thus provide protection at a younger age. These are usually given at 6 weeks of age.
• The final injection is given at 12 weeks old. The puppy or kitten is not considered to be fully protected until 4–5 days after this injection as it takes time for the secondary response to become effective.
• In areas where there is a high incidence of canine parvovirus, a third injection may be given at 16–18 weeks to ensure adequate protection.
• Annual boosters are recommended to maintain protective levels of immunity. The regime depends on the antigen as some pathogens are more immunogenic (stimulate immunity) than others:
  — Leptospirosis, killed parvovirus and cat 'flu vaccines are poorly immunogenic and should be given annually.
  — Distemper, live parvovirus and canine adenovirus are highly immunogenic. Immunity lasts for life but, in the absence of stimulation by the naturally occurring disease, antibody levels may fall. Boosters are recommended every other year.
  — Kennel cough vaccine should be given every 6 months and should be given 2–3 weeks before the dog is put into kennels.
  — Rabbits are vaccinated against myxomatosis and viral haemorrhagic disease at 9–12 weeks old. Boosters are given annually.

Vaccination certificates

Every animal must be given a certificate after vaccination has been completed. This provides proof of its immune status and the certificate may need to be shown before the dog or cat is put into kennels, enters a show, is exported and imported as part of the PETS scheme, or prior to mating by a stud dog or cat.

The certificates are usually provided by the vaccine manufacturers and have the practice details printed on them. All information entered on to the certificate must be correct and should include:

- name and address of owner
- name, species, age, breed, colour and sex of animal
- type of vaccine used
- batch no. – in case of adverse reactions – helps to identify a faulty batch
- date
- recommended date of next vaccination or booster
- signature of the veterinary surgeon.

This information must also be kept on the practice records in case the certificate is lost.

Storage of vaccines

To maintain efficacy vaccines must be stored in a fridge at temperatures of +2°C to +8°C. If transported they must be kept in a coolbox and returned to the fridge as soon as possible.

Stock control

All vaccines are marked with an expiry date, which should be strictly noted, as they may have a reduced effect after that date. Rotate the stock to ensure that older bottles are used first.

INFECTIOUS DISEASES OF THE DOG

DISTEMPER

Aetiology: Morbillivirus related to rinderpest and measles.

Incubation period: 7–21 days.

Pathogenesis: Aerosol infection or ingestion. Virus replicates in tonsils and local lymph nodes leading to viraemia. Spreads to epithelial cells of respiratory and alimentary tract. Also affects nervous system, skin and bone marrow.

Clinical signs: Pyrexia after 1 week, other signs develop later. Anorexia, coughing (differentiate from kennel cough), vomiting, diarrhoea, serous-mucopurulent nasal and conjunctival discharges, tonsillitis and pneumonia. Several weeks later there may be hyperkeratosis of the nose and pads (hardpad), nervous signs including fits and chorea (skin twitches), and enamel hypoplasia seen in recovered puppies.

Treatment: No specific methods – treat symptomatically – antibiotics, i.v. fluids, antitussants, antiemetics, anticonvulsants. Good nursing care. Euthanasia may be recommended.

Prevention: Vaccination with modified live vaccines. Booster every other year.

Other comments: Highly contagious. Epidemics could occur in areas where the immunity of the local population has fallen due to lack of routine vaccination.

INFECTIOUS CANINE HEPATITIS (ICH)

Aetiology: Canine adenovirus – CAV-1.

Incubation period: 5–9 days.

Pathogenesis: Ingestion following direct or indirect contact with vomit, faeces, saliva or urine. Virus replicates in tonsils and local lymph nodes leading to viraemia, followed by further replication in vascular endothelial cells of many organs including the kidney, eye and in the hepatocytes of the liver.

Clinical signs: Presents as acute disease – pyrexia, followed by death within 24 hours. If dog survives, it may show lethargy, anorexia, thirst, vomiting, diarrhoea, conjunctivitis, photophobia, petechial haemorrhages and jaundice. Persistent infection may result in glomerulonephritis, corneal and uveal inflammation (blue eye). Recovered cases may become carriers – shedding the virus in urine for up to 6 months.

Treatment: i.v. fluids, antibiotics, antiemetics. Good nursing care.

Prevention: Vaccination. Live CAV-1 vaccine causes mild disease and blue eye. Use live CAV-2 vaccine which protects against CAV-1 and CAV-2 infections. CAV-2 is a cause of kennel cough.

KENNEL COUGH (infectious
tracheobronchitis or canine contagious
respiratory disease – CCRD)

Aetiology: *Bordetella bronchiseptica*, CAV-2, para-influenza virus, herpes virus, reovirus, secondary bacterial infections.

Incubation period: 5–7 days.

Pathogenesis: Aerosol infection between dogs in direct contact or within the same air space. Pathogens replicate in tonsils, local lymph nodes and epithelium of the upper respiratory tract.

Clinical signs: Dry hacking cough, often precipitated by exercise or excitement. May be followed by gagging or retching. Most cases remain bright and well. In severe infections, there may be pyrexia, mucopurulent nasal ocular discharges, anorexia and bronchopneumonia.

Treatment: Antibiotics and antitussives.

Prevention: Vaccination – no vaccine incorporates all the causal organisms. Use of CAV-2 to protect against ICH will also cover kennel cough. *Bordetella bronchiseptica* is given as an intranasal sub-unit vaccine as the best protection is produced by local antibodies and cell-mediated immunity in the nasal mucosa. Boosters should be repeated every 6 months and should be given 2–3 weeks before the dog is put into kennels.

Other comments: Kennel cough is highly contagious and spreads rapidly through groups of dogs kept in close contact, e.g. in boarding kennels. Consideration should be given to the design of kennels – including reduced numbers of dogs in one air space and good ventilation rates. Owners of kennels must adopt a strict vaccination policy.

LEPTOSPIROSIS

Aetiology: *Leptospira canicola* and *Leptospira icterohaemorrhagiae*, other leptospires have been reported.

Incubation period: Up to 7 days.

Pathogenesis: Penetration through broken skin and mucous membranes. Transplacental and venereal infection also occur. Spread by direct or indirect contact with infected urine or contaminated water. Replication in local lymph nodes, blood, renal nephrons and liver.

Clinical signs: Depend on species of leptospire:

- *L. canicola* – affects the kidney and causes acute renal failure. Initial oliguria followed by polyuria, polydipsia, acute vomiting, renal pain, azotaemia. Raised blood urea and serum creatinine.
- *L. icterohaemorrhagiae* – affects the liver and may cause sudden death in unvaccinated animals. Acute vomiting, anorexia, jaundice, anterior abdominal pain, collapse, petechial haemorrhages. Elevated liver enzymes.

Recovered cases may excrete leptospires in urine for weeks or even years.

Treatment: Antibiotics, i.v. fluids, antiemetics. Dietary management. Good nursing care.

Prevention: Vaccination with killed vaccine. Annual boosters.

Other comments: Important zoonosis – Weil's disease in humans – take precautions to prevent spread from infected urine. Also occurs in rats and cattle, although cats may become infected. Most significant source of infection is from contaminated water. Avoid water sports in lakes and ponds inhabited by rats.

LYME DISEASE

Aetiology: *Borrelia burgdoferi.*

Incubation period: Variable – spirochaete can lie dormant for several months or years in infected animal.

Pathogenesis: Transmitted by Ixodid ticks – notably *Ixodes dammeri* found on deer. Affects humans and many species of animal.

Clinical signs: Many animals show no evidence of disease. Pyrexia, anorexia, rash, depression, enlarged lymph nodes, chronic arthritis and lameness, encephalitis.

Treatment: Antibiotics, analgesics. Remove ticks.

Prevention: Avoid entering tick-infested areas. Apply tick repellents. Remove ticks as soon as possible. Vaccine available in USA.

Other comments: This disease is not common in the UK except in areas of heathland such as the New Forest and Cumbria. Changes in environmental conditions and to import/export regulations may lead to infected ticks entering the country and the risk of widespread endemic disease in tick-infested areas.

PARVOVIRUS

Aetiology: Canine parvovirus 2.

Incubation period: 4–7 days.

Pathogenesis: Infection by ingestion of the virus following direct or indirect contact with faeces. Viral replication occurs in lymph nodes of the gastrointestinal tract and then virus particles are carried by the blood to all rapidly dividing cells including bone marrow, lining of the intestine, lung, liver and kidney.

Clinical signs: In neonatal puppies it may cause sudden death due to myocardial disease. Severe haemorrhagic gastroenteritis, acute vomiting, anorexia, dramatic weight loss, abdominal pain, dehydration. Death may occur within 72 hours. Recovery may be complicated by malabsorption. Haematology – severe leucopenia and raised packed cell volume.

Treatment: i.v. fluid therapy, antibiotics, antiemetics. Good nursing is essential – isolation and barrier nursing.

Prevention: Vaccination – live attenuated vaccine gives better protection, but killed vaccine can be used for pregnant bitches. At-risk puppies may be vaccinated at 6 weeks, repeat at 8 weeks, 12 weeks and if necessary at 16 weeks. Antiserum may be used for young puppies in an outbreak. Boosters recommended every other year.

Other comments: Virus particles are found in faeces during the incubation period and may survive on fomites for up to 6 months. Stringent hygiene precautions are essential to prevent spread, particularly within the practice. Vaccine, available since the early 1980s, has led to a level of immunity within the dog population. Epidemics may occur in areas where immunity is low due to lack of routine vaccination.

INFECTIOUS DISEASES OF THE DOG AND CAT

RABIES

Aetiology: Rhabdovirus (bullet-shaped RNA) belonging to the genus *Lyssavirus*.

Incubation period: Variable – depending on factors such as site of bite, dose and strain of virus, species of animal; 1–6 months but occasionally longer.

Pathogenesis: Affects all warm-blooded animals. Virus is excreted in saliva and is usually transmitted by a bite or contamination of an open wound. The virus remains in the area of the bite, then replicates in the muscles. It then travels along peripheral nerves until it reaches the central nervous system and eventually reaches every organ via nerves. Rabies virus is only vulnerable to antibody attack when in the 'muscle phase'.

Clinical signs: there are three phases, which may be difficult to differentiate:

- **Prodromal phase** – slight pyrexia, change in temperament – friendly animals become aggressive and unpredictable; timid animals become very friendly. May last for 1–3 days, before progressing to the furious or dumb phases.
- **Furious phase** – these periods last for a short time or for several days. Hyperexcitability, aggression, snap and bite at imaginary objects, tendency to chew and eat unusual objects such as stones and wood, wander for miles then return home apparently quite normal. Progressive paralysis, difficulty in swallowing, worried expression on face due to facial paralysis, drooling and frothing of saliva. Death within 7 days usually during a seizure.
- **Dumb phase** – much more common. May lead from furious phase or from the prodromal phase. Gradual paralysis, incoordination, convulsions, coma and death.

Treatment: None. This is a **notifiable** disease – the Department of the Environment, Food and Rural Affairs (DEFRA) must be informed of any suspected case. Animal is destroyed and case is confirmed by histological examination of brain material.

Prevention

- Dogs and cats returning to the UK under the Pet Travel Scheme from a specified list of countries must be vaccinated with killed vaccine and blood-tested to confirm efficacy. This must be done at least 6 months before travelling.

- Quarantine regulations still apply to animals returning to the UK from remaining countries.
- Anyone working with animals that could develop rabies, e.g. in quarantine kennels or zoos, must be vaccinated.
- Post-exposure vaccination for humans – vaccination must be given as soon as possible to kill the virus in the 'muscle phase'.
- Oral vaccines given in bait to wildlife such as foxes have significantly reduced numbers of cases in France.

SALMONELLA

Aetiology: mainly *Salmonella typhimurium*.

Pathogenesis: Source of infection is most often contaminated meat. 1–5% of normal cats and dogs shed the organism in their faeces without showing any clinical signs.

Clinical signs: Variation in signs and may be asymptomatic – acute or chronic gastroenteritis, pyrexia, depression, vomiting, pneumonia, conjunctivitis. Reproductive problems including stillbirth, abortion, fading puppies or kittens. Transient bacteraemia may result in multiple abscesses in lungs, liver, spleen and lymph nodes.

Treatment: Avoid the use of antibiotics as this may select resistant strains and prolong the excretion of the organisms in faeces, particularly in cats. If antibiotics are used always precede with a sensitivity test. Treat symptomatically. Good nursing care.

Other comments: Salmonellosis can be spread to humans from dogs and cats, but where owners and their pets are both infected it is more likely to have come from a common source.

INFECTIOUS DISEASES OF THE CAT

CHLAMYDIOSIS

Aetiology: *Chlamydia psittaci*.
Incubation period: 3–10 days.
Pathogenesis: Ocular discharges containing *Chlamydia* are transmitted by direct contact. The pathogens enter via the conjunctiva and nasal mucosa.

Clinical signs: Persistent conjunctivitis, mild nasal discharge, sneezing, coughing, mild pyrexia. Symptoms may persist for some months and may recur at intervals. Co-infection with respiratory viruses and secondary infection with bacteria cause a more severe disease which may progress to mild pulmonary involvement.

Treatment: Ophthalmic ointment containing tetracyclines. Systemic antibiotics if necessary. Treat all in-contact cats. Isolate infected cat and take hygiene precautions to prevent transmission of infection.

Prevention: Vaccination using live or killed adjuvenated vaccine.

Other comments: May become enzootic in colonies of young cats and kittens and is particularly associated with rehoming facilities.

FELINE LEUKAEMIA VIRUS (FeLV)

Aetiology: Retrovirus.

Incubation period: Variable. A few weeks to several months.

Pathogenesis: Virus is excreted in saliva, urine, faeces and milk. Transmission by direct contact including biting and licking. Also vertical transmission to foetal and neonatal kittens via the placenta and in milk. Ingested virus replicates in the lymph nodes of the oropharynx, and a primary viraemia spreads the virus to other lymphoid tissues including the bone marrow (Fig. 2.13). Further replication and a secondary viraemia establish a persistent infection. In the initial stages, some cats may eliminate the infection, although latent infection within the bone marrow may persist. Once the infection is established, clinical disease will develop and the cat is a source of infection to other cats.

Susceptibility to infection depends on the age of the cat – kittens affected in utero will die young; kittens affected at 7–8 weeks have a 70–80% chance of developing a persistent viraemia; adults have a 10% chance of becoming viraemic.

Clinical signs: Associated with infection of the haemopoietic system and include lymphosarcoma, non-regenerative anaemia, glomerular

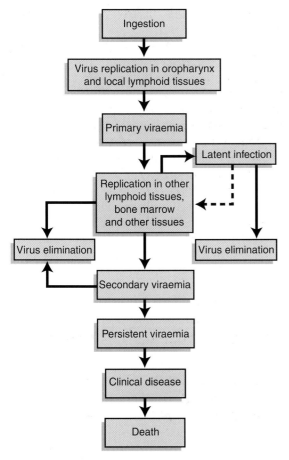

Figure 2.13 Pathogenesis of feline leukaemia virus infection. (Reproduced with permission from Bennett and Gaskell 1996.)

- all cats going to stud
- stud toms every 3 months
- any cat known to have been in contact with a FeLV-positive cat
- new kittens/rehomed adults introduced into a FeLV-free multicat household.

Other comments: ELISA tests may give false positives – if cat is healthy but FeLV positive, infection should be confirmed by virus isolation or immunofluorescence.

FELINE INFECTIOUS ANAEMIA (FIA)

Aetiology: *Haemobartonella felis.*

Incubation period: Unknown. Carrier state is thought to exist.

Pathogenesis: Method of transmission is not known, but it is likely to be spread by biting insects such as fleas and lice. Vertical transmission may also occur. This intracellular rickettsia binds to the red blood cells and they are then removed from the circulation by phagocytosis.

Clinical signs: May be asymptomatic. Cat may show symptoms if affected by stress or concurrent disease such as FeLV. Acute haemolytic anaemia, heart murmur, pyrexia, tachycardia, splenomegaly, weakness and collapse. Blood smear may show organisms attached to red blood cells.

Treatment: Antibiotics – tetracyclines, blood transfusion. Treat flea infestations.

FELINE INFECTIOUS ENTERITIS OR FELINE PANLEUCOPENIA

Aetiology: Parvovirus.

Incubation period: 2–10 days.

Pathogenesis: Virus is excreted in saliva, vomit, faeces and urine. It is transmitted by direct or indirect contact – may survive on fomites for up to a year – and enters body by ingestion. Transplacental infection may cause feline ataxia syndrome in kittens. Virus replicates in intestinal lymph nodes and attacks all rapidly dividing tissues including intestinal epithelium and bone marrow.

Clinical signs: Lethargy, pyrexia, anorexia, vomiting. After a few days there will be profuse

nephritis, immunosuppression, polyarthritis, and reproductive problems such as stillbirth, abortion and foetal resorption. 40% of affected cats will eliminate the virus and recover; 30% develop a low immunity and show symptoms; 30% may have a latent infection which may be shed or may become viraemic again due to stress, corticosteroid therapy or other infections.

Treatment: None. Nursing care to alleviate symptoms. Isolation and barrier nursing to prevent spread to other cats in the household.

Prevention: Vaccination using killed adjuvenated, sub-unit and genetically engineered vaccines. ELISA test to identify peripheral antigen in the following cats:

watery diarrhoea or dysentery causing severe dehydration. Mortality rate is 25–75%. Haematology shows a panleucopenia.

Treatment: i.v. fluid therapy, antibiotics, antiemetics and antidiarrhoeal drugs. Hygiene precautions to prevent spread to any in-contact cats. Pay attention to spread by fomites.

Prevention: Vaccination – modified live or killed adjuvenated. Provides high levels of immunity. Boosters given every other year. Avoid use of live vaccines in pregnant queens.

Other comments: Highly infectious and may be enzootic in unvaccinated populations of feral cats. Recovered cases may become carriers.

FELINE INFECTIOUS PERITONITIS (FIP)

Aetiology: Coronavirus.

Incubation period: Variable.

Pathogenesis: Oronasal infection. Virus replicates in lymph nodes of the gut and then travels to the blood vessels, peritoneum, pleura, meninges, kidneys and eyes.

Clinical signs: Outcome depends on immune status of the cat:

- strong immunity: only the gut is affected causing mild diarrhoea
- mild immunity: symptoms develop slowly and are of dry FIP. May affect central nervous system, abdomen, liver, kidney, eye and causes splenic dysfunction, paresis, ataxia, convulsions and death
- weak immunity: acute wet FIP develops. Ascites, hydrothorax, pericardial effusion, depression, anorexia, weight loss, diarrhoea and death.

Treatment: None. Good nursing care to alleviate symptoms.

Other comments: Very variable disease. Some cats may eliminate the virus; others become persistent carriers.

FELINE IMMUNODEFICIENCY VIRUS (FIV)

Aetiology: Retrovirus (related to human immunodeficiency virus or HIV).

Incubation period: Variable. A few weeks to months.

Pathogenesis: Virus is secreted in saliva, and mainly transmitted by biting and scratching. Neonatal kittens may become infected via milk. Infection is more common in free-ranging and feral male cats. Viral replication occurs in local lymph nodes and spreads to bone marrow and other lymphoid tissues.

Clinical signs: Causes immunosuppression and, as with HIV, clinical signs are related to secondary infection with other micro-organisms and may include chronic gingivitis, chronic upper respiratory tract disease, anorexia, loss of weight, anaemia, FIP, FeLV, and FIA. Most often seen in older cats that may have been infected for years.

Treatment: None. Treat secondary infections symptomatically.

Prevention: Identify by ELISA test – can give false positives. Laboratories also use immunofluorescence assay. Try to prevent spread from infected cats by stopping cats from roaming. Test before going to stud or cat shows. Normal hygiene precautions in catteries and rehoming establishments.

FELINE UPPER RESPIRATORY TRACT DISEASE

Aetiology: Feline calicivirus (FCV) and feline herpesvirus (FHV).

Incubation period: 2–10 days.

Pathogenesis: Aerosol infection. Indirect or direct contact. Virus enters by intranasal, oral and conjunctival routes. Virus replication takes place in all the surrounding tissues.

Clinical signs: FCV causes a milder infection – transient pyrexia, mild sneezing and conjunctivitis, slight lethargy, ulcers on tongue, soft and hard palate. FHV is more severe – depression, marked sneezing, anorexia, pyrexia, ocular and nasal discharges, dyspnoea and coughing. Secondary bacterial infection may lead to chronic infection and damage to intranasal structures.

Treatment: Antibiotics, i.v. fluids or enteral feeding in severe cases. Nursing care – clean nasal and ocular discharges, provide smelly foods to encourage eating, decongestants to clear airways. Home nursing may stimulate a quicker recovery! Isolate affected cat if in a multicat household.

Prevention: Vaccination – range of types and routes of administration.

Other comments: Infection with either virus may lead to a carrier state but after FCV infection the virus is shed continuously – may be lifelong; after FHV the virus is shed intermittently, usually as a result of stress.

TOXOPLASMOSIS

Aetiology: *Toxoplasma gondii.*
Incubation period: 2–5 weeks.
Pathogenesis: This protozoan uses a wide range of intermediate hosts to complete its lifecycle. The cat is the end host, i.e. one in which sexual reproduction occurs. Oocysts, shed in cat faeces, become sporulated and are then infective after 3 days. They are ingested by an intermediate host where they encyst in the body musculature. Cats eating uncooked infected meat complete the lifecycle.

Clinical signs: *T. gondii* reproduces in the small intestine of the cat and this may cause mild diarrhoea. It is more commonly asymptomatic. If cysts develop in other organs, the cat may show lethargy, anorexia, vomiting, jaundice, but this is rare. Congenital infection of kittens may contribute to fading kitten syndrome.

Treatment: Antibiotics.

Prevention: Do not feed uncooked or undercooked meat to cats; clean litter trays daily to prevent oocysts from reaching the infective stage; prevent cats from hunting as wild birds and rodents may be intermediate hosts.

Other comments: This is an important zoonosis and may particularly affect pregnant women and their unborn children. To prevent spread:

- wear gloves when cleaning litter trays or gardening
- wash all vegetables
- cook meat thoroughly and keep separate from uncooked meat
- wash hands after handling cats, raw meat and litter trays

- pregnant women should avoid working with sheep which are intermediate hosts.

INFECTIOUS DISEASES OF THE RABBIT

MYXOMATOSIS

Aetiology: Poxvirus.
Pathogenesis: Transmitted by insect vectors such as the mosquito and the stick tight flea *Spilopsylla cuniculi.* Depending on virulence, the virus may cause a peracute infection and death or production of skin tumours. A respiratory form has also been reported.

Clinical signs: In acute cases, the rabbit is lethargic, pyrexic and depressed. The eyes become red, swollen and watery; the lips, genitalia and anus are oedematous. Progresses rapidly to death. In the less virulent form, skin tumours develop in large numbers.

Treatment: Often unsuccessful. i.v. fluid therapy, antibiotics. Nursing care to alleviate symptoms.

Prevention: Vaccination – live vaccine – given subcutaneously or intradermally at the base of the ear. Control insect vectors and prevent contact with wild rabbits.

Other comments: This disease is endemic in the wild rabbit population.

VIRAL HAEMORRHAGIC DISEASE

Aetiology: Calicivirus.
Incubation period: 1–2 days.
Pathogenesis: highly infectious with high morbidity (70–80%) and mortality (100%). Only affects rabbits over 2 months of age. Spread by direct or indirect contact. Virus is ingested in faeces and from contaminated fomites, but may also enter via nasal and conjunctival mucous membranes. Replication leads to viraemia and subsequent generalised failure of intravascular coagulation mechanisms.

Clinical signs: Rapid course of disease – pyrexia, depression, lethargy, anorexia. Some may show signs of tachypnoea, cyanosis, diarrhoea, convulsions, epistaxis and death. Many cases develop so rapidly that the rabbit is found dead without having shown any apparent symptoms.

Treatment: None. Nursing care to relieve symptoms.

Prevention: Vaccination – killed adjuvenated vaccine. Given at 10–12 weeks old. Annual boosters recommended. Buy young rabbits from vaccinated stock only.

ZOONOSES

A zoonosis is a disease that can be passed from vertebrate animals to humans. Details of zoonotic diseases in dogs, cats and rabbits can be found in Table 2.6. Anyone working with animals, whether in a zoo, kennels or veterinary practice, is at risk of contracting one of these diseases and must take sensible precautions to minimise this risk. It is also important to warn owners of the existence of such diseases and advise them of the ways in which they can prevent the transmission of infection from their pets to themselves or their families.

Sensible precautions include:

- Increase awareness of the existence of zoonoses – anyone who works with or owns animals should understand the risk of infection and how to avoid it.
- Do not eat or smoke after handling animals.
- Wash hands after handling animals.
- Wear protective clothing when working with animals.
- Do not take protective clothing home – this prolongs exposure to pathogens on the clothes.
- Do not allow animals to foul in public places or in areas of the garden used by children.
- Never let animals share your food, lick your plate or lick your face.
- Never feed raw meat to animals.
- Do not store raw meat for animals in the same place as meat for human consumption.

Table 2.6	Some examples of zoonotic diseases with relevance to the dog, cat and rabbit		
Disease	Species	Causal organism	Symptoms in humans
Rabies	Warm blooded animals	Lyssavirus	Affects CNS and PNS – progressive paralysis, hydrophobia, death
Leptospirosis – Weil's disease	Dog, rat, cattle – rare in the cat	*Leptospira icterohaemorrhagiae L.canicola*	Flu-like symptoms – may take several months to recover
Toxocariasis	Dog	*Toxocara canis* – roundworm	Associated with retinal lesions. May be misdiagnosed as retinoblastoma – a malignant tumour
Scabies	Dog, cat	*Sarcoptes scabiei* – mange mite	Irritant red rash – particularly around waist
Toxoplasmosis	Cat	*Toxoplasma gondii*	Flu-like symptoms. Reproductive problems in women. Foetal abnormalities – may affect the eyes or the brain
Ringworm	Dog, cat, rabbit	*Microsporum canis, Trichophyton mentagrophytes*	Irritant patches of broken hairs and flakey skin. Secondary infection leads to oozing and suppuration
Fleas	Dog, cat, rabbit	*Ctenocephalides felis, Spilopsyllus cuniculi*	Irritant spots – scratching leads to secondary infection
Giardiasis	Dog, cat	*Giardia duodenalis*	Acute and chronic diarrhoea. May be contracted from same source
Cat scratch fever	Cat	*Bartonella hensilae*	Pustule develops. Local lymphadenitis. Perinaud's ocular glandular syndrome

CNS, central nervous system; PNS, peripheral nervous system.

- Consult your doctor if you suspect you have been in contact with a zoonotic disease.
- Keep your tetanus vaccination up to date.

NOTIFIABLE DISEASES

Under the Animal Health Act 1981, certain diseases are classified as **notifiable.** Most of these diseases affect farm animals and have a significant effect on public health, animal welfare and agricultural economics. The only notifiable disease relating to dogs and cats is rabies.

If a notifiable disease is suspected or diagnosed, it must be reported immediately to the police and to DEFRA. Procedures relating to the prevention of spread to other animals and laid down in the Animal Health Act 1981 will then be put into action.

REFERENCES

Cooper B, Lane DR (eds) 1999 Veterinary nursing, 2nd edn. Butterworth-Heinemann, Oxford, pp 365, 371, 375
Bennett M, Gaskell RM 1996 Feline and canine infectious diseases. Blackwell Science, Oxford, p 48

Masters J, Bowden C (eds) 2001 Pre-veterinary nursing textbook. Butterworth-Heinemann in association with BVNA, Oxford, pp 12, 169

FURTHER READING

Bennett M, Gaskell RM 1996 Feline and canine infectious diseases. Blackwell Science, Oxford
Cooper B, Lane DR (eds) 1999 Veterinary nursing, 2nd edn. Butterworth-Heinemann, Oxford
Flecknell P (ed) 2000 Manual of rabbit medicine and surgery. BSAVA, Gloucester
Hillyer EV, Quesenberry KE 1997 Ferrets, rabbits and rodents. Clinical medicine and surgery. WB Saunders, Philadelphia
Ikram M, Hill E 1991 Microbiology for veterinary technicians. American Veterinary Publications, California
Moore M (ed) 1999 Manual of veterinary nursing. BSAVA, Gloucester

CONTENTS

3

Common medical diseases

Katie Dunn   Stephen J Baines

PART 1

The alimentary tract
(Tables 3.1 and 3.2)

Katie Dunn

ANATOMY AND PHYSIOLOGY

The alimentary tract starts at the mouth and comprises the oesophagus, stomach and intestines. Its primary function is the ingestion, digestion and absorption of nutrients.

In the mouth the food particles are broken down into smaller pieces by the action of the teeth and are mixed with saliva by the tongue. Saliva helps lubricate the food to make swallowing easier but also contains enzymes that start the process of digestion. The food/saliva mix forms a bolus which is passed to the back of the mouth where the swallowing reflex passes the food through the pharynx into the oesophagus. The oesophagus is a muscular tube running between the pharynx and the stomach. It is normally closed at the pharynx by a sphincter, and at the distal end by the angle of entry of the oesophagus into the stomach. The stomach has three distinct areas:

- the cardia (entrance)
- the fundus (body or main part)
- the pylorus (which exits into the first part of the intestine).

Mucus and hydrochloric acid are secreted by specialised cells in the stomach wall and these secretions are mixed with the food. Enzymes which break down fat (lipase) and proteins (pepsinogen) are also secreted. Rhythmical contractions help

Table 3.1 Important questions to ask the owner of a vomiting animal

Question	Reason for question and interpretation of answer
Is the animal bright?	Depression may be associated with systemic disease causing vomiting (as opposed to primary gastrointestinal disease)
How long has the patient been vomiting?	Most cases of simple vomiting resolve within 24–48 hours. Vomiting persisting beyond this time will require further investigation
How frequent is the vomiting?	Vomiting may be associated with a particular time, when the patient has an empty stomach or soon after eating. Frequent vomiting can be very debilitating and distressing and if this is persistent the patient should be admitted for observation and further tests
What is the animal vomiting?	Patients with problems of gastric emptying will vomit whatever has been in the stomach. Systemic illness is often associated with the vomiting of bile
Is there any blood?	Blood in the vomit suggests upper gastrointestinal tract ulceration. This is a concerning finding if there are significant quantities of blood
Is water being kept down?	Vomiting of water is a concerning sign. Patients unable to keep fluids down will require intravenous fluid therapy
Does the animal want to eat and drink?	Anorexia may be associated with nausea or systemic disease. Patients with gastric emptying problems may not want to eat if their stomach is still full from the previous meal
Is the animal known to scavenge – or has there been a recent diet change?	Exposure to unusual or rotten foods can result in acute gastroenteritis (GE). Signs are usually self-limiting. Repeated bouts of GE may be the result of persistent scavenging or can sometimes be traced to a single food source, e.g. milk intolerance. Lead walking or muzzling to prevent scavenging can aid diagnosis

Table 3.2 Important questions to ask the owner of an animal with diarrhoea

Question	Reason for question and interpretation of answer
How long has the diarrhoea been going on?	Most cases with uncomplicated diarrhoea resolve within a few days. As diarrhoea becomes more chronic it can become self-perpetuating
Is there any vomiting?	Vomiting associated with diarrhoea may indicate generalised involvement of the gastrointestinal tract. However, vomiting can be associated with colitis without gastric disease
How frequent is the diarrhoea?	Frequent episodes of diarrhoea may be associated with large bowel inflammation. If significant volumes of diarrhoea are passed frequently fluid loss can be substantial and replacement should be considered
What is the nature of the diarrhoea (watery, pasty)?	Watery diarrhoea (particularly in young or old animals) requires more urgent attention. Fluid and electrolyte losses can be substantial and intravenous fluid therapy may be required
Is there any blood?	Fresh blood in the diarrhoea indicates large bowel ulceration. Blood from lesions in the small intestine will be digested (melaena) by the time it appears in the faeces
What colour is the diarrhoea?	Black diarrhoea indicates the presence of melaena. Pale faeces may be associated with high fat content (maldigestion)
Is the animal losing weight?	Weight loss with diarrhoea suggests maldigestion or malabsorption of food. This always requires further investigation
Does the animal want to eat and drink?	Depression and inappetance associated with diarrhoea are concerning signs. Most animals with uncomplicated diarrhoea are otherwise bright and healthy. Small intestinal diarrhoea may be associated with increased appetite due to poor digestion/absorption.

to mix the stomach contents and further break up food particles. Food is only allowed to exit the stomach when it has been broken down into small particles. The liquid leaving the stomach contains gastric acid and must be neutralised on entering the intestine.

The small intestine is concerned with digestion and absorption of nutrients. It is the longest area of the alimentary tract and its surface area is increased many thousands of times by multiple folds and finger like projections (villi) from its wall. It can be divided into three sections:

- duodenum (into which the pancreatic duct and bile duct empty)
- jejunum
- ileum.

Secretions from the pancreas enter the duodenum and these start to break down proteins and carbohydrates in the food. Bile salts are also released from the liver and these act like a detergent assisting the breakdown of fats. The intestine also secretes a mixture of bicarbonate to neutralise the acid secretions from the stomach, disaccharidases (to break down disaccharide sugars to simple sugars) and peptidases (to break down peptides to amino acids). Once the protein and carbohydrates have been broken down into smaller molecules these can be absorbed across the intestinal wall. Fatty acids from the breakdown of fat enter the body through the thoracic duct. Remaining gut contents pass from the small intestine through the ileocaecocolic valve into the large bowel.

The large bowel can be divided into:

- caecum
- colon
- rectum.

The main function of the large bowel in cats and dogs is the absorption of water. Around 95% of the water that enters the large bowel is resorbed; it is easy to see why disease of this area can have serious consequences for fluid balance. The colon is also used to store faeces before elimination from the body.

PATHOPHYSIOLOGY

Diseases of the gastrointestinal tract can be classified according to their major presenting sign (see Box 3.1).

Vomiting

Causes

Vomiting is the process of emptying the stomach towards the mouth. It can occur as a result of diseases of the stomach or small intestine, or of systemic diseases having effects on the vomiting

Box 3.1	Diseases of the gastrointestinal tract		
Vomiting	**Diarrhoea**	**Regurgitation**	**Constipation/tenesmus**
Gastric foreign body	Small intestinal foreign body	Oesophageal foreign body	Large intestinal foreign body, fur
Infectious disease	Infectious disease	Megaoesophagus	balls or bones
Gastric tumour	Intestinal tumour	Oesophageal tumour	Megacolon
Gastritis	Malabsorption	Oesophagitis	Large intestinal tumour
Systemic disease	Dietary indiscretion	Oesophageal stricture	Neurological disease
Hepatic failure	Inflammatory disease	Vascular ring anomaly	Perineal hernia
Renal failure	Parasitic infections		Fractured pelvis
Pyometra	Chronic lead ingestion		
Pancreatitis			
Colitis			
Gastric dilatation			
Motion sickness			
Chronic lead ingestion			

> **Box 3.2** Typical signs associated with vomiting
>
> May be preceded by lip smacking, salivation and signs of distress
> Active abdominal effort
> May contain digested food and bile
> Often occurs many hours after eating
> Stomach contents are usually acid but if small intestine contents expelled the pH may be increased

> **Box 3.3** Typical signs associated with regurgitation
>
> Often occurs suddenly without warning
> No effort required – animal lowers head and volumes of material expelled
> Food contents undigested
> Can occur soon after feeding but contents may remain in oesophagus for many hours
> Oesophageal contents should have a neutral pH

centre in the brain. Vomiting is very common in dogs and cats because it evolved as a protective mechanism to prevent absorption of toxic substances. When an animal vomits the stomach muscle is relaxed and contents are expelled through an open cardiac sphincter by contractions of the abdominal muscles.

Signs

The signs of vomiting are familiar to us all but it is vital to be able to differentiate vomiting from regurgitation (see Boxes 3.2 and 3.3).

Diagnostic tests

Acute vomiting is often treated symptomatically without diagnosis. In more severe or chronic cases investigations may include blood tests to rule out a systemic disease, e.g. kidney failure, and to monitor the metabolic effects of the vomiting, i.e. dehydration or electrolyte abnormalities. Radiographs may be useful to detect radio-opaque foreign bodies, and contrast radiographic studies may show other foreign bodies, obstructions and motility disorders. Ultrasonography can be useful for detection of intussusception and tumours. Endoscopic examination of the stomach and small intestine may reveal lesions in the stomach

or intestine walls and biopsies can be taken to provide a definitive diagnosis.

Treatment

Symptomatic management in acute cases should include withholding of all food and provision of adequate fluid intake, either orally or intravenously if oral fluids are not kept down. If vomiting persists then identification and treatment of the primary cause are essential. Since many causes are infectious attention to hygiene is essential when nursing the patient with signs of gastrointestinal disease.

Diarrhoea

Causes

Diarrhoea is defined as increased liquidity of faeces and is often associated with an increased faecal volume and frequency of defecation. It can arise for four reasons:

1. interference with nutrient digestion or absorption (increased solute in gut draws in water)
2. excessive fluid secretion into the gut
3. mucosal damage resulting in increased permeability of the gut (solute and fluid leak in together)
4. altered motility of the gut (in most cases of diarrhoea the gut is hypomobile).

Signs

Abnormally soft faeces are passed. Depending on the cause of the diarrhoea the patient may be bright or systemically ill with abdominal pain, pyrexia or anorexia. Other signs may be associated with diarrhoea which may help to differentiate whether the problem is in the small or large bowel (see Box 3.4). These signs are not specific and it is common for a mixture of signs associated with the large and small bowel to be seen. Vomiting may be seen with either large or small intestinal disease. Melaena (black faeces) due to partially digested blood implies bleeding into the upper gastrointestinal tract. Fresh blood in the faeces (haematochezia) is seen if bleeding is occurring in the lower bowel.

Box 3.4 Characteristics of diarrhoea depending on origin	
Large intestine	**Small intestine**
Frequent defecation	Increased faecal volume (due to failure of absorption)
Small volume of faeces passed	Normal (or increased) frequency of defecation
Urgency to pass faeces	Weight loss but increased appetite
Straining/pain on defecation	Pale fatty faeces (rare)
Fresh blood or mucus in faeces	

Diagnostic tests

In many cases of diarrhoea a definitive diagnosis is never made and the condition often responds to symptomatic treatment. More chronic cases require further investigation. The history often provides a clue as to the likely location of the problem, i.e. small or large bowel. Identification of a systemic disease causing gastrointestinal (GI) signs may be possible and measurement of trypsin-like immunoreactivity (TLI) cobalamin folate can give an indication of the presence of related diseases. For definitive diagnosis a gut biopsy is often required. Endoscopic or colonoscopic examination may be useful and may permit biopsy of the intestine without laparotomy. Breath hydrogen measurements can be made to help confirm a diagnosis of small intestinal bacterial overgrowth (SIBO), or culture of intestinal juice samples collected at laparotomy or endoscopy can give an indication of the bacterial load present. Radiographic examination is rarely helpful but ultrasound may be useful for identification of thickened gut wall in infiltrative disease.

Treatment

Most cases are self limiting but if patients have systemic signs of illness or are not improving on symptomatic treatment after 2–3 weeks, further investigations are required. Symptomatic treatment includes:

- Fast 24–48 hours (reduces osmotic diarrhoea by reducing solute in gut and reduces food

supply to abnormal bacteria). Fasting for longer periods is not recommended as this may also starve the cells in the gut wall resulting in reduced mucosal integrity and gut function.
- Feed easily digestible diet (low fat and high biological value protein) for 5–7 days followed by gradual reintroduction of normal diet.
- Maintain fluid and electrolyte balance.
- Adsorbents such as kaolin are not advisable without definitive diagnosis.

Dietary considerations

Addition of fibre in colonic disease increases colonic muscle tone and contractions and increases water resorption. Fermentable (soluble) fibre also binds irritant fatty acids and can be digested by colonic bacteria to provide fuel for the cells in the colonic wall.

Constipation

Constipation is defined as a difficulty in passing faeces which may be due to impaction of the colon or rectum with faecal material. Patients with constipation may show straining (**tenesmus**) but tenesmus can occur with many conditions other than constipation. High-fibre diets reduce the risk of constipation but this is not an appropriate treatment once constipation is present. Multiple enemas or manual evacuation under general anaesthetic may be required to shift the blockage.

Exocrine pancreatic function

The pancreas secretes all enzymes needed to digest protein, carbohydrate and fat:

- Pancreatic **lipase** breaks down triglycerides to fatty acids (with the help of bile salts).
- **Amylase** breaks down starch to sugars.
- **Proteases** break down proteins to polypeptides.

Lack of pancreatic enzymes can occur as a result of congenital pancreatic atrophy or damage (often secondary to pancreatitis). This prevents normal digestion and osmotic diarrhoea develops.

Faeces are usually foul-smelling, greasy and affected animals are polyphagic with weight loss.

SPECIFIC DISEASES

Acute pancreatitis

Cause

Normally pancreatic enzymes are held in specialised storage pouches (zymogen granules) in the pancreas, to stop them digesting the pancreatic tissue. If these enzymes are released by inflammation or trauma in or around the pancreas, pancreatitis develops. In cats, pancreatitis is commonly associated with inflammatory bowel disease (IBD) or cholangiohepatitis.

Signs

In dogs, acute disease is typically associated with vomiting and abdominal pain. This can be an acute life-threatening disease with rapidly developing dehydration and shock. Complications such as peritonitis and ascites may develop. In cats, the disease is often more chronic and the only signs may be anorexia and depression. The vague signs in cats can make diagnosis difficult.

Diagnostic tests

Clinical signs of pancreatitis often suggest the diagnosis. In dogs the disease can be diagnosed by measurement of enzymes released by the pancreas (amylase and lipase) which are usually found in high concentrations in animals with pancreatic disease. Radiographs may show some peritoneal fluid in the cranial abdomen but ultrasound is more sensitive for the detection of pancreatic inflammation.

Treatment

Nil by mouth for 3–5 days (until vomiting ceases) – feeding stimulates further pancreatic secretions and makes the problem worse.

Intravenous fluids are given to replace fluid loss and supply maintenance requirements while nil by mouth. Antibiotics are given, particularly in cats, where infection ascending the pancreatic duct from the bowel may be important.

Analgesia – usually pethidine (morphine and non-steroidal anti-inflammatory drugs (NSAIDs) should be avoided).

Dietary considerations

Low-fat diet is recommended to reduce the requirement for fat digestion and the stimulus for pancreatic secretion.

Exocrine pancreatic insufficiency (EPI)

Cause

A condition caused by insufficient production of pancreatic enzymes resulting in poor digestion of food. Usually a congenital problem (common in the German Shepherd dog) in which the pancreas fails to develop normally but can also develop later in life in cats and dogs as a result of damage to the pancreas (which may be after a severe episode of pancreatitis). As a result of the undigested food remaining in the bowel it is common for bacterial overgrowth to occur.

Signs

Weight loss despite a good appetite with production of large volumes of greasy, smelly faeces. Occasionally vomiting and a poor-quality greasy haircoat.

Diagnostic tests

Blood tests to measure the levels of TLI, which in EPI will be low.

Treatment

Control of the disease relies on being able to supply the missing pancreatic enzymes. A powdered form of the pancreatic enzymes (Pancrex) is added to the food. Coconut oil supplements may also be given to improve weight gain. Antibiotic therapy may be required in the first instance to control the SIBO.

There is controversy surrounding the use of antacids, e.g. H_2-blockers in dogs with EPI. In humans these are used to reduce gastrin production and hence acid secretion in the stomach. The acid environment can deactivate the pancreatic enzymes added to the diet. Increasing the pH allows a greater proportion of the pancreatic enzyme replacement to reach the small intestine, theoretically enhancing its activity. Studies in dogs have shown conflicting results and some people think that antacids may actually reduce digestion.

Dietary considerations

Restriction of fat in the diet reduces the load on digestion and the risk of SIBO. Protein should be of high biological value. Highly digestible carbohydrate is used to provide energy. High-fibre diets are avoided as these can reduce the efficacy of the pancreatic enzymes. Water-soluble vitamins may be lost in the diarrhoea and absorption of zinc and copper is often reduced so dietary supplementation of these may be beneficial.

Gastric dilation and volvulus (GDV)

This condition is a true medical emergency and is usually seen in large deep-chested dogs, e.g. German Shepherd dogs and Setters.

Cause

The aetiology is not known but there are many predisposing factors:

- rapid ingestion of a large meal
- vigorous exercise with a full stomach
- increased production of gas from highly fermentable food
- reduced expulsion of gas
- delayed gastric emptying due to a motility disorder.

Signs

Affected animals are often uncomfortable and have a sudden increase in abdominal size with attempted vomiting. Breathing problems may develop as the disease progresses due to com-pression of the thorax by the pressure in the abdomen. Cardiovascular collapse occurs in untreated animals.

Diagnostic tests

The signs of GDV are usually fairly obvious. Abdominal radiographs may be useful in deciding whether the stomach has twisted or is just distended.

Treatment

Fluid therapy is essential to counteract vascular collapse. This should be given at a flow rate suitable for treating shock. The pressure in the stomach must be relieved either by passing a stomach tube or by trocharisation with a needle. Surgical treatment to fix the stomach to the body wall (gastropexy) so that GDV cannot recur is essential. Necrosis of the gastric wall will occur rapidly at high pressures and surgical examination allows any necrotic areas to be dealt with. Additional treatment with antibiotics to control infection and H_2-blockers, e.g. cimetidine to reduce gastric acid secretion, will reduce the risk of gastric ulceration or rupture.

DRUGS COMMONLY USED IN THE TREATMENT OF GASTROINTESTINAL DISEASE

Vomiting

Antiemetics

Metoclopramide and domperidone promote gastrointestinal motility and stimulate contractions in the upper GI tract. Metoclopramide also inhibits the vomiting reflex and can be administered i.v. as well as p.o. and so is very useful in the symptomatic management of vomiting. Other classes of antiemetic are used to control the feeling of nausea associated with motion sickness and some forms of chemotherapy.

Antacids (cimetidine/ranitidine)

These drugs act to reduce gastric acid secretion and hence the acidity of the stomach. When the stomach wall is inflamed a high acid environment can cause discomfort and vomiting.

Gastric protectant (sucralfate)

Gastric protectants bind to damaged areas of gut wall forming a protective barrier. They can be used to reduce discomfort and aid ulcer healing whenever there is suspicion of GI ulceration. Sucralfate forms a physical barrier between the gut lumen and the gut wall cells and may reduce the absorption of some other drugs if they are administered at the same time.

Diarrhoea

Adsorbent (kaolin)

Kaolin is a powder usually administered as a suspension. Toxins and bacteria in the intestine are attracted to and captured by the grains of powder and are then carried through the GI tract and eliminated from the body. This reduces the absorption of substances from the gut.

Laxatives

Lactulose is an osmotic laxative metabolised in the colon to form acids which draw water into the bowel causing osmotic diarrhoea. Liquid paraffin passes through the GI tract unchanged and acts as a lubricant for faeces. Microlax enemas are ready prepared doses of laxative which are administered per rectum. Increasing the fibre content of the diet can help some cases of constipation and fibre supplements, e.g. peridale and nutrifyba, may be used.

THE LIVER (see Table 3.3)

ANATOMY AND PHYSIOLOGY

The liver is situated in the cranial abdomen lying immediately behind the diaphragm next to the stomach. It receives a normal blood supply from the systemic circulation as well as all the blood in the veins draining from the gut (hepatic portal system). The liver has a variety of functions concerned with detoxification and because many toxins are taken out of the blood and concentrated in the liver for processing, the liver cells are very prone to toxic damage. However, up to 80% of the liver can be damaged without altering its function and it has an ability to regenerate even when large numbers of cells have been lost.

The liver filters and removes bacteria from the intestine and breaks down drugs, chemicals and environmental contaminants. Ammonia (produced by breakdown of protein in the gut) is converted to urea in the liver. The liver is the major site of glucose homeostasis and converts excess glucose to glycogen for storage. It can metabolise fatty acids and synthesise some lipids which are used elsewhere. Triglycerides, iron and some vitamins

Table 3.3 Important questions to ask the owner of an animal with suspected liver disease	
Question	Reason for question and interpretation of answer
Is the animal bright?	Depression may be associated with hepatic encephalopathy. Active hepatitis may be painful and make the animal systemically unwell
Is the animal vomiting?	Vomiting can be associated with hepatic inflammation (causing gastric irritation), or due to toxaemia associated with liver dysfunction
Does the animal want to eat and drink?	Anorexia and depression are concerning signs in patients with liver disease. Fluid therapy may be considered if the animal is not drinking
Has the animal lost weight?	Weight loss is common in animals with liver disease
Are there any behavioural changes or nervous signs, e.g. seizures?	Hepatic encephalopathy resulting in neurological signs may be seen with severe liver disease
Is urine colour normal?	Animals with jaundice often excrete large amounts of pigment in their urine. This makes the urine appear dark or concentrated. Owners often notice the changes in urine before skin discoloration

are also stored here. Proteins such as albumin and clotting factors are synthesised in the liver. Bile is produced in the liver and stored in the gall bladder before release into the intestine after eating. Bile acts like a detergent (breaking down fats for digestion) and so if insufficient bile is produced faeces will be greasy and maldigestion occurs. Bilirubin from breakdown of red blood cells is taken up by the liver and excreted in the bile.

PATHOPHYSIOLOGY

Jaundice is yellow discoloration of the skin due to the accumulation of bilirubin in the tissues. Jaundice occurs if the capacity of the liver to excrete bilirubin in the bile is exceeded. Liver damage can cause swelling or obstruction of the bile ducts resulting in reduced bile flow, or if hepatocytes are severely damaged, then uptake and secretion of bilirubin may be reduced.

Ascites is not uncommon in liver disease and results from one of two mechanisms:

- Portal hypertension – due to abnormal liver structure the pressure within the portal circulation is increased and fluid leaks out of the vessels into the peritoneal space.
- Hypoproteinaemia – if protein production is reduced in severe liver disease the oncotic pressure (which keeps fluid in the circulation) is reduced and fluid leaks from all vessels.

Causes

Almost all categories of disease can affect the liver (see Table 3.4). Liver disease may be primary (disease or damage primarily involving the liver), or secondary (other diseases having effects in the liver, e.g. hyperadrenocorticism causing steroid hepatopathy, or metastatic neoplasia).

Signs

Liver damage is often very severe before clinical signs become apparent. The signs associated with disease of the liver are often quite vague: anorexia, lethargy, weight loss, polyuria/polydipsia,

Table 3.4 Potential causes of liver disease

Type of cause	Example
Toxic	Some drugs, blue green algae, copper accumulation
Infectious	Canine hepatitis virus, leptospirosis
Congenital	Portosystemic shunt
Neoplasia	Haemangiosarcoma, hepatoma, secondary metastasis
Degenerative	Cirrhosis
Inflammatory/ immune mediated	Cholangiohepatitis
Trauma	Bruising, rupture or torsion
Metabolic	Hyperadrenocorticism, diabetes mellitus

vomiting and diarrhoea. There are some more specific signs such as cranial abdominal pain, icterus, and hepatic encephalopathy. The term **hepatic encephalopathy** is used to describe a group of neurological signs seen in severe liver dysfunction. These include ataxia, depression, circling, head pressing, blindness and seizures. Signs are often most pronounced after eating a high-protein meal but some individuals may be permanently affected. Toxic compounds from the gut, including ammonia, are not metabolised by the liver and enter the circulation from where they reach the brain.

Diagnostic tests

Blood tests are very useful in the investigation of liver disease. Liver enzyme measurements can give an indication of ongoing damage but other tests, e.g. bile salt assay, are needed to assess the function of the liver. Diagnostic imaging can be useful in investigating liver disease. Radiographs will provide information about the size of the liver but ultrasonography is more useful to give an indication of the internal structure of the liver and to identify focal or diffuse lesions. Unfortunately, in most cases, definitive diagnosis is not possible without liver biopsy.

Treatment

If the underlying cause of the liver damage can be corrected then liver regeneration and recovery of function are possible. Supportive care may be necessary in the meantime to keep the animal alive whilst liver regeneration takes place. In many cases the underlying condition is progressive despite treatment. Supportive care aimed at reducing the workload on the liver, and hence reducing clinical signs, may be the only option.

In most diseases antibiotics are indicated to assist in removal of bacteria from the portal circulation and to reduce the bacterial load in the gut which will in turn reduce ammonia production. If hepatic encephalopathy is present lactulose may be given to bind ammonia in the gut lumen and prevent it getting into the circulation.

If gastric ulceration is present sucralfate can be used as a local protectant and histamine blockers, e.g. ranitidine, may be required to reduce gastric acidity.

The presence of a coagulopathy is a poor sign. This can be managed acutely by administering fresh plasma and vitamin K_1 injection if necessary but the outcome is poor.

NUTRITIONAL CONSIDERATIONS

Since the liver is a highly metabolic centre a diet for liver disease would ideally be one that is easy for the liver to handle. The ideal hepatic support diet has reduced protein content, but contains protein of high biological value. Calories should be supplied in the form of carbohydrates and fat may need to be moderately restricted. Water-soluble vitamins (B, C and E) should be supplemented in the diet and extra zinc may also be required. Fluid therapy may be required in acute cases.

SPECIFIC DISEASES

Cirrhosis

Causes: endstage of long-term liver damage with little repair, resulting in fibrosis of liver tissue.

Signs: progressive anorexia and weight loss, melaena, haematemesis, ascites.

Diagnosis: blood screens indicate liver dysfunction with low plasma proteins and raised bile salts; diagnostic imaging may show small dense liver. Biopsy is required for definitive diagnosis.

Treatment: long-term supportive care.

Portosystemic shunt

Causes: congenital abnormality, inherited in some breeds, e.g. Yorkshire terrier. Abnormal blood supply results in blood from portal system bypassing the liver altogether and entering circulation.

Signs: poor growth and appetite as a puppy, may develop hepatic encephalopathy and ascites.

Diagnosis: blood screens indicate liver dysfunction. Diagnostic imaging (radiography and ultrasonography) to demonstrate small liver and presence of shunt; nuclear medicine techniques, i.e. scintigraphy may also be used to demonstrate shunting of blood around the liver.

Treatment: surgical ligation of aberrant vessel if possible, otherwise long-term medical supportive therapy.

Cholangiohepatitis

Causes: primarily a disease of cats but can be seen in dogs. Ascending bacterial infection from intestine passing up bile duct to biliary system; additional immune-mediated aetiology has been suggested.

Signs: jaundice, anorexia, weight loss, fever.

Diagnosis: blood screens indicate active hepatic inflammation; biopsy is needed for definitive diagnosis.

Treatment: antibiotics and supportive care; many cases require immunosuppression with prednisolone to dampen inflammation.

Acute hepatitis

Causes: infectious agents, e.g. feline leukaemia virus (FeLV), feline immunodeficiency virus (FIV) in cats, canine leptospirosis or adenovirus hepatitis in dogs. Parasitic disease or toxic agents, e.g. blue-green algae poisoning or many drugs in cats can also cause acute disease.

Signs: vomiting, anorexia, abdominal pain and pyrexia. Jaundice may develop.

Diagnosis: laboratory tests indicate liver damage but often underlying cause is not found.

Treatment: supportive management and removal of inciting cause or specific treatment of underlying disease if identified.

DRUGS COMMONLY USED IN THE MANAGEMENT OF LIVER DISEASE

Gastric protectant (sucralfate)

Gastric protectants bind to damaged areas of gut wall forming a protective barrier. They can be used whenever there is suspicion of gastro-intestinal ulceration to reduce discomfort and aid ulcer healing. They may reduce the absorption of some other drugs if these are administered at the same time because sucralfate forms a physical barrier between the drug and the gut wall cells.

Water-soluble vitamins

In animals with polyuria/polydipsia, water-soluble vitamins are lost in large quantities in the urine. This loss can exceed the dietary intake and result in deficiency if supplementation is not provided.

Antacid/H$_2$-blocker (ranitidine/cimetidine)

These drugs reduce gastric acid production and help to reduce discomfort associated with gastro-intestinal ulcers.

Osmotic laxative (lactulose)

Usually used for management of hepatic encephalopathy. Lactulose is metabolised in the colon to form acids which draw water into the bowel causing osmotic diarrhoea. The acid environment also traps ammonia in the gut, thus reducing the ammonia levels in the blood. High ammonia is one of the contributing factors in the development of hepatic encephalopathy.

Antibiotics

Oral antibiotics should reduce the bacterial population in the colon, therefore reducing ammonia production. Antibiotics may also be useful to remove bacteria which cross the gut wall and enter the portal circulation because these are normally removed by the liver.

Ursodeoxycholic acid

This is used in patients with cholestasis because it protects the cells in the biliary system from damage.

CARDIOVASCULAR SYSTEM (Table 3.5)

ANATOMY AND PHYSIOLOGY

The function of the heart is to pump blood around the body under pressure. It is basically a muscular pump comprising three layers:

- endocardium – inner lining layer
- myocardium – heart muscle
- epicardium – outer layer.

The heart is contained within a sac (the **peri-cardium**). Unlike other muscles the heart muscle contracts rhythmically without stimulation from a nerve. Electrical activity starts in an area of specialised tissue (the **sino-atrial (SA) node**) from where it is conducted to the atrioventricular node (located at the junction of atria and ventricles). From here the electrical activity passes through the **bundle of His** to the **Purkinje fibres** which distribute the impulse to the contracting muscle cells. This active contraction of the myocardium (systole) pumps blood out of the heart into the circulation. At the end of the contraction the heart relaxes (diastole) and passively fills with blood returning from the circulation.

Deoxygenated blood enters the right atrium and from there passes to the right ventricle. Blood is pumped around the lungs where it is oxygenated and returns to the left atrium. Oxygenated blood leaves the left atrium through the aorta and is pumped around the body. Major blood vessels branch off the aorta and these subdivide many times until they become small vessels (**capillaries**) within the tissues (see Fig. 3.1). In the capillaries the red cells are in close contact with other tissue cells and oxygen is able to cross blood vessel walls into the tissue. Deoxygenated blood leaving

Table 3.5 Important questions to ask the owner of an animal with heart disease	
Question	Reason for question and interpretation of answer
Has the animal previously had signs of heart disease, e.g. murmur?	Animals may have compensated heart failure for many years before developing clinical signs of disease. However, remember that the presence of a murmur does not indicate heart failure
Is the animal able to exercise normally?	Heart disease is often associated with exercise intolerance or collapse at exercise
Have there been any changes in appetite or water intake?	Patients in heart failure are often inappetant and cachexic. In early stages of failure the patient may become polydipsic
Have there been episodes of collapse or weakness?	Collapse or weakness can be the signs of poor circulation (reduced cardiac output)
Does the animal settle to sleep easily at night?	Nocturnal restlessness is common in congestive heart failure – patients in heart failure find it difficult to breathe when lying down
Is there any breathing difficulty or coughing?	Respiratory difficulties may be associated with pulmonary oedema. Coughing is more commonly a sign of respiratory disease but can be seen due to the pressure of a large heart on the bronchus. Any patient with respiratory difficulty should be examined with urgency

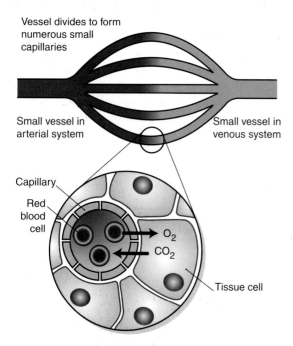

Vessel divides to form numerous small capillaries

Small vessel in arterial system

Small vessel in venous system

Capillary

Red blood cell

O_2

CO_2

Tissue cell

Figure 3.1 Capillaries: oxygen transfer at tissue.

the capillary network enters small veins and these vessels join up to form progressively larger veins which drain into the vena cava and finally back into the heart. As blood flows through the capillaries some fluid is forced out of the vessel into the interstitial space (between cells). This fluid is drained back into lymph capillaries and lymph vessels via which it travels through a filtering system in the lymph nodes and finally enters lymph ducts which drain into the vena cava or right jugular veins.

The primary function of the cardiovascular system is to supply adequate blood flow to meet the body's metabolic demands. Cardiac output is obviously tightly controlled and this maintains blood pressure in normal circumstances. Cardiac output depends on heart rate and the amount of blood ejected from the heart with each contraction (stroke volume). If, for any reason, blood pressure starts to fall, e.g. reduced cardiac output, the body initially compensates by increasing heart rate. This means that although a smaller volume of blood is pumped with each heart contraction, because there are more contractions in a given time, the amount of blood pumped remains constant. Thus:

- Heart rate is altered by stimulation of the sympathetic nervous system (increases rate) and parasympathetic nervous system (slows rate).
- Stroke volume is affected by the force of contraction (ability of myocardium to contract).

The heart responds automatically to changes in venous return. The more blood returned to the heart the harder the next contraction, so the more blood is ejected.

If demand for blood flow increases or cardiac output falls (due to low blood pressure or damaged heart) then the compensatory mechanisms are automatically activated.

There are two important regulatory mechanisms for cardiac function:

- Sympathetic nervous system
- Renin–angiotensin–aldosterone system (RAAS)

Stimulation of sympathetic nerves causes:

- increased heart rate and stronger contractions (increases cardiac output)
- peripheral vasoconstriction (diverting blood to essential organs)
- venoconstriction (reducing the amount of blood pooling in venous system)
- renin release from kidneys (stimulating the RAA system).

Stimulation of the RAAS

- Renin release stimulates the conversion of angiotensin to angiotensin I which is, in turn, converted by angiotensin-converting enzyme (ACE) to angiotensin II.

- This causes aldosterone release from the adrenal glands, retention of salt and water, and vasoconstriction (Fig. 3.2).

By these means cardiac output is maintained and compensated heart failure exists. No signs of heart disease are present at rest but signs may develop at times of increased stress, e.g. exercise or excitement. However, although the animal may appear normal the underlying problems continue and heart failure progresses:

- Fluid retention due to RAA activation results in increased return of blood to heart and hence increased stretch of myocardium, causing it to hypertrophy.
- Increased heart rate and strength of contraction result in increased oxygen demand of myocardium which cannot be met and hypoxia develops.
- Increased venous return due to sympathetic stimulation of veins results in increased pressure in the ventricles. There is more resistance to blood entering the ventricle and blood eventually dams back into the veins resulting in congestion and oedema.

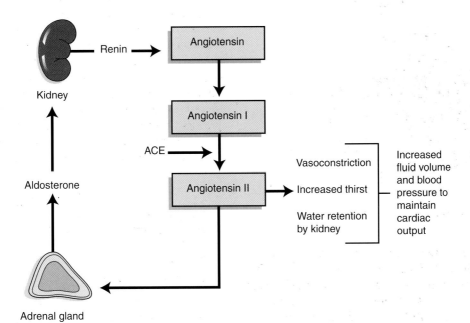

Figure 3.2 Stimulation of the renin–angiotensin–aldosterone system. ACE, angiotensin-converting enzyme.

- Arterial constriction increases resistance to blood flow making it harder to pump blood out into the circulation.
- Vasoconstriction reduces blood flow to non-essential organs causing weakness.

As blood starts to pool in vessels at high pressure fluid starts to leak out. This is **decompensated heart failure.**

The most common type of heart failure is congestive or backward heart failure. This can affect primarily the left or right sides of the heart but usually progresses to involve both sides.

Right-sided congestive heart failure (CHF) results in congestion of the venous circulation in the liver and spleen which often causes ascites. Congestion of organs results in reduced function.

Left-sided CHF causes congestion of vessels in the lungs and fluid leaking from here causes pulmonary oedema. Oedema and pulmonary congestion reduce oxygen transfer in the lungs. High heart rate and the hypertrophied heart muscle increase the oxygen demand of the myocardium. The imbalance leads to reduced pumping efficiency and dysrhythmias.

PATHOPHYSIOLOGY

Congestive heart failure

Cause

Pooling of blood in the venous system because of:

- Systolic failure, which is reduced efficiency of the myocardium to contract (e.g. dilated cardiomyopathy).
- Diastolic failure, which is reduced ability of the myocardium to relax and therefore fill with blood (e.g. hypertrophic cardiomyopathy, pericardial disease).
- Volume overload, where excess volumes of blood entering the chamber cause myocardial stretching (e.g. mitral regurgitation, patent ductus arteriosus).
- Pressure overload, where resistance to outflow of blood increases the force of contraction needed and muscle hypertrophy increases pressure in the ventricle (e.g. aortic stenosis, hypertension).

- Dysrhythmias, which reduce efficiency of pumping action (e.g. atrial fibrillation, ventricular tachycardia).

Signs

- Exercise intolerance
- cough
- dyspnoea
- syncope/collapse
- weight loss (cardiac cachexia)
- pale mucous membranes (due to poor blood supply to the peripheral circulation)
- ascites
- restlessness.

Diagnostic tests

Auscultation of the heart for the presence of murmurs (as well as rhythm and heart rate) is essential. Normal heart rate is 70–140 beats/min (often with a sinus dysrhythmia) in the dog and 140–220 beats/min in the cat. Often the first sign of cardiac disease is an increase in heart rate and loss of sinus dysrhythmia. It is important to palpate the pulse at the same time as auscultating the heart since some dysrhythmias result in a difference between pulse rate and heart rate. The quality of the pulse, i.e. strength and consistency of each pulse, can also be important.

The colour of the mucous membranes may be altered – cyanotic (blue) with pulmonary oedema or pale if cardiac output is reduced.

Thoracic radiographs are important to assess the size and shape of the heart as well as the presence of pulmonary oedema or pleural fluid.

Ultrasonography provides information about the internal cardiac anatomy:

- valves
- septa
- vessels
- myocardium.

Ultrasound can be used to assess myocardial thickness and also contractility. Flow rates through vessels and valves can be measured and fluid in the pericardial sac can be seen.

Electrocardiography (ECG) provides crude information about cardiac chamber size but is important in the detection, recognition, classification and monitoring of dysrhythmias.

Treatment

Early heart disease (where there are no signs of failure but a murmur is detected) require that a diagnosis of the underlying cause be made and corrective treatment be started if possible. An ECG should be performed to rule out the presence of dysrhythmias. If corrective therapy is not possible it is likely that the heart failure will progress so the patient should be checked regularly (3–6 months) to monitor for signs of disease.

A reduced calorie diet should be prescribed to control weight (at this stage salt restriction is not necessary).

As signs of heart failure develop exercise restriction should be imposed. Regular checks must be continued and may need to be more frequent. If pulmonary oedema and congestion are a problem ACE inhibitors and diuretics may be introduced as appropriate.

Supportive care, such as the drainage of pleural or peritoneal effusions that are compromising respiration, and increasing oxygen in the environment are important considerations.

Dietary considerations

The value of salt restriction in CHF is still under discussion. Reduced salt diets are probably beneficial in patients with severe CHF. There is some evidence that low salt diets may cause further stimulation of the RAA system which may be counterproductive in early heart disease.

SPECIAL CIRCUMSTANCES
Acute heart failure

Acute heart failure is the sudden development of signs of decompensated forward failure. Forward failure occurs if the heart is unable to pump enough blood to meet metabolic demands but is normally rare as the main aim of the compen-satory mechanisms is to try to maintain blood pressure, CO and tissue perfusion. Severe cases presented in acute decompensated heart failure must be cage rested and protected from stressful events. Intravenous diuretics may be needed to relieve pulmonary oedema and vasodilators may also help. If myocardial function is poor or heart rate very fast digoxin may be required.

SPECIFIC DISEASES
Congenital heart disease

Patent ductus arteriosus (PDA)

One of the most common congenital heart diseases in the dog.

Cause: failure of fetal circulation to close after birth. Overcirculation of pulmonary vasculature results in volume overload to left side of heart.

Signs: often no clinical signs, murmur detected at routine examination, e.g. vaccination. May be presented in early stages of heart failure.

Diagnosis: detection of classical murmur. Thoracic radiographs shows enlarged left side of heart with dilation in region of pulmonary artery/aorta on dorsoventral projection. Ultrasound may show turbulence around the openings of the ductus into aorta and pulmonary artery.

Treatment: ligation of duct before development of CHF results in good prognosis. Once CHF is present, treatment is symptomatic.

Pulmonic stenosis

Cause: congenital narrowing of pulmonary valve or the artery leaving heart.

Signs: often murmur detected at routine examination but can progress to right-sided CHF.

Diagnosis: thoracic radiographs show enlargement of right side of heart. Ultrasound examination shows thickening of right heart wall. The narrowing of the vessel may be detected using Doppler ultrasound and this can help establish the severity of the stenosis.

Treatment: severe cases require dilation of the artery. Symptomatic medical treatment in non-surgical cases.

Aortic stenosis

Cause: narrowing of outflow of left side of heart (or abnormal development of the aortic valve) causes resistance to outflow resulting in hypertrophy of the left heart. A common congenital disease in the dog.

Signs: depending on severity of stenosis, signs may be present at a young age or develop in adulthood. Fainting due to output failure with progressive left heart CHF. Collapse or sudden death due to cardiac dysrhythmia.

Diagnosis: thoracic radiograph may show dilation of aorta after the stenosis. Ultrasound can be used to visualise the stenotic area/valve and Doppler studies to measure flow rates through stenotic area. ECG examination frequently shows cardiac dysrhythmias, e.g. ventricular premature complexes (VPCs).

Treatment: symptomatic treatment with anti-dysrhythmic drugs and beta blockers. Mild cases may not require treatment.

Ventricular septal defect

Cause: relatively common in cat but rare in dog. Failure of heart to develop properly results in a connection between the left and right sides. Blood flows from left to right, therefore pulmonary vasculature returns too much blood and left sided volume overload develops.

Signs: murmur progressing to left-sided CHF.

Diagnosis: thoracic radiograph shows generalised cardiomegaly. Ultrasound may show turbulent blood flow in the heart chambers near the defect – occasionally the defect is large enough to be seen with ultrasound.

Treatment: may be no signs, in which case treatment is unnecessary. Symptomatic treatment if CHF develops.

Acquired heart disease

Dilated cardiomyopathy (DCM)

Mainly seen in young adult large/giant breed dogs, especially Dobermann Pinschers.

Cause: myocardium thinned resulting in loss of contractility. Can be the result of taurine deficiency, often idiopathic.

Signs: left and right CHF, typically ascites and pulmonary oedema in dogs and pleural effusions and pulmonary oedema in cats.

Diagnosis: thoracic radiographs show increased cardiac size and evidence of heart failure, e.g. pulmonary oedema. Ultrasound demonstrates thin myocardium and poor contractility. ECG often shows dysrhythmias, particularly atrial fibrillation.

Treatment: symptomatic medical treatment for CHF. Taurine supplementation in some cases.

Hypertrophic cardiomyopathy (HCM)

More common in cats than dogs.

Cause: thickening of heart wall which may be idiopathic or the result of hypertrophy due to increased myocardial work, e.g. hypertension of hyperthyroidism in cats.

Signs: CHF.

Diagnosis: thoracic radiograph may show heart enlargement. Ultrasound shows thickening of heart wall. ECG commonly shows dysrythmias, e.g. VPCs.

Treatment: treat underlying cause if possible; otherwise symptomatic management of CHF.

Endocardiosis

Most common acquired disease in dogs, particularly in Cavalier King Charles Spaniels.

Cause: degenerative condition of the atrio-ventricular valves (usually the mitral valve) causing faulty valve function and blood flow leaking through valves when closed.

Signs: cardiac murmur progressing over years to CHF (usually left-sided).

Diagnosis: thoracic radiograph shows left sided heart enlargement, particularly left atrium. Ultrasound demonstrates distortion of valves and turbulent blood flow with leakage of blood through valves when closed.

Treatment: symptomatic management of CHF.

Pericardial effusion

Often seen in middle sized and large breed dogs.

Cause: fluid accumulation inside pericardial sac prevents heart from filling with blood in diastole.

Signs: lethargy and dyspnoea due to right-sided CHF. Muffled heart sounds and weak pulses with pale mucous membranes. Heart sounds muffled due to fluid in sac around heart. Ascites often develops.

Diagnosis: thoracic radiograph may show enlargement of cardiac silhouette. Ultrasound allows visualisation of fluid in pericardial sac and may identify cause of effusion, e.g. tumour.

Treatment: drainage of fluid (pericardiocentesis).

Vascular disease

Hypertension

Infrequently diagnosed until recently, as blood pressure was not routinely measured in veterinary medicine.

Cause: primary, or secondary to systemic disease, e.g. renal failure or Cushing's disease in dogs and hyperthyroidism in cats.

Signs: often signs of underlying disease, blindness associated with retinal haemorrhage.

Diagnosis: measurement of blood pressure.

Treatment: treat underlying disease, medical therapy to reduce blood pressure.

Dysrhythmias

Atrial fibrillation

More common in giant breeds where it may be asymptomatic.

Cause: often associated with diseases causing large atria, e.g. dilated cardiomyopathy.

Signs: often signs of underlying disease; may be asymptomatic.

Diagnosis: auscultation and pulse palpation, ECG.

Treatment: treat underlying cause, aim to reduce heart rate with calcium channel blockers or digoxin.

Ventricular premature contractions

Cause: usually myocardial hypoxia or irritation.

Signs: may be asymptomatic unless occurring frequently when result in output failure.

Diagnosis: ECG.

Treatment: treat underlying cause; if progress to ventricular tachycardia can treat with lidocaine (lignocaine) or procainamide.

Heart block

Cause: abnormal conduction of impulse from atria to ventricle resulting in disordered contractions and poor cardiac output.

Signs: may be no signs, signs of output failure (collapse), CHF.

Diagnosis: auscultation and pulse monitoring may give indication, ECG for diagnosis.

Treatment: depending on type of block and underlying causes. Treatment ranges from none to medical therapy to cardiac pacemaker implantation.

DRUGS COMMONLY USED IN THE MANAGEMENT OF HEART DISEASE

Positive inotropes

The most commonly used group of drugs in this class are the cardiac glycosides and the best known of these is digoxin. These drugs increase the force of contraction of the heart muscle. They also slow the heart rate and so can be very beneficial in diseases like dilated cardiomyopathy. At high doses they can cause side effects such as nausea.

Calcium channel blockers (diltiazem)

Calcium channel blockers help the heart muscle to relax in diastole and so are useful in diseases such as HCM where the stiffness of the myocardium makes it difficult for the heart to fill.

Local anaesthetics (lidocaine (lignocaine))

Local anaesthetics are given intravenously in some kinds of dysrhythmia. They reduce the sensitivity of the heart muscle so that abnormal contractions are reduced. As they can only be given intravenously they are useful only in short-term control of severe dysrhythmias.

Anti-dysrhythmics (procainamide)

Anti-dysrhythmic agents can be given by tablet for long-term control of abnormal contractions, e.g. VPCs. Procainamide stabilises the cell membrane of cardiac cells thereby slowing electrical conduction through the heart.

Diuretics (furosemide (frusemide), spironolactone)

Diuretics are used to promote renal excretion of fluids and hence reduce oedema. Furosemide (frusemide; loop diuretic) is the most commonly used diuretic in veterinary practice. It inhibits the resorption of salt and water filtered by the kidneys so that more fluid is lost in the urine. Because electrolytes are also lost in the urine following diuretic administration serum concentrations of potassium may fall with prolonged treatment. Spironolactone can be given in cases where potassium concentrations are low because it does not cause potassium loss. High doses of diuretic can reduce blood volume and hence cardiac output (CO).

Vasodilators

These drugs reduce the workload of the heart by:

- Dilating systemic veins, thereby reducing pressure in the veins and making it less likely that oedema will form.
- Dilating arterioles, making it easier for the heart to pump blood forward.

Beta blockers (propranolol)

These drugs slow heart rate and are particularly useful in cats with HCM. They may also reduce the force of heart contraction so are not routinely given to patients with poor heart muscle contractility, e.g. dilated cardiomyopathy.

Angiotensin-converting enzyme inhibitors (ACEi) (enalapril, rimapril, benazepril)

These drugs are useful to overcome some of the adverse effects caused by the body's natural response mechanisms to heart failure. They reduce the production of angiotensin II and hence fluid retention.

RESPIRATORY TRACT (Table 3.6)

ANATOMY AND PHYSIOLOGY

The respiratory system is, for convenience, divided into upper (nasal passages, sinuses and trachea) and lower (bronchi and pulmonary system) tracts. Clinical signs of disease in the two systems are completely different but signs of respiratory distress are often very obvious. Many animals generally live quiet lives and can have quite severe respiratory compromise before showing any clinical signs.

The upper respiratory tract (URT) is concerned with warming, filtering and humidifying the air entering the body and can be used as an area for heat loss. The lower respiratory tract (LRT) is primarily concerned with gas exchange. Air is drawn into the respiratory system by active effort – flattening the diaphragm and pulling out of the ribs which causes expansion of the chest cavity. This action expands the lungs and they fill with air. As air enters the lungs oxygen diffuses across the alveoli walls into the blood and carbon dioxide moves in the opposite direction. Exhalation is a passive process in which muscle relaxation causes contraction of the thoracic cavity and lung collapse resulting in air expulsion.

The respiratory rate is adjusted according to levels of carbon dioxide and oxygen in the blood. These values are measured by receptors in the walls of arteries (carotid and aortic bodies) and receptors in a part of the brain (medulla), which monitor the pH of blood. Information from these receptors is fed to the medullary respiratory centre which adjusts the respiratory rate if required.

The normal resting respiratory rate is 10–30 breaths/min for the dog and 20–30 breaths/min for the cat.

In normal animals the respiratory tract is lined with cilia which propel secretions towards the upper respiratory tract. This is the **mucociliary clearance system.** Alveolar macrophages help to remove unwanted secretions from the LRT.

Table 3.6 Important questions to ask the owner of an animal with signs of respiratory disease

Question	Reason for question and interpretation of answer
Is the patient dyspnoeic at rest or only on exertion?	Many patients are able to compensate for quite severe respiratory distress by reducing the workload of the respiratory system. They may have few signs of disease at rest but if forced to exert themselves they may rapidly become breathless. It is always a concern if breathing difficulties are obvious at rest, particularly in cats
Is the breathing fast or slow?	Rapid, shallow breathing may be associated with pain and a reluctance to stretch the lungs and move structures in the chest. Slow, deep breathing may be associated with obstruction to airflow
Is the breathing laboured?	If patients have obstructed airways they have to put a lot of effort into their breathing
Is there increased noise on breathing?	Harsh breathing sounds may be associated with upper airway disease (nasal chambers and larynx); rattling or wheezing noises often come from lower in the respiratory tract. It may be possible to localise an area where breathing sounds are loudest
If the animal is coughing: When does this occur? What does the cough sound like? Is it productive?	Coughing can be associated with specific situations. Bronchospasm may be triggered by breathing cold air or by exposure to aerosol sprays in cats with asthma. Tracheal collapse is exacerbated by excitement and patients with excessive mucus production may cough after they have been lying still for a period of time and large volumes of mucus have accumulated
Have there been any discharges from nose?	Nasal discharge usually indicates nasal disease; however, severe lower respiratory tract infections can result in purulent nasal discharge, particularly in recumbent animals
Has the patient been restless or unable to settle?	In some respiratory conditions it is harder or easier for the animal to breathe when in certain positions, e.g. patients with pulmonary oedema often find it easier to breathe when standing up
Is patient unwell, e.g. anorexic, lethargic, unwilling to exercise?	Signs of systemic illness may indicate a more generalised or severe disease. Pyrexia as a result of bacterial or viral infection may be present. Some systemic illnesses alter respiratory patterns (due to metabolic acidosis/alkalosis) without causing respiratory changes
Has the animal collapsed or lost consciousness?	Collapse or loss of consciousness is rarely associated with primary respiratory disease. These are more usually features of cardiac disease and the possibility of an underlying cause of respiratory disease should be sought
Vaccination status and potential exposure to infectious agents, e.g. recent kennelling, are also relevant	Many respiratory diseases in dogs and cats are caused by infectious agents. Vaccination may reduce the severity of many of these diseases but it does not always provide 100% immunity so infectious disease cannot be ruled out even in vaccinated pets. Recent exposure to potential sources of infection or signs of disease in in-contact animals does increase the likelihood of an infectious cause

PATHOPHYSIOLOGY

Inflammation of the respiratory tract activates receptors in the larynx, trachea and bronchi resulting in coughing, an active reflex designed to remove secretions from the respiratory tract. There are many causes of coughing, some of which are:

- irritation of upper airways

- pulmonary oedema (usually secondary to congestive heart failure)
- pulmonary haemorrhage
- pneumonia.

Dyspnoea is an increased effort in breathing caused by:

1. Reduced lung volume for air exchange:
   a. Pulmonary

(i) pulmonary oedema
(ii) pulmonary haemorrhage
(iii) pneumonia
(iv) neoplasia
(v) poisoning (paraquat)
b. Extrapulmonary
(i) pleural fluid or air
(ii) mediastinal fluid
(iii) mass pressing on trachea or bronchi (neoplasia or large left atrium)
(iv) diaphragm pressing on thorax (GDV, hepatomegaly, ascites)
2. Airway obstruction:
a. laryngeal spasm or collapse
b. tracheal collapse
c. bronchospasm (feline asthma)
d. lungworm/oslerus
e. tonsillitis/pharyngitis/tracheitis
f. foreign body.

When handling any patients with respiratory distress great care should be taken not to struggle with them. Dyspnoeic patients can easily fatally decompensate. If possible, examination and further investigations may be delayed until the patient has recovered from the journey to the surgery. Cage rest and oxygen administration can dramatically improve the condition of many dyspnoeic patients. In many circumstances it is much safer to administer a low dose of sedation to these animals than to struggle with them.

UPPER RESPIRATORY TRACT DISEASE

The URT is divided into the nasal passages, sinuses, nasopharynx and trachea.

Cause

The causes of upper respiratory disease are many (see Box 3.5).

Signs

Nasal discharge is the most common sign of URT disease. This may be unilateral (from one nostril) or bilateral (from both). Localised nasal disease usually produces a unilateral discharge whereas

Box 3.5 Causes of respiratory disease	
Lower respiratory tract diseases	**Upper respiratory tract diseases**
Pulmonary disease	***Nasal disease***
Pulmonary oedema	Chronic rhinosinusitis
Pulmonary neoplasia	(cat' flu)
Pneumonia	Nasal foreign body
Paraquat poisoning	Nasal neoplasia
Lung worm/parasitic	Nasal aspergillosis
disease	***Laryngeal disease***
Extrapulmonary disease	Nasopharyngeal polyps
Fluid in pleural space	Laryngeal paralysis
(hydrothorax,	***Upper airway disease***
chylothorax, pyothorax,	Canine
haemothorax)	tracheobronchitis
Pneumothorax	Chronic bronchitis
Ruptured diaphragm	Allergic bronchitis
	Tracheal collapse

systemic disease or LRT disease more often produces bilateral discharge. Sneezing, retching and coughing may occur in diseases of the LRT or URT.

Classification of nasal discharge may give a clue as to its cause. Initially inflammation of the rhinariun results in serous or mucoid discharge; secondary bacterial or fungal infection produces purulent discharge. Haemorrhagic discharge (epistaxis) can be caused by fungal erosion, neoplasia or a defect of haemostasis (a primary bleeding problem).

Diagnostic tests

Physical examination of the patient is most important to establish the nature of any discharges. Palpation of the external surface of the nose and percussion of the sinuses may reveal pain or swelling. Auscultation of the larynx and trachea can help to detect obstructive URT disease.

Full physical examination is important to identify whether the disease is systemic or confined to the respiratory tract.

Radiographs of skull, nasal passages and larynx may be appropriate investigations. Endoscopic examination of the trachea and nasal passages (with biopsy or flushing) can provide a definitive diagnosis but requires general anaesthesia.

Transtracheal washes may be performed in some conscious animals.

Treatment

URT disease is rarely a life-threatening condition. If an underlying cause is established this can be treated, but in all cases symptomatic treatment will be necessary. Nasal discharges should be cleaned to maintain nasal patency. If secretions are thick the animal can be placed in a humidified environment, i.e. a shower room, to assist secretion removal. Laryngeal or tracheal obstructive diseases are often exacerbated by exercise, excitement and heat, so a quiet environment with cool moist air-flow should be provided. Pay attention to appetite in animals with nasal obstruction, particularly in cats, because if sense of smell is impaired a patient may not eat.

SPECIAL CIRCUMSTANCES
Acute respiratory distress

Management of acute respiratory distress is a medical emergency. Proceed as follows:

1. Ensure airway is patent which may require:
   a. placement of endotracheal tube
   b. placement of tracheostomy tube
   c. suction to remove secretions.
2. Increase oxygen content in environment by use of:
   a. face mask (may increase struggling and be counter-productive)
   b. naso-oesophageal tube (usually well tolerated)
   c. endotracheal tube (in anaesthetised or unconscious patients)
   d. oxygen cage (often wasteful of oxygen).
3. Ensure pulmonary function is adequate to maintain animal, i.e. enforced cage rest to reduce respiratory demands.
4. Depending on aetiology of respiratory dysfunction it may be necessary to:
   a. drain fluid from thoracic cavity (thoracocentesis)
   b. provide manual ventilation if respiration has failed.
5. Drug therapy may involve the use of:
   a. diuretics for pulmonary oedema
   b. mucolytics to liquidise secretions for removal
   c. bronchodilators.

LOWER RESPIRATORY TRACT DISEASE
Cause

The causes of lower respiratory disease are many (see Box 3.5).

Signs

Clinical signs of LRT disease are coughing and dyspnoea. In severe disease cyanosis may develop. Patients may collapse, particularly if put under increased stress. Auscultation of the airways and air movement in the lung are very important. Heart and lung sounds may be muffled or quiet if pleural fluid is present. In cases where the lung tissue is solid (pneumonia or pulmonary oedema) air will not be moving, so breath sounds will be absent. In dogs percussion of the chest may give an indication of the presence and location of pleural fluid or solid lung tissue.

Diagnostic tests

Radiographs of the chest are very useful to evaluate the lungs and airways. Pleural fluid is easily detected on radiographs but may mask other conditions such as masses in the chest.

Ultrasonographic examination is invaluable in cases with pleural fluid for the identification of underlying causes, e.g. masses in the pleural or mediastinal space.

Endoscopic examination of the respiratory tract allows visualisation and collection of samples for analysis. Tissue biopsies can also be collected using rigid or flexible endoscopy. Bronchoalveolar lavage is used to collect samples of cells for cytological examination. This may provide information as to whether there is a parasitic, allergic, bacterial or neoplastic aetiology to the condition.

Blood gas analysis can be useful to assess how well gas exchange is occurring. Animals with pulmonary disease will have low arterial blood oxygen and increased concentration of carbon dioxide.

Treatment

Treat underlying cause, e.g. antibiotics for infection or medical therapy for CHF.

SPECIFIC DISEASES

Upper respiratory tract diseases

Cat 'flu (chronic rhinosinusitis)

Cause: infection with feline herpes and/or calicivirus and often secondary bacterial infection.
Signs: sneezing, ocular and nasal discharge, fever, mouth ulcers.
Diagnosis: clinical signs, oropharyngeal swab for virus isolation.
Treatment: symptomatic, good nursing care, antibiotics for secondary bacterial infection, vaccination available. Isolation of affected individuals is important to prevent spread.

Canine tracheobronchitis (kennel cough)

Cause: infection with *Bordetella bronchiseptica*, respiratory viruses or a combination of agents.
Signs: harsh, non-productive coughing, fever. Complications may develop, e.g. pneumonia, nasal discharge.
Diagnosis: clinical signs and history.
Treatment: may be none required or antibiotics and antitussives; vaccination available. Isolation to prevent spread is important.

Nasal neoplasia

Cause: adenocarcinomas most common in the dog but lymphosarcoma may be seen in the cat.
Signs: epistaxis, respiratory noise, nasal discharge, sneezing.
Diagnosis: nasal chamber radiography shows destruction of turbinates and soft tissue density; biopsy required for definitive diagnosis.

Treatment: radiotherapy may provide remission in some cases, chemotherapy for lymphosarcoma.

Laryngeal paralysis

Cause: damage to recurrent laryngeal nerve, usually idiopathic in large breed dogs.
Signs: noisy breathing particularly after exercise, exercise intolerance, cough, altered tone of bark.
Diagnosis: signs, examination of larynx under light general anaesthetic.
Treatment: surgical 'tie back' of laryngeal cartilages.

Lower respiratory tract diseases

Chronic bronchitis

Cause: chronic damage to or irritation of airways.
Signs: persistent or intermittent coughing for months. If bronchitis is severe there may be exercise intolerance and dyspnoea.
Diagnosis: signs, bronchoscopy and bronchoalveolar lavage for cytology.
Treatment: antibiotics, bronchodilators, mucolytics and chest coupage to remove secretions.

Allergic bronchitis (feline asthma)

Cause: hypersensitivity resulting in bronchospasm and airway obstruction.
Signs: wheezing, paroxysmal coughing with neck extended.
Diagnosis: chest radiography, bronchoscopy and bronchoalveolar lavage for culture and cytology.
Treatment: avoid known allergens, give steroids and bronchodilators if necessary.

Pulmonary oedema

Cause: usually secondary to CHF.
Signs: moist, productive cough, exercise intolerance, cyanosis if severe.
Diagnosis: chest radiography.
Treatment: diuretics to remove oedema and treat underlying cause.

Pneumonia

Cause: bacterial or viral, occasionally fungal infection.

Signs: dyspnoea, cough, fever, lethargy, anorexia, cyanosis if severe.

Diagnosis: chest radiography (shows increased density in lungs), bronchoscopy and bronchoalveolar lavage for culture and cytology.

Treatment: antibiotics or fungal therapy, nursing care, oxygen therapy.

Pulmonary neoplasia

Cause: primary usually adenocarcinomas. Often metastatic spread from tumours elsewhere.

Signs: may be none, chronic cough, haemoptysis.

Diagnosis: chest radiography, lung biopsy.

Treatment: lung lobe removal if localised primary tumour, otherwise palliative treatment only.

Extrapulmonary diseases

Pleural fluid

Cause: pyothorax (infection), transudate (right sided heart failure, hypoproteinaemia), haemothorax (coagulopathy, trauma), modified transudates (neoplasia in chest, ruptured diaphragm), chylothorax.

Signs: dyspnoea, exercise intolerance, muffled lung sounds.

Diagnosis: chest radiography (shows collapse of lung lobes with fluid in pleural space), thoracocentesis for aspiration of fluid. Ultrasonography to identify underlying masses.

Treatment: drainage of fluid if large quantities present and treat underlying cause.

Pneumothorax

Cause: usually trauma, rarely primary lung lesion, e.g. neoplasia or bulla, can be idiopathic.

Signs: dyspnoea, hyperresonance of chest.

Diagnosis: chest radiography shows collapsed lung with air in pleural space.

Treatment: drainage of air, correction of underlying problem.

DRUGS COMMONLY USED IN THE MANAGEMENT OF RESPIRATORY TRACT DISEASE

Bronchodilators

Agents like theophylline are used to open the large airways to facilitate air movement. Most useful where there is bronchospasm.

Antitussives (cough suppressants)

The name literally means an agent which suppresses coughing. The most commonly used are codeine and butorphanol. These can be used to reduce severe coughing which can be distressing for animal and owner. These agents must not be used where a productive cough is present (as the cough in these cases is beneficial in removing secretions from the lower respiratory tract).

Mucolytics

These agents are used to loosen and liquify mucus in the respiratory tract making it easier for the body to remove. The most commonly used is bromhexine hydrochloride (Bisolvon).

Diuretics

Diuretics may be indicated in cases with pulmonary oedema, particularly when it is due to heart failure.

Antibiotics

Antibiotics used for the treatment of respiratory tract disease should have good penetration into the respiratory system.

Tracheotomy tube placement

Indications

This is indicated in laryngeal collapse, paralysis or obstruction.

Placement

- In an emergency surgical preparation may be minimal.

- Place the animal on its back with head and neck extended.
- Local or general anaesthesia may be used depending on the circumstances.
- A midline skin incision is made below the larynx and the trachea is exposed.
- A flap is made by cutting approximately 60% of the way round two or three tracheal rings and an appropriately sized tracheostomy tube is passed through the hole into the trachea.
- Inflate cuff (if cuffed tube is used).
- The tube is secured around the neck using ties.
- Vaseline may be applied on the skin under the tube opening to prevent scalding.

Complications

Blockage

The tracheotomy tube is the sole airway for the patient and if it becomes blocked the patient will be unable to breathe. Regular maintenance of the tube is essential. Ideally a suction system should be available to allow debris and secretions to be removed through the tube. A small amount of sterile saline can then be flushed into the tube every hour to clear any mucus and secretions that have accumulated, and then aspirated using the suction system. The external portion of the tube can be wiped down to remove debris. Take care not to occlude the tube inadvertently when handling the patient.

Dislodgement

Premature removal of the tube can result in respiratory obstruction.

Infection

The site will always be contaminated so broad-spectrum antibiotic cover is given routinely.

Subcutaneous oedema

If the tube does not provide a tight seal air can escape into the subcutaneous tissues. This is rarely a significant problem and will disperse naturally once the leak is sealed.

Removal

Before removal check the airway function by temporary tube obstruction. Once the tube has been removed the hole will seal by secondary intention.

Thoracic drain placement

Indications

- To remove fluid or air which requires repeated drainage from the pleural space.
- To administer medications to the pleural space, e.g. antibiotics in pyothorax.

Placement

- Good restraint is important so most patients require sedation or general anaesthesia (very collapsed patients may not).
- Clip and surgically prepare area of skin incision over 5th–11th intercostal spaces.
- Infiltrate with local anaesthetic (if not using general anaesthetic).
- Make a stab incision half way up the chest wall at 10th intercostal space.
- Preplace a purse-string suture around incision and leave suture ends long.
- Use a curved haemostat to create a tunnel under the skin from the stab hole to the 6th intercostal space.
- Force the haemostat into the chest cavity at the level of 7th or 8th intercostal space and open jaws wide.
- Ensure drain is clamped then grab the chest tube with a second haemostat and pass through tunnel into thoracic cavity.
- Release chest drain and push it into the thorax and remove both haemostats.
- Alternatively a chest drain introducer can be used – a stylet is inserted into the drain for introduction into the pleural space. This is removed once the drain is in place and the drain plugged with a Christmas tree adaptor and a 3-way stopcock attached.
- Place a cloth over the hole in the chest wall, open the chest drain and attempt to aspirate from the chest – the drain may need to be

moved slightly to permit drainage (air introduced during the procedure will be removed at this point).

- For additional security apply a gate clamp to the drain.
- Affix drain to skin using Chinese finger-trap suture with free ends of purse-string suture (alternatively apply tape butterfly to drain and suture to skin).
- Place antiseptic soaked gauze over drain exit from body wall and protect drain using a body bandage.
- Radiograph chest to confirm correct drain position (ideally cranioventral thorax) and to check effectiveness of initial aspiration.
- Aspirate from drain as necessary but monitor patient closely for all the time the drain is in place.

Complications

Pneumothorax

Leakage of air through an unsecured drain or around the drain will result in pneumothorax and lung collapse. Placing a clamp on the drain in addition to the plug ensures that air cannot enter should the plug be dislodged. Patients should always be closely monitored while a drain is indwelling and radiographs may be necessary if dyspnoea increases.

Infection

Strict attention to asepsis when placing the drain is important. Always clean the external portion of the drain before and after aspirating. Many patients will be given systemic antibiotics to guard against the risk of introducing infection into the pleura space.

Trauma to structures within the chest

Clumsy drain placement can result in laceration of lung lobes (leading to persistent pneumothorax), or haemothorax due to puncture of the intercostal artery, lung vessel or even the heart. This damage almost always occurs during drain placement but patients must always be monitored

closely for signs of deterioration after the drain is in place.

Dislodgement

Ensure the drain cannot be interfered with by bandaging and use of an Elizabethan collar if necessary.

Removal

The drain should be removed after no air has been aspirated for 12–24 hours or fluid production is less than 2 ml/kg bodyweight. Remove drain swiftly and close skin incision immediately by tightening purse-string suture.

URINARY TRACT (Table 3.7)

ANATOMY AND PHYSIOLOGY

The main urinary tract functions are:

- removal and storage of waste products from the blood
- regulation of fluid balance
- stimulation of red blood cell production through erythopoietin release.

The urinary tract comprises:

- Two kidneys which are situated in the retroperitoneal space (outside the peritoneum covering the abdominal cavity), either side of the midline, just beneath the lumbar spine. The left kidney is positioned slightly caudal to the right. In the dog the kidney position is relatively fixed but in the cat the kidneys are more mobile and may be palpated in a variety of locations.
- A ureter joining each kidney to the bladder. The ureters run from the hilus on the medial aspect of each kidney and end in a 'J'-shaped curve where they join the bladder. The ureters enter through the bladder wall at an angle near the bladder neck; it is this anatomy which helps prevent flow of urine from the bladder up the ureters when the bladder is full.

Table 3.7 Important questions to ask the owner of an animal with urinary problems

Question	Reason for question and interpretation of answer
Is urination abnormal – more or less frequent?	The primary problem in an incontinent animal may be sudden polydipsia which overwhelms failing continence mechanisms, e.g. bitch with pyometra may be presented for nocturnal incontinence
Is the volume of urine greater or less than normal?	If urine volume is increased and patient is not dehydrated it must be polydipsic. Absence of urine is serious – this may indicate obstruction to urine flow or a failure of urine production (acute renal failure)
Is there pain associated with urination?	Painful urination is associated with inflammation or obstruction of urinary tract. Primary incontinence, e.g. sphincter mechanism incontinence (SMI), is not painful
Is the animal voiding urine each time it strains?	If patient is not passing urine on each attempt it may have urinary tract obstruction or ruptured bladder. These cases should be seen immediately
Does the urine appear abnormal, i.e. discoloured, or have an unusual/pungent smell?	Incontinence does not result in abnormal urine. Discoloration and/or smell is commonly associated with urinary tract infection
Is the animal well in itself?	Signs of ill health may indicate systemic disease, infection, or renal failure
Is the animal drinking more than normal?	Polydipsia may be associated with a primary renal failure or a systemic disease
Is there any incontinence? If so, is this at rest or is urine dripping constantly?	Incontinence when the patient is relaxed is more often associated with SMI. Ectopic ureters can be associated with continual urine dripping
Is there a preputial discharge in males?	Preputial discharge may be associated with prostatic disease
When was last season in females?	Signs of incontinence may be associated with pyometra in the bitch. Pyometra typically develops within a few weeks of a season. Polydipsia secondary to diabetes mellitus may also develop in the high progesterone phase of the reproductive cycle (within 2 months of a season in the bitch)
Has there been recent surgery?	Patients with compensated renal failure may be 'tipped' into overt renal failure by dehydration in the perioperative period. There is a risk of damage to the urinary tract during abdominal surgery (particularly urethral ligation during ovariohysterectomy)
Ask owner to bring urine sample to surgery	Examination of a urine sample provides a lot of information in the investigation of a patient with urinary tract disease

- The bladder, when empty, is a few centimetres long with a wall around 4 mm thick. When distended it can fill about one third of the abdominal space and the wall is considerably thinner. The trigone of the bladder is the division between the body of the bladder and the bladder neck which narrows into the urethra.
- The urethra which connects the bladder neck to the outside world. In the male the urethra runs from the bladder to the tip of the penis. In the female the urethra empties into the vestibule.

The kidneys have a large reserve capacity and more than two thirds of total renal function must be lost before any clinical signs are apparent. This means that the whole of one kidney and one third of the other can be non-functional and the animal still has no changes associated with renal dysfunction on routine screening tests.

The kidneys comprise two functional units, the glomeruli and the tubules. In the normal animal the kidneys receive about 20% of the blood coming from the heart. The blood is forced through the glomeruli and fluid containing dissolved substances is forced out of the blood into the kidney tubules. Water and the required electrolytes are then actively absorbed out of the glomerular filtrate leaving behind metabolic waste products such as urea. Kidneys also excrete phosphorus. Blood concentrations of calcium and phosphorus are closely regulated. High levels of phosphorus in the blood stimulate the production of parathyroid hormone and this causes calcium to be mobilised from body stores. If levels of calcium and phosphorus are both high calcium is deposited in the soft tissues including the kidneys. Parathyroid hormone can also cause direct damage to the kidney. The water and electrolytes re-enter the bloodstream and the remaining waste products are excreted as urine into the ureters and are collected in the bladder for voiding at a convenient time.

The bladder can distend widely to store large volumes of urine. Exit from the bladder into the urethra is controlled by two sphincters, one with conscious (voluntary) control and the other unconscious or automatic control:

- internal sphincter (involuntary control)
- external sphincter (voluntary control).

The urethra is normally flattened to prevent flow of urine. This is achieved by smooth and striated muscle and elastic tissue in the urethral wall. The length of the urethra is also important in preventing urine leakage. Males have longer urethras than females which means that urinary incontinence is less common in males.

As the bladder fills with urine its walls are stretched and this is detected by sensors which send a signal to the brain indicating the need for urination. Dogs pass 20–80 ml urine/kg per day and cats 10–15 ml/kg per day.

The kidneys also produce a hormone called **erythropoietin** which stimulates the production of red blood cells in the bone marrow. Hormone production is increased when oxygen levels in the blood are low, which usually indicates anaemia or hypoxia.

The urinary system is, for convenience, divided into upper (kidneys and ureters) and lower (bladder and urethra) tracts.

The upper urinary tract is concerned with the production of urine. The lower tract is primarily concerned with urine storage and voiding.

Clinical signs of disease in the two systems are often completely different. Cats which do not use a litter tray may have severe changes in urinary habits before the owner notices – unless the cat is urinating in the house it may not be presented for investigation.

PATHOPHYSIOLOGY
Upper urinary tract disease

The upper urinary tract comprises kidneys and ureters.

Cause

Damage to the kidneys may be caused by infection (from the blood or ascending the ureters), toxaemic or ischaemic damage, calculus formation, or increased pressure as a result of obstruction to urine flow.

Signs

Renal disease may result in azotaemia (raised blood urea concentration) which may be associated with uraemic signs, e.g. anorexia, weight loss, vomiting, polyuria and polydipsia if renal function is compromised. Abdominal pain (colic) may be seen with pyelonephritis and renal or ureteric calculi. Changes in the nature of urine, i.e. altered colour or concentration, can be seen with upper urinary tract disease.

Diagnostic tests

Kidneys can easily be palpated in the cat and changes in size, shape and the presence of pain are easily assessed. In large or fat dogs renal palpation is much more difficult and physical assessment may not be possible.

Radiography can be useful for the evaluation of the size and shape of the kidneys, but two views of the abdomen (a lateral and dorsoventral projection) are needed. Ultrasonography is a better method for examination of the kidneys as it also provides information about the structure of the kidney. Kidney function cannot be assessed by either of these methods. Crude tests of renal function should include blood screens to check for the presence of azotaemia and measurement of urine specific gravity (to check the ability of the kidneys to concentrate urine), but these will only detect renal damage if kidney function is severely compromised. Other functional tests such as measurement of the excretion of sodium and potassium in the urine are more accurate for detecting milder renal dysfunction.

Treatment

Renal damage is not reversible. Management is aimed at preventing further damage to the system and, if renal function has been reduced, supporting the patient to reduce the amount of work expected of the kidneys.

Lower urinary tract disease

The lower urinary tract (LUT) comprises the bladder and urethra. In the bitch and queen the urethra is short and comparatively wide whereas in the male the urethra is longer. This explains why complications associated with urethral disease are much more common in the male.

Cause

Infection is relatively common in the LUT, as is damage caused by calculi. Neoplasia of the bladder and urethra is increasingly common.

Signs

Diseases of the lower urinary tract typically result in problems with urination. Urination frequency may be decreased or increased, urination may be painful or impossible and haematuria is common.

Diagnostic tests

In most animals a full urinary bladder can be palpated and the presence or absence of a full bladder may be a useful clinical finding. A rectal examination should be performed in dogs as bladder stones or prostatomegaly may be detected.

Investigation of the LUT requires collection of a urine sample for analysis and usually some kind of diagnostic imaging technique. Plain radiography can provide information about the size and position of the bladder but contrast studies are needed to assess the urinary tract itself. Ultrasound examination is particularly useful in assessment of the bladder but cannot be used to visualise the urethra. Urine samples should be examined for the presence of crystals, blood or other cells and cultured to determine the presence of infection.

Treatment

Where possible the underlying cause of the LUT disease should be identified and treated. Symptomatic treatment of infection or inflammation should then be considered. All patients with LUT disease should be closely monitored to ensure that they are able to urinate voluntarily. Obstruction to voiding can result in an over-distended bladder which may cause excessive stretching or rupture of the bladder and potentially damage the kidneys. If the animal is unable to urinate voluntarily a urethral catheter should be passed or the bladder drained by cystocentesis. It is unwise to leave urinary catheters in situ for any period of time since they provide a focus for infection and cause inflammation in the urethra. Urethral inflammation may result in spasm (and obstruction) when the catheter is removed, creating a vicious cycle of inability to void urine voluntarily.

SPECIFIC DISEASES
Acute renal failure

Cause

There are a number of causes of acute renal failure (ARF):

- reduction of blood flow to kidneys
- obstruction to elimination of urine
- progression from chronic renal failure
- primary severe damage to the kidneys, e.g. toxic.

Signs

Signs of ARF relate to uraemia and are therefore similar to chronic renal failure. Urea and creatinine rises will be rapid in acute failure (whereas in chronic disease they will have been elevated for a significant period of time). In many cases urine production is low or absent.

Diagnostic tests

Blood samples show sudden azotaemia and there is usually reduced urine production. Further tests are directed towards identifying the primary cause.

Treatment

- Correct fluid and electrolyte balance.
- Promote urine output.

Management of severe electrolyte imbalances is urgent, particularly high potassium which can cause fatal dysrhythmias. Affected animals should be given potassium-free intravenous fluids.

To stimulate urine flow, fluids should be given at 6 ml/kg per hour – however it is important to monitor urine output closely because if urine is not produced overhydration will occur. Monitoring central venous pressure is the best method of assessing whether a patient is being over-hydrated. If no urine has been produced diuretic drugs (furosemide (frusemide) or mannitol) may be given. Oliguric patients may be stimulated to produce urine and in the initial stages diuresis will occur with the production of very dilute urine and intravenous fluids should be continued to prevent dehydration.

Dietary considerations

Appetite is often suppressed and provision of nutrition may be very difficult due to the presence of nausea and vomiting. Nasogastric tube placement for delivery of high biological value protein food is useful; calories may be further supplemented by administration of glucose in fluids.

The underlying cause of the acute failure may not be identified. However, if poisoning with nephrotoxic agents is the cause peritoneal dialysis may be useful to eliminate these from the body.

Chronic renal failure

Cause

Chronic renal failure (CRF) is a slowly progressive development of azotaemia. It is most often seen around 7 years of age but young animals may be affected because of congenital renal disorders. In older animals it may be due to nephrotoxic or ischaemic damage, pyelonephritis and glomerulonephritis, although most cases are idiopathic.

Signs

A loss of 75% of kidney function is required for signs to develop. Signs are progressive and usually start with polydipsia/polyuria and depression, inappetance progressing to anorexia, weight loss, oral ulcers and vomiting. Severely affected individuals may have seizures. Halitosis is often one of the signs that prompts the owner to seek veterinary advice.

Diagnostic tests

Laboratory demonstration of azotaemia with inappropriately dilute urine (urine specific gravity 1.008–1.012) will usually be sufficient to confirm the diagnosis in a patient with classical signs. Other features on blood screen are non-regenerative anaemia and high phosphate concentrations. Cats commonly also have low serum potassium concentrations.

By the time of diagnosis the underlying cause of the renal damage may not be identifiable.

Treatment

Administration of intravenous fluid therapy may help to remove urea and other metabolic waste products from the body. High urine output may also flush vital electrolytes from the body which the compromised kidney is unable to reclaim from the urine.

Dietary considerations

Appetite is often significantly suppressed in CRF and every attempt should be made to encourage patients to eat. Offering palatable food warmed to body temperature is helpful but syringe or nasogastric tube feeding may be necessary. Appetite stimulants can be used. Patients may be inappetant due to nausea and in these cases the use of antacids or antiemetics may be necessary.

There is some controversy over the correct diet for a patient with renal dysfunction. High levels of protein in the diet may result in increased urea content in the blood and for this reason low-protein diets have been advocated in renal dysfunction. In fact, animals with renal dysfunction certainly require sufficient protein in their diet to prevent the breakdown of body protein stores and, since many patients with renal disease have poor appetites, adequate nutrition can be a problem. Patients should be fed a moderately restricted protein diet with highly digestible proteins and this can be given at high levels unless clinical signs associated with uraemia are seen. Once clinical signs are seen the protein content of the diet should be reduced to the maximum level which does not cause clinical signs. Anabolic steroids may help to prevent the breakdown of body proteins. Water-soluble vitamins are lost in urine and supplementation with B vitamins in particular is required.

Restriction of dietary phosphorus is important and this helps to reduce parathyroid hormone levels and slow renal disease. If this fails to control high phosphorus blood levels then drugs which bind phosphorus, e.g. aluminium hydroxide, may also be required. Sodium restriction may help reduce hypertension. Potassium supplementation may be required in cats who are often hypokalaemic.

Feline lower urinary tract disease (FLUTD)

Cause

The cause of FLUTD is unclear. Some studies have suggested a viral infection may be involved; others think that it is a type of stress response in some individuals.

Signs

Signs are very similar to those of cats with urethral obstruction, i.e. haematuria and dysuria with frequent attempts at micturition. The bladder in non-obstructive FLUTD is small, painful and may feel thickened. The signs tend to come and go without treatment – most cats recover within a week only to relapse a few weeks later.

Diagnostic tests

Diagnosis is based on the ruling out of other causes of LUT disease in the cat. Urine is sterile and radiographic and ultrasonographic examinations are normal (except for a thickened bladder wall).

Treatment

It is difficult to assess treatment since the condition gets better and worse independent of therapy. Anti-inflammatory drugs, e.g. glucocorticoids, may help.

Urinary tract infection

Cause

Urinary tract infection is very common in bitches but usually remains confined to the LUT. Most infections result from ascending infection and are caused by common bacteria such as *Escherichia coli* and *Staphylococcus* spp. Infection usually results from a lesion in the urinary tract such as trauma caused by uroliths or stones; retention of urine (so that bacteria are not flushed out of the tract); or a reduced immune system such as in patients with concurrent illness, e.g. diabetes mellitus or hyperadrenocorticism.

Signs

Many urinary tract infections are silent, i.e. cause no clinical signs. Where signs are present these are typically of LUT inflammation. Care must be taken to differentiate signs of inflammation from obstruction. The bladder will usually be empty on palpation if inflammation is present because voiding occurs frequently; conversely, if there is urinary obstruction urine cannot be voided and the bladder will be distended.

Diagnostic tests

Urine culture is essential in the diagnosis of this condition (particularly in cats to distinguish between infection and FLUTD). Whilst voided urine or samples collected by urinary catheterisation are acceptable for culture, urine samples should ideally be collected by cystocentesis. This is the only method of collecting a sample without contamination from the urogenital tract below the bladder. It is essential to collect a urine sample for culture *before* any treatment is administered. If inappropriate antibiotic therapy is given it may fail to control clinical infection but will almost certainly prevent growth of bacterial culture from a urine sample and this makes selection of an appropriate treatment more difficult.

Treatment

Urine culture and sensitivity testing allow identification of appropriate antibiotic therapy for management of infection. Treatment should be continued for 10–14 days for LUT infection and at least 3–4 weeks if pyelonephritis is suspected. Treatment should be given for at least 7 days after all clinical signs have resolved to prevent recurrence of infection as soon as treatment stops. Ideally urine culture should be repeated 7 days after the end of treatment to confirm resolution of the infection.

In chronic or recurrent cases antibiotics may need to be given for 6 months or more to resolve the infection.

Urolithiasis (urinary stones, calculi)

Cause

Uroliths form when there is a high concentration of minerals in the urine. Uroliths can be made of different types of minerals. The most common stones are:

- struvite (containing magnesium)
- calcium oxalate
- calcium phosphate
- urate.

Some breeds have metabolic defects which increase the likelihood of certain stones, e.g.

Dalmations often have urate stones. Struvite stones are commonly associated with urinary tract infections and calcium-containing stones are often the result of high levels of calcium in the urine.

Signs

Uroliths may form in the kidney or in the bladder and signs are usually related to the location of the stone. Recurrent urinary tract infections are common as the stones form a focus for bacteria to congregate. Kidney stones may cause colic, whilst those in the bladder commonly result in infection and haematuria. Occasionally stones get trapped in the ureter or urethra which not only prevents the passage of urine but is excruciatingly painful. Blockages caused by uroliths must be removed as soon as possible to prevent permanent damage to the kidneys.

Diagnostic tests

Some uroliths can be seen on plain radiographs (radiopaque) but others are not visible (radiolucent). These can be seen as filling defects if radiographic contrast studies of the urinary tract are performed. Most uroliths can be identified using ultrasound provided their location can be viewed with the ultrasound probe. Examination of a urine sample from a patient with uroliths may show crystals (traces of minerals) but, although it is likely that these will be the same composition as the urolith, this is not always the case. The only definitive method for identifying a urolith is to remove it and send a sample for laboratory analysis.

Urine pH should be measured in all animals with uroliths as this may help to determine what sort of stone is likely to develop.

Treatment

Uroliths causing obstruction to the urinary tract must be removed. Uroliths most commonly become lodged in the urethra of male animals, particularly around the **os penis** in the dog where the urethra is narrowed. It may be possible to pass a urethral catheter and gently push the stones back into the bladder; alternatively inserting a catheter into the urethra and then flushing saline through may dilate the urethra and wash the stones out. Sedation and pain relief must be given to ensure that the patient is relaxed during this procedure if it is to have any chance of success. If all else fails surgical removal is required. Patients that have been obstructed for some time may develop acute renal failure.

Dietary considerations

Uroliths which are not causing clinical signs or those safely located in the bladder can be treated more conservatively. Depending on the type of stone it may be possible to alter the diet so that the concentration of the stone-forming mineral in the urine is reduced, or to change the pH of the urine to make it more acid or alkaline (depending on the type of urolith) and promote the stone to dissolve. There are commercial diets which will promote the correct environment for removal or prevention of specific types of urolith but it is essential that investigation be performed to investigate the cause of the urolithiasis and to address this problem where possible.

Nephrotic syndrome

Cause: progression of glomerulonephropathy to end stage.

Signs: lethargy, weight loss, ascites, limb oedema, polydipsia/polyuria.

Diagnosis: proteinuria and hypoalbuminaemia, increased urea and creatinine.

Treatment: high biological value protein, restricted salt and phosphorus, anabolic steroids, corticosteroids, antibiotics.

Cystitis

Cause: trauma, calculi, diabetes mellitus, hyperadrenocorticism, obstruction, neoplasia, bacterial infection.

Signs: increased frequency and pain on urination and straining, wetting in house, haematuria.

Diagnosis: urinalysis, radiography, blood samples for diagnosis of underlying cause.

Treatment: treat underlying cause, antibiotics, urine acidifiers, increase voiding and water intake.

INCONTINENCE

Urethral sphincter mechanism incompetence (USMI)

Cause

USMI is caused by reduced urethral tone which may increase as a result of response to hormones produced at first season. It can develop after first season due to reduction in circulating oestrogens. It may be associated with abnormal (caudal) bladder position.

Signs

Seen more often in females than males and often in large breeds, with leakage of urine, often when lying down.

Diagnosis

Measurement of pressures, flow or resistance in urinary tract is rarely done in practice. Diagnosis is usually made on the basis of signs and history and ruling out other causes of incontinence by contrast radiographic urinary tract studies, e.g. intravenous urography.

Treatment

Spayed bitches may respond to phenylpropanolamine combined with oestrogen. In some cases surgery to relocate bladder or increase urethral resistance may help.

DRUGS COMMONLY USED IN TREATMENT OF URINARY TRACT DISEASE

Diuretics

These are used to promote urine production and can be used if production is low, e.g. ARF. Furosemide (frusemide: loop diuretic) is the most commonly used diuretic in veterinary practice. It inhibits the resorption of salt and water filtered by the kidneys so that more fluid is lost in the urine. Mannitol (osmotic diuretic) increases the concentration of the glomerular filtrate thereby drawing water into the urine.

Aluminium hydroxide (phosphate binder)

This binds phosphate in the genito-urinary tact so that it cannot be absorbed. This reduces phosphate levels in the blood and so reduces the amount of phosphate which has to be excreted by the kidney. Aluminium hydroxide is also used to neutralise gastric acid and may alleviate some of the vomiting in CRF.

Antacids (cimetidine/ranitidine)

These drugs act to reduce gastric acid secretion and hence the acidity of the stomach. When the stomach wall is inflamed a high acid environment can cause discomfort and vomiting.

Nandrolone (anabolic steroid)

The anabolic action of this hormone helps to prevent the breakdown of body proteins and so reduces urea formation from protein digestion in the gut. It may also promote red cell production.

Vitamin B

Water-soluble vitamins are lost in urine in large amounts if large volumes of urine are produced (as in CRF). Supplementation of these vitamins in the diet or by injection may be necessary to prevent deficiency. They also have an appetite-stimulating effect in some animals which can be beneficial.

Incontinence

Phenylpropanolamine (alpha receptor blocker)

This drug stimulates the alpha adrenergic receptors causing increased tone in the urethra and therefore reducing incontinence. It may take days to weeks to have effect and has to be continued long term to be effective.

Urinary catheter placement

Indications

- Empty bladder before surgery or investigations.
- Collect a urine sample for analysis.
- Empty bladder when patient is unable to, e.g. in flaccid bladder or obstructive urinary tract disease.
- Measure urine output, e.g. in monitoring acute renal failure.
- Administer drugs or radiographic contrast agents.

Placement

- Premeasure the distance from the external urethral opening along the urethra to the bladder.
- Select a catheter that is the correct length (if the catheter is too short it will not reach the bladder; too long and the excess length within the bladder can knot, making removal through the urethra impossible).
- Select appropriate gauge of catheter – which should be the largest catheter that will easily pass (if catheter is too small patient may urinate around catheter).
- Catheter and lubricant must remain sterile throughout procedure.
- Clip away hair from, and clean, penis or vulva to prevent introduction of contaminant bacteria into urethra.
- Gently introduce the lubricated catheter via the urethra into the bladder (introduction in the bitch is made easier if the urethral opening is viewed using a vaginal speculum).
- Urine can be drained from the bladder and the catheter flushed with sterile saline.
- If the catheter is to remain indwelling it must be plugged or a urinary collection bag attached to create a sealed sterile unit.
- Urine flow will promote flushing of potentially harmful bacteria so patients should be walked regularly to promote voiding (intravenous fluid rates can be increased to encourage urine flow).

Complications

Infection

Non-sterile placement of an indwelling catheter will result in infection. Infection can still enter after sterile placement and so regular cleaning of the catheter exit is important. There is some debate as to the merits and disadvantages of routinely giving antibiotics to patients with indwelling urinary catheters. It is possible that this practice could promote growth of antibiotic-resistant bacteria in the bladder, but others feel that it is necessary to give antibiotics to guard against ascending renal or systemic infection.

Inflammation

Placement of urinary catheters always results in some inflammation of the urethra. Often this is mild but in some animals it can cause spasm of the urethra after the catheter has been removed. Urethral spasm can prevent the animal from urinating and this can result in a vicious cycle of removal of catheter and inability to pass urine resulting in placing a new catheter. In general the urinary catheter should be left indwelling for as short a time as possible.

Urethral damage

Clumsy catheterisation or the use of force can occasionally result in tearing the urethra (or even bladder). Small tears may go unnoticed and seal without any treatment. Large tears can result in urine escape into the peritoneal cavity and serious uroperitonitis.

Blockage

Catheters may become kinked or blocked with debris or calculi if they are not regularly flushed. A blocked catheter should be removed immediately and a new catheter placed if necessary. If urine stagnates in the catheter the risk of infection is high.

Removal

Unintentional removal of the entire urinary catheter is inconvenient but not too serious (a new catheter may need to be placed). A more serious complication would be the removal of the external portion of the catheter, leaving the urethral portion in place. Indwelling catheters should be protected by suturing to the skin and the use of an Elizabethan collar.

Table 3.8 Important questions to ask the owner of a female animal with suspected genital tract disease	
Question	Reason for question and interpretation of answer
Is the animal entire or neutered?	Some conditions can only be seen in entire animals, e.g. ovarian cancer cannot occur after the ovaries have been removed. Other conditions are more common in the entire animal, e.g. pyometra
When was the last season?	Many reproductive diseases are linked to the reproductive cycle, i.e. pyometra is more likely to occur a few weeks after the last oestrus
Is there a vaginal discharge? If so, what is it like?	Clear or bloody discharge may be associated with a normal season. Purulent (yellow or reddish brown) discharge implies vaginal or uterine infection. Following whelping the normal green vaginal discharge should cease within a few days – persistent discharge may indicate puppy or placental retention. Bloody discharge after whelping suggest subinvolution of placental sites
Is the animal unwell?	Pyometra is often associated with signs of ill health. Many hormonal diseases do not affect health initially. Paraneoplastic conditions, e.g. bone marrow suppression with ovarian tumours, may also cause ill health
Are the seasons regular?	If seasons are close together it is likely that ovulation is not occurring. Absence of seasons may be associated with many other diseases, e.g. hypothyroidism. Menopause is *not* a common cause of cessation of seasons in a bitch or queen

GENITAL TRACT (Tables 3.8 and 3.9)

MALE ANATOMY AND PHYSIOLOGY

The male reproductive system comprises:

- testes
- epididymis
- vas deferens
- prostate gland
- penis and prepuce.

The testes lie outside the body (in the scrotum) which, in the dog, is between the hind legs, and in the cat lies beneath the anus. The testes start their development within the body cavity sited just behind the kidneys and from there they migrate through the inguinal ring and into the scrotum. This journey is normally complete by around 3 months and if the testes fail to arrive in the scrotum by this time the animal is classed **cryptorchid.**

The testes produce spermatozoa and hormones, e.g. testosterone and oestrogens. Testosterone is responsible for the development of secondary sexual characteristics. Spermatozoa produced in the testes are stored in the epididymis until ejaculation when they empty into the urethra through the vas deferens. The urethra runs through the prostate gland and is protected within the corpus cavernosum (a spongy erectile tissue) within the penis.

The prostate gland in the dog is sited at the bladder neck and in the cat is further down the urethra. The prostate gland often enlarges in older entire males and can compress the urethra running through it or the colon which lies immediately dorsal. The prostate gland produces seminal fluid which forms part of the ejaculate. The canine penis contains a bone (**os penis**) and is contained within the prepuce and suspended from the midline ventral abdominal wall. The feline penis points backwards and has spiked barbs at its tip.

FEMALE ANATOMY AND PHYSIOLOGY

The female reproductive tract comprises:

- ovaries
- fallopian tubes
- uterus
- vagina
- vestibule
- clitoris.

The ovaries are found just caudal to the kidney, attached to the body wall by the suspensory ligament. Their blood supply comes from the ovarian artery which is a direct branch of the aorta. The main functions of the ovaries are to produce eggs and hormones:

- progesterone – produced by corpus luteum to maintain pregnancy
- oestradiol – produced by ovarian follicle to prepare for pregnancy
- relaxin – produced by corpus luteum to relax the ligaments around the birth canal.

The eggs are produced in follicles which rupture releasing the ova and these are taken up into the fallopian tubes. The ruptured ovarian follicle develops into the corpus luteum.

Table 3.9 Important questions to ask the owner of a male animal with suspected genital tract disease

Question	Reason for question and interpretation of answer
Is the animal neutered?	Some conditions can only be seen in entire animals, e.g. testicular cancer cannot occur after the testes have been removed. Other conditions are more common in the entire animal, e.g. prostatic disease
Has a preputial discharge been seen?	Prostatic disease may result in preputial discharge. This should not be confused with the fairly 'normal' preputial discharge seen in many dogs as a result of superficial infection in the prepuce
Any difficulties with urination/defecation?	Conditions causing enlargement of the prostate gland often compress the rectum or urethra causing secondary signs of straining

The uterus has two long horns leading to the body and cervix. The uterus has a smooth muscle wall and is lined by epithelium (endometrium).

Hormonal cycles in the bitch

The bitch first 'comes into season' at 6–18 months of age. In the bitch the reproductive hormone cycle follows the same course whether or not she is mated or becomes pregnant (see Box 3.6). The ovarian follicle develops over a period of 4–28 days and this is the period of vulval bleeding during which the bitch is said to be 'in season' or 'on heat' (pro-oestrus). At the end of this period the follicle ruptures and the eggs are released (ovulation) – the oestrus period (when the bitch will accept mating) lasts between 7 and 10 days. Whether or not the bitch is pregnant the corpus luteum develops and progesterone levels now rise and remain at a peak for about 6 weeks, before declining over the next 2 weeks. Bitches have two distinct breeding periods each year with a reproductively inactive period (anoestrus) in between.

Hormonal cycles in the queen

Oestrus in the cat is brought about by increasing day length and so the young queen usually starts to cycle the first spring after she is 6 months old. The queen has quite a different cycle from the bitch. Follicles develop while the queen is showing oestral behaviour but ovulation does not occur without mating. After ovulation progesterone concentrations begin to rise and remain high for about 4 weeks – if the queen is pregnant progesterone remains high for a further 4 weeks but in a non-pregnant queen it begins to fall and oestrus recurs. Queens have a single breeding season which lasts from early spring to autumn.

SPECIFIC DISEASES IN THE FEMALE
(Box 3.7)

Pyometra (cystic endometrial hyperplasia)

This is a far more common condition in the bitch than the queen since the prolonged progesterone phase of the cycle only occurs in queens which have ovulated. In normal queens ovulation only occurs after mating; however, spontaneous ovulation can occur and the condition can also develop after administration of progestogens. Pyometra can occasionally occur after ovariohysterectomy if the uterus is not removed sufficiently close to the cervix.

Cause

After oestrus in the bitch, progesterone levels rise and remain high. This stimulates thickening of

---

Box 3.6 Canine reproductive cycle

Proestrus
Follicles enlarge and mature. Vulva enlarges and bloody discharge is present
Oestrus
Discharge reduces and becomes clear, ova are released
Metoestrus
Corpus luteum forms in site of ruptured follicle, vulval swelling subsides
Dioestrus
Time of activity of corpus luteum or pregnancy
Anoestrus
No ovarian activity

Box 3.7 Causes of reproductive tract disease

Female reproductive tract diseases	Male reproductive tract diseases
Ovary	Prostate
Ovarian cyst	Benign prostatic
Ovarian tumour	hypertrophy
Uterus	Prostatic cyst
Pyometra	Paraprostatic cyst
Uterine tumour	Prostatic infection
Vagina	Prostatic tumour
Vaginal tumour	Testicles
Vaginal prolapse	Orchitis
Vaginitis	Testicular tumours
Vaginal hyperplasia	Cryptorchidism
Vulva	Penis
Transmissible venereal	Penile tumour
tumour	Transmissible venereal
	tumour
	Paraphimosis

the endometrium and an increase in the number of glands in the endometrium. Excess fluid may accumulate in the uterus as a result of secretion from the glands and, if bacteria enter, infection can develop. Pyometra can be induced by the use of progestogens and oestrogen hormones for medical conditions. Ultimately the uterus becomes a large pus-filled sac and bacterial toxins enter the bloodstream and cause the typical clinical signs.

Signs

Pyometra is more common in middle-aged to older bitches. Signs typically develop within a few weeks of oestrus. The most common presentation is as a result of polyuria/polydipsia but lethargy, anorexia and vomiting are also common. About one third of cases have a vaginal discharge but in most cases the cervix remains closed and the discharge is retained within the uterus.

Diagnosis

Diagnosis is usually based on the clinical signs. An enlarged uterus may be palpated but is more commonly recognised on radiographs or using ultrasound.

Treatment

The treatment of choice is ovariohysterectomy. Some bitches may require medical stabilisation before surgery but this should not delay surgery for more than 12 hours. Fluid therapy is essential throughout surgery and the post-operative period. Antibiotic therapy should also be given. Some cases have been treated medically with drugs (prostaglandins) which empty the uterus; however, complications and risks associated with the use of these drugs are high.

False pregnancy (pseudopregnancy)

This is classically a condition of dogs. Cats can occasionally develop pseudopregnancy after an unsuccessful mating but this usually results in an absence of oestrus rather than any clinical signs.

Cause

No one knows why some bitch pregnancy and others do not, undergo the same hormonal c ...ether they are pregnant or not. False pregnancy can almost be regarded as a normal physiological occurrence in the bitch. However, if a bitch develops signs of a false pregnancy following one oestrus she is likely to continue to develop similar (or more severe) signs after all subsequent oestrus cycles.

Signs

Clinical signs develop between 6 and 12 weeks after the end of oestrus and may last for many months. Initially the changes are largely behavioural with nest making and 'adoption' of objects as puppies. Mammary development and lactation occur later and mastitis may develop.

Diagnosis

The condition is easily recognised although there may be some confusion in the owner's mind as to whether the bitch is actually pregnant or not.

Treatment

The majority of cases will resolve spontaneously given time. Stimulation of lactation by removal of milk is likely to prolong the condition so the use of an Elizabethan collar to prevent the bitch licking herself may be advisable. Drugs to suppress lactation can be given.

Severe or persistent cases may require hormonal treatment (oestradiol benzoate or methyltestosterone) but treatment may have to be prolonged and withdrawn gradually to be effective.

Ultimately the most successful course of action is neutering to prevent further recurrence. It is important that bitches are not neutered until all signs have resolved (and not for at least 3 months after the end of oestrus). Neutering while the condition continues may result in persistence of clinical signs.

Mastitis

Cause

Mastitis is seen in lactating animals (after whelping or in pseudopregnancy), and is caused by blocked milk ducts or bacterial infection.

Signs

Hot, swollen, painful mammary glands are seen. There may be signs of systemic illness, e.g. anorexia, depression or pyrexia.

Diagnosis

Diagnosis is by examination of mammary glands. Milk samples can be collected for bacterial culture but often broad-spectrum antibiotics are given.

Treatment

Treat by regular emptying of affected gland and hot compresses. Use antibiotics if there is systemic infection.

SPECIFIC DISEASES IN THE MALE
(see Box 3.7)

Prostatic disease

Cause

Prostatic disease is common in older entire male dogs. The prostate tends to increase in size as dogs get older due to hormonal stimulation. Bacterial infection results from infection ascending the urethra which runs through the centre of the prostate gland. Cysts or tumours may develop inside the prostate.

Signs

Enlargement of the prostate can cause compression of the colon resulting in faecal tenesmus with the production of thin strings of faeces. Infection and neoplasia may result in haematuria. Pain and weakness or swelling of the hindlimbs

can occur with severe prostatic disease. Systemic signs such as weight loss, anorexia and fever may be seen with neoplasia or infection.

Diagnosis

The enlarged prostate gland can often be palpated on rectal examination or occasionally by abdominal palpation. Benign hypertrophy usually results in a smooth, non-painful, symmetrically enlarged prostate. Prostate infections are usually painful on palpation and prostatic tumours are often asymmetrical and may become secondarily infected. Enlarged prostate glands can be visualised on radiographs or ultrasonographic examination. Ultrasonographic examination also allows assessment of the structure of the prostate and biopsies may be collected using ultrasound guidance.

Treatment

Most prostatic conditions can be improved by castration. If infection is present then antibiotics will also be required; some severe infections develop pockets of infection which may require surgical drainage. Prostatic cysts require drainage or removal. Treatment of prostatic tumours is difficult and the tumours often metastasise readily, however radiotherapy may relieve clinical signs for a while.

Paraphimosis

Cause: the erect penis becomes too enlarged to slide back inside the prepuce. Once the prepuce becomes tight at the root of the penis it acts like a tourniquet and blood can flow into the penis under pressure but cannot escape and the condition gets worse.

Signs: swollen, red penis permanently protruded.

Diagnosis: visual examination is sufficient to identify the problem.

Treatment: reduce swelling by cold pack application, lubrication of the penis and gentle massaging of the prepuce back over the penis. This is an emergency situation – if the penis cannot be reduced it may be necessary to cut the prepuce to get the penis retracted.

Testicular tumours

There are three tumours commonly associated with the testicle:

- Sertoli cell tumour
- interstitial cell tumour
- Leydig cell tumour.

Although these have a roughly equal incidence, the most important of these in the clinical setting is the Sertoli cell tumour.

Sertoli cell tumour

Cause: usually related to a retained testicle.

Signs: enlarged testicle (often with atrophy of the other testicle). Feminisation signs are usually present, e.g. attractiveness to male dogs, hair loss is common and bone marrow suppression can occur due to high oestrogen levels.

Diagnosis: based on clinical signs, hormone assays are possible to show increased oestrogen concentrations but in most cases diagnosis is made by histological assessment of the mass after removal of both testicles.

Treatment: surgical removal of the tumour is indicated. Pre-surgical screens for pulmonary metastases should be made. In rare cases bone marrow suppression is irreversible after surgery.

DRUGS COMMONLY USED IN THE MANAGEMENT OF GENITAL TRACT DISEASES

Females

Antiprolactins

Bromocriptine and cabergoline are used for management of pseudopregnancy and pregnancy termination.

Proligesterone

Acts like progesterone – used for oestrus control and treatment of false pregnancy.

Oestradiol benzoate

Can be used in the male to treat prostate hypertrophy. Treatment of misalliance in females. Oestrogens all carry a risk of bone marrow suppression.

Methyl testosterone

Acts to reduce prolactin which is thought to cause many of the signs of false pregnancy (behaviour changes and lactation). Also used for suppression of oestrus in the bitch.

Males

Delmadinone acetate (Tardak)

A progestogen given as a depot injection with long-lasting effects. Used in the management of many forms of prostate disease and as a chemical form of castration (for control of hypersexuality and sexual behaviour problems). It produces reduced libido but not infertility. Response to treatment usually suggests that castration will provide a similar but permanent response. Some dogs fail to respond to injection but do respond to surgical castration.

THE EYE (Table 3.10)

ANATOMY AND PHYSIOLOGY

Although the shape and size of the eye vary greatly between the species and between breeds of dog the basic anatomy is always the same.

The eyelids comprise a fibrous layer covered with skin on the outside and conjunctiva (a mucous membrane layer) on the inside. The upper eyelid has a row of small eyelashes (cilia) at its edge. A third eyelid is positioned in the medial corner of the eye and this is also covered with conjunctiva. The eyelids protect the surface of the globe and spread the tear film across the eye to keep it moist.

Conformational abnormalities of the eyelids are common in dogs and these include:

Table 3.10 Important questions to ask the owner of a dog with eye disease

Question	Reason for question and interpretation of answer
Is the eye swollen?	Protrusion of the globe may be due to enlargement of the globe itself or due to pressure behind the globe pushing it forward (retrobulbar mass). Check carefully to see if the eye itself appears enlarged
Is there a discharge – if so what colour?	Purulent ocular discharge indicates infection in the eye. Serous (clear) discharges are common in eyes with increased tear production (due to irritation or pain), or may be the result of tear overflow due to blocked drainage from the eye
Does the eye appear cloudy or clear?	Cloudiness of the eye may be due to cloudiness of the cornea or changes within the globe (pus in the globe or lens opacity)
Is there history of trauma to the eye, e.g. cat fight?	Trauma is a common cause of acute-onset eye disease, particularly in the cat
Does the animal appear to be blind?	Sudden-onset blindness is usually relatively easy to identify. However if animals have become blind over a longer period of time they often adapt very well to gradual loss of vision and are able to get around in a familiar environment. The owner may be unaware of how poor the pet's eyesight has become

- ectropion (where the eyelid rolls out to expose the conjunctival surface)
- entropion (where the eyelid turns in so that the skin is in contact with the cornea)
- distichiasis (where abnormal hairs grow on the conjunctival surface of the lid and rub against the cornea).

These abnormalities can all result in corneal damage and ulceration.

Tears are produced in the lacrimal gland and drain through small holes (puncta) in the lower eyelid into the nasolacrimal duct. If the puncta or duct is blocked or excessive amounts of tears are produced tears will flow over the lid and drain down the face. The tear film is required to protect the cornea and if the tear film is insufficient, e.g. in keratoconjunctivitis sicca (dry eye), corneal ulceration may occur.

The globe itself has three layers (Fig. 3.3):

- The outer layer is a protective coat and comprises the fibrous sclera at the back and the clear cornea at the front.
- The middle layer is vascular and pigmented, comprising the choroids, tapetum, ciliary body, suspensory ligament and iris.
- The inner layer of the eyeball contains the cells sensitive to light.

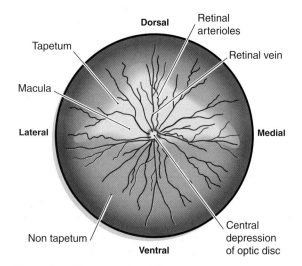

Figure 3.3 The ocular fundus of the right eye of the dog as viewed with an ophthalmoscope. (Reproduced with permission from Evans 1993.)

The globe is filled with fluid which is maintained at a constant pressure. Fluid is produced in the ciliary apparatus and flows through the pupil into the anterior chamber from where it drains out at the angle between the iris and the cornea.

PATHOPHYSIOLOGY

Cause

Pathology may affect any structure within the eye.

Signs

Many eye diseases present with a red and painful eye. Signs of pain include blepharospasm, photophobia, fear of being touched around the head (which may manifest as aggressive behaviour in some animals), depression and anorexia. Ocular discharges are common and these may be clear initially but may become purulent if infected. Vision deficits can be hard to detect in small animals unless they are very severe as animals often learn to find their way around familiar environments using their sense of smell. The first indication of vision loss may be a reluctance to explore new environments and lack of confidence when going out at night. Total blindness is not a common presentation.

Diagnostic tests

Ophthalmoscopy

An ophthalmoscope is used for examining the internal structures of the eye. The scope allows the examiner to focus on the retina or the lens within the eye. Examination should be performed in a darkened room so that the patient's pupils are maximally dilated and it may be necessary to give a few drops of a drug (mydriatic) into the eye to keep the pupil dilated. Most animals tolerate examination well but if the eye is very painful then local anaesthetic drops may also be needed. Since the examination requires the examiner to put the face close to the patient's head potentially aggressive dogs should be muzzled to prevent injury.

Fluorescein staining

This test is used for the detection and monitoring of corneal ulcers. The cornea is normally covered by a protective layer of epithelium. This layer is impervious to fluorescein dye. If the epithelium is perforated (ulcerated), the stroma is exposed and fluorescein will stick to the surface of the eye causing a patch of green staining.

Fluorescein drops can also be put in the eye to test the patency of the nasolacrimal duct. In the normal eye the tears drain through the nasolacrimal duct into the nose. Detection of the green fluorescein dye at the nostrils means that drainage is occurring. If the duct is obstructed tears will overflow on to the face and dye will not be detected at the nostril.

Schirmer tear test

This test measures the volume of tear production in the eye. Small absorbent test strips are placed just beneath the eyelid and left in place for a minute. The liquid tear film soaks up the strip and the distance it has travelled up the strip in a minute gives an indication of how well tears are being produced. The normal result in dogs is around 14 mm in 1 minute (less than 10 mm wetting is abnormal). In dry eyes the strip may remain completely dry.

Tonometry

This is the method of measuring the pressure within the eye. In some eye conditions, e.g. glaucoma, pressure increases and this can be detected with tonometry before permanent damage is done to the eye. Local anaesthetic is applied to the eye and the tonometer tip is placed on the cornea. This applies pressure and measures how much the cornea indents. The scale on the instrument converts the result to measurement of intraocular pressure in mmHg.

Treatment

Nursing care and hygiene are vitally important when dealing with eye disease. Ocular discharges should be cleaned from the eye as often as possible. Some eye conditions are extremely painful. This can result in blepharospasm or behavioural changes (aggression, timidity or depression). Analgesia can be provided in the form of NSAIDs or opioids – but treatment of the underlying cause is always the most effective method of pain control.

Protection of the eye

The eye is an extremely delicate structure and it is important that further damage is not caused by the patient rubbing at a sore eye. The use of an Elizabethan collar can be helpful in some cases but patients with particularly sore eyes, i.e. glaucoma, may become distressed by the presence of something at the edge of their field of vision.

Temporary protection can be achieved by sewing conjunctiva or eyelids across the corneal surface but this makes monitoring difficult as the lesion cannot be visualised. Alternatively contact lenses are available and these form a clear protective barrier.

Application of eye treatment

- It is hard to restrain a patient and to administer medication to the eye so ask someone to hold the patient for you.
- Shake suspension or warm ointment before use.
- Hold the patient with its nose tilted upwards.
- Approach the eye from the side and hold the bottle or tube a few centimetres above the eye surface.
- Allow one drop of solution or a strip of ointment to fall on to the surface of the cornea.
- Do not touch the eye with the applicator.
- Allow the animal to blink to spread the treatment evenly over the eye surface.

SPECIFIC DISEASES (Figs 3.4 and 3.5)

Glaucoma

Cause: increase in pressure within the globe itself; may be idiopathic or due to something blocking fluid drainage, e.g. tumour, dislocated lens.

Signs: painful red eye; there may be corneal oedema and clouding of the eye. If the condition is untreated the globe swells, the pupil dilates and retinal damage results in blindness.

Diagnosis: signs, demonstration of increased pressure within the eye using tonometry.

Treatment: analgesia, reduction of fluid production within the eye (carbonic anhydrase

CORNEAL OEDEMA

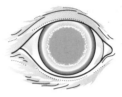

Glaucoma
If caused by glaucoma there may be vessel engorgement and visual disturbance

LIPID DEPOSITION

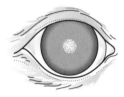

Lipid dystrophy
Central crystalline deposition

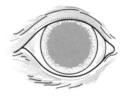

Arcus lipoides cornea – at the limbus
Associated with hypothyroid or lipid metabolic abnormality

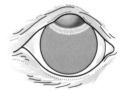

Lipid keratopathy
Associated with corneal vascularisation or limbal mass

Figure 3.4 The white eye. (From *Veterinary Ocular Emergencies* by Williams (2002). Reprinted by permission of Elsevier Science Ltd.)

inhibitors) and miotics. Treat underlying cause if possible.

Conjunctivitis

Cause: inflammation of the conjunctiva for any reason, e.g. infection (bacterial, chlamydia in cats or viral), allergy, neoplasia, trauma.

Signs: redness in mucous membrane surrounding eye, increased vascularisation, ocular discharge.

Diagnosis: signs.

Treatment: manage underlying cause. Ointments or creams containing antibiotic (to treat

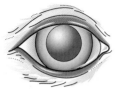

Conjuctivitis
Redness of lid and globe
Conjunctiva
Diffuse redness

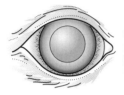

Uveitis
Intense redness increasing
near limbus
Little or no lid redness

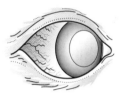

Classic acute glaucoma
Individual engorged vessels
– little redness in between
here with lens luxation

Figure 3.5 Form and appearance of redness.
(From *Veterinary Ocular Emergencies* by Williams (2002).
Reprinted by permission of Elsevier Science Ltd.)

secondary infection) and glucocorticoids (to reduce inflammation).

Corneal ulcer

Cause: damage to corneal surface usually as a result of a scratch; may be related to viral disease, e.g. herpes infection in cats.

Signs: painful eye with ocular discharge and increased blepharospasm.

Diagnosis: visual inspection of cornea, fluorescein drops.

Treatment: mild cases may resolve spontaneously if there is no secondary infection. Treat every few hours with topical antibiotic solution. More severe cases may need soft contact lenses or third eyelid flap to protect eye whilst healing.

Retinal disease

Cause: infection or inflammatory, hereditary degenerative conditions, e.g. progressive retinal atrophy, traumatic (retinal detachment), taurine deficiency in cats.

Signs: blindness or reduced vision.

Diagnosis: inspection of retina with ophthalmoscope.

Treatment: may be able to stop progression of disease in some cases but unlikely to reverse changes already present.

Uveitis

Cause: inflammation of the iris due to trauma or viral infections, neoplasia. May be associated with infectious canine hepatitis in dogs and feline infectious peritonitis (FIP) in cats.

Signs: painful red eye, photophobia, pupil contracted, colour change in iris.

Diagnosis: examination of the eye.

Treatment: steroids and mydriatics.

Keratoconjunctivitis sicca (dry eye)

Cause: insufficient tear production can be caused by damage to tear production as a result of inflammation, immune-mediated disease or drugs.

Signs: sticky purulent discharge on surface of eye, corneal ulceration.

Diagnosis: insufficient tear production measured on Schirmer tear test.

Treatment: replacement of tears with synthetic tears, ciclosporin drops if immune-mediated damage, management of underlying cause.

Cataract

Cause: most cataracts in dogs are inherited. Other causes are damage or degenerative changes to the lens which allow water to enter lens capsule.

Signs: opacity seen in eye, poor night vision progressing to blindness.

Diagnosis: visual inspection of the eye is important – taking care to differentiate cataract from clouding of other areas of the eye and senile sclerosis (a normal ageing change which causes blueness of the lens).

Treatment: no specific treatment – cataracterous lenses can be removed if vision is severely impaired.

Pannus

Cause: common condition in some dog breeds, e.g. GSD. The cornea becomes invaded by pigment and vascular tissue.

Signs: thickening and clouding of cornea, often with serous discharge but no pain.

Diagnosis: clinical examination is usually distinctive, but other conditions, e.g. corneal ulcer, should be ruled out.

Treatment: corticosteroids topically or injected under conjunctiva, or ciclosporin drops. Treatment must be continued lifelong.

DRUGS COMMONLY USED IN THE MANAGEMENT OF EYE CONDITIONS

Carbonic anhydrase inhibitors

These reduce the production of aqueous humour and hence reduce pressure in the eye. Dorzolamide can be used for the reduction of intraocular pressure in glaucoma but must be given at least three times daily.

Mydriatics

These are used for dilation of the pupil. Prolonged dilation may be needed to relieve the spasm associated with iritis/uveitis and in this case atropine may be used. Atropine may cause severe salivation in cats. Examination of the retina can be facilitated by the administration of a short-acting drug such as tropicamide.

Miotics

Used topically to penetrate the cornea and cause pupil contraction. Pilocarpine is used in veterinary medicine for the treatment of glaucoma.

Local anaesthetics

Topical local anaesthetics for use in the eye include tetracaine (amethocaine) and proxymetacaine. These reduce discomfort associated with eye conditions to allow a complete ocular examination (e.g. looking under the third eyelid for a grass seed). Tetracaine (amethocaine) provides quite strong anaesthesia and can be used for minor, superficial surgical procedures to the eye.

Artificial tears

Artificial tear solutions must be applied regularly (at least hourly) for aqueous drops or six times daily for gel solution. Ointment lubricants can be applied last thing at night.

Antibiotics

Often broad-spectrum drugs are used without culture and sensitivity testing. Usually given topically for eye disease. Doxycycline can be effective in treatment of *Chlamydia* infection in cats if given orally.

Corticosteroids

Often used for their anti-inflammatory effects but must never be used in an infected eye. If infection is present this should be treated appropriately before steroid application. There is little indication for the use of combined corticosteroid and antibiotic treatments. Specific indications for the immunosuppressive effects of steroids are in immune-mediated disease such as pannus.

Fluorescein

This is a dye used to reveal corneal lesions and to check patency of tear drainage. It comes as impregnated sterile strips for placing in the eye or as single use dropper bottles. Once these bottles have been opened unused contents should be discarded because of the risk of contamination and cross infection.

Ciclosporin

Most commonly used in the treatment of keratoconjunctivitis sicca. Topical application stimulates tear production and its immune-suppression effect reduces the damage to tear producing apparatus in immune-mediated eye conditions.

Formulations

Drops

Aqueous drops are rapidly removed from the eye and must be applied frequently for continuous therapy. Viscous formulations persist for longer. Drops are often easier to administer than ointments.

Ointments

Oily formulations persist in the eye and this means that administration can be less frequent. Most treatments need to be applied 4–6 times daily.

THE SKIN (Table 3.11)

ANATOMY AND PHYSIOLOGY

The skin covers the body surface to protect against invasion by micro-organisms and damage from ultraviolet radiation. It has many sensory receptors and provides early warning of potential damage for the body tissues. Other important functions are in the regulation of body temperature and vitamin D synthesis. The skin has three important layers:

- Epidermis (surface layer) – hair follicles, sebaceous and sweat glands (but no blood supply). Specialised sebaceous glands are found in certain areas of the skin:
  — tail gland – sebaceous glands concentrated on the dorsal surface of the tail base which tend to produce more secretions in older animals which may result in matted, greasy hair.
  — circum-anal glands – scent glands located around the anus in male dogs.
  — anal sac glands – found in the lining of the anal sacs, they secrete a foul smelling scent used for marking faeces.

Table 3.11	Important questions to ask the owner of an animal with skin disease
Question	Reason for question and interpretation of answer
Has the animal had similar signs previously? If so, what time of year did signs occur? Did the signs respond to treatment?	Some skin conditions are seasonal, e.g. atopy. Previous response to treatment may give a clue to the cause of the problem but remember that many conditions will wax and wane irrespective of treatment and this may be mistaken for response to treatment. Also treatment may help to reduce secondary changes without treating the underlying cause, i.e. response to antibiotics in pyoderma secondary to hypothyroidism
Is the animal scratching or grooming more than usual?	Some types of skin disease are classically not pruritic, e.g. endocrine alopecia, however secondary infection is common in all types of skin disease and this infection can result in pruritus
Is there any hair loss?	Hair may be lost during the normal shedding process and then not regrow – this is the case with many endocrine diseases. In pruritic conditions the act of scratching or grooming may cause hair loss or damage
How old was the animal when signs were first noticed?	Pruritic skin disease in animals less than 6 months old is far more likely to be due to parasitic conditions (or possibly food allergy) than in older animals where atopy would be a more common diagnosis. Most of the endocrine conditions causing non-pruritic alopecia, e.g. Cushing's and hypothyroidism, occur in older animals and non-pruritic signs in a younger animal may be due to fungal infection or demodex
Is the patient well in itself?	Skin disease may be a presentation of underlying systemic disease, e.g. hepatocutaneous syndrome or an endocrine disease. Most animals with primary skin disease are bright and well otherwise, the exception being severe generalised disease and deep infections
Do any in-contact pets have similar signs?	If in-contact pets have similar signs an infectious cause (usually parasitic) is more likely
Does the owner have any lesions?	Some of the infectious causes of skin disease, e.g. ringworm and parasites such as cheyletiella, can be zoonotic

- Dermis – nerve supply for sensation.
- Hypodermis – fat, muscle, blood supply and connective tissue.

The foot pads in the dog and cat have thickened epidermis and dermis and lack hair but they do contain sweat glands.

PATHOPHYSIOLOGY

Dermatological cases account for about one in every five cases seen in small animal practice.

Cause

There are many types of pathology that can cause skin disease (see Box 3.8).

Signs

The skin has a limited range of responses to disease. Many skin diseases are pruritic (or result in secondary bacterial infection which is pruritic) and, as a result of scratching, the skin may be further damaged. In chronic cases it can be very difficult to differentiate the forms of skin disease because ultimately all skin diseases start to look the same.

The skin is a very unusual organ in that the whole of it is on display and can be examined. Remember that a full clinical examination should be performed in all cases with skin disease to rule out an underlying medical cause for the problem.

Simple visual inspection of animals with skin disease can be very useful. It is helpful to draw a diagram marking out the location of lesions – this can be particularly useful for monitoring response to therapy. Try to pinpoint which areas of the skin are most affected – and establish whether the lesions affect most of the body or are confined to specific areas. Ideally a bright light and a magnifying glass should be used to examine the skin. Many of the larger parasites, e.g. lice, fleas, cheyletiella, will be seen using this method. Flea faeces may also be seen even if adult parasites are not present.

The haircoat should be examined and its quality assessed. See if the hairs pull out easily – if there are areas of hair loss the hairs around the edge should be examined to see if they are broken (if so the animal may be causing hair loss by biting at itself).

Diagnostic tests

Brushing the debris from skin on to a moistened piece of white paper (wet paper test) is a rapid patient-side test for the recent presence of fleas. Flea faeces, which is essentially dried blood, will dissolve and form red streaks on the paper.

Hair pluckings can be examined under the microscope. It is possible to see louse eggs attached to the hairshaft and fungal spores (in ringworm infections). Damage to the hairshaft caused by biting and scratching may be more obvious under the microscope.

Adhesive tape

Adhesive tape samples are taken by applying a piece of adhesive tape to a clipped area of skin

---

Box 3.8   Causes of skin disease

Parasitic skin disease	Miscellaneous	Immune mediated skin disease
Fleas	Neoplasia	Atopy (inhaled allergen)
Lice	Lymphosarcoma	Contact allergy
Mites	Mast cell tumour	Dietary allergy
Demodex	Fungal: ringworm	Autoimmune skin disease, e.g. pemphigus
Sarcoptes	Yeast: *Malassezia*	Drug reaction
Cheyletiella	Hormonal skin disease	
Harvest mites	Hyperadrenocorticism	
	Hypothyroidism	
	Oestrogen imbalance	

and then removing it. This is stained using Diff Quick and stuck on to a microscope slide for examination.

Skin scrapings

Skin scrapes are easily collected and are vital to detect parasitic skin disease caused by mites. The skin area to be scraped is clipped and moistened with oil. A scalpel blade is then placed at right angles to the skin surface and gently scraped over the surface abrading the skin. Scrapings should be continued deep enough to cause capillary bleeding. This increases the chance of detecting parasites of the deeper layers, e.g. demodex. Multiple skin scrapings should always be taken and these should be collected from the edge of active lesions. Samples are placed on microscope slides and spread for examination.

Bacterial culture

Secondary bacterial infections are common in all forms of skin disease and bacteriological testing allows selection of appropriate antibiotic therapy. Swabs should be taken from any active lesions for culture and sensitivity examination. If pustules are present these can be gently opened with a needle and the purulent contents squeezed on to a sterile swab for culture. Samples should be plated on to culture plates immediately or placed in transport media for transport to laboratory.

Fungal examination

Some cases of *Microsporum canis* ringworm will glow green (fluoresce) when examined under a UV lamp. Remember that not all cases of ringworm will fluoresce and so a negative result on this test does not rule out a diagnosis of ringworm. This technique can be used to identify affected hairs so that they can be collected for fungal culture. Fungal culture can also be performed on samples from skin biopsy (for deep fungal infection), nail samples, and skin brushings. Fungi are slow growing, so culture can take up to 3 weeks.

Biopsy

In many cases skin biopsy for histological examination is necessary for definitive diagnosis. Selection of the biopsy site is very important. If there are multiple lesions samples should be collected from several sites. Samples should be taken from the edge of an active lesion. Punch biopsies can often be obtained under sedation and local anaesthetic, although general anaesthesia is required to obtain good samples from the face or feet. Once the biopsy has been collected it should be pinned to a piece of cardboard (to prevent skin curling) before placing in a bottle of fixative.

Dietary considerations

Dietary exclusion trials are often used to rule out a diagnosis of food allergy in patients with suspected allergic skin disease. Dietary exclusion trials are a waste of time unless they are performed with care. A novel protein and carbohydrate source should be selected (based on discussion with the owner). The old standard diet of chicken and rice is a poor choice as so many pets have been exposed to these food sources in normal life. Try to select a diet that the patient has never experienced (venison, ostrich), is likely to eat and the owner can afford, prepare and obtain over a prolonged period. The novel diet must be fed, to the exclusion of everything else with water only to drink, for a period of around 6 weeks (although response time is variable and may be between 3 and 12 weeks). It is preferable not to use other supplements for the diagnostic period but, if the patient is likely to remain on the diet for a long period, vitamin supplements may be needed. Specially prepared prescription diets are available but are not ideal for making the diagnosis of food allergy. They can be very useful for long term feeding of food allergic pets after a diagnosis has been made.

The novel diet is usually begun at the same time as other diagnostic and therapeutic strategies. Food-allergic dogs should start to improve within a few weeks of the dietary change (although some may take up to 12 weeks to respond). Pruritus should decrease and no new skin lesions develop. However, there are other reasons why animals may improve whilst on the diet:

- Some pruritic skin conditions are seasonal and wax and wane naturally.
- Concurrent treatment to resolve bacterial infections may reduce the level of pruritus.

In order to confirm the diagnosis the patient should be put back on its normal diet at the end of the exclusion diet trial to confirm that the pruritus recurs. However, it can be quite difficult to convince the owner of the need for this challenge test in a patient that seems to be cured.

Other tests

Further investigations may be appropriate at this point depending on the suspected diagnosis. Intradermal skin testing may be helpful in the identification of allergic skin disease but should only be performed by a specialist who performs the test on a regular basis. There are some tests which can be performed on blood samples (enzyme-linked immunosorbent assay (ELISA) test) to indicate potential causes of atopy. False-positive reactions are common with this test, but a negative result makes a diagnosis of atopy less likely.

Treatment

Treatment of secondary bacterial infection is important. If self-trauma has been a problem then further damage should be prevented by the use of Elizabethan collars or foot bandaging to prevent skin damage caused by a hind leg brought up to scratch.

SPECIFIC DISEASES

Pyoderma

Cause

Bacterial infection can be classified according to the layers of the skin affected: surface, superficial or deep (see Box 3.9). Bacteria involved in skin infection can be normal inhabitants of the skin (**commensals**), transient inhabitants not normally

Box 3.9	Classification of bacterial infections	
Surface	**Superficial**	**Deep**
Pyotraumatic dermatitis (hot spots, wet eczema) Skin fold pyoderma (lip, muzzle, tail)	Impetigo (puppy pyoderma)	Furunculosis Deep folliculitis Nasal pyoderma

able to grow on the skin, or pathogenic (able to invade normal skin and cause disease). Any condition which interrupts the skin barrier, e.g. inflammation or self-trauma due to pruritus, permits the entry of surface bacteria and can result in the development of pyoderma. Pathogenic bacteria or reduced systemic immune response are more likely to lead to deep bacterial infection.

Signs

Bacterial skin disease often results in pustules or discharging sinuses. It can be very pruritic and self-trauma is common.

Diagnostic tests

Bacterial infections cause pustular skin lesions. They cause pruritus which commonly results in self-trauma. Deep infections may develop sinus tracts and discharging sinuses. Peripheral lymph node enlargement and systemic illness may also be seen.

Identification of underlying causes is the most important part of the diagnostic investigation. Identification of bacteria involved is usually relatively straightforward through skin swabbing and culture. Sensitivity testing can be invaluable, particularly in cases that have already failed to respond adequately to treatment, to aid in the selection of appropriate antibiotic therapy. It is important to establish the extent of the infection, i.e. superficial or deep, in order to provide the correct treatment.

Treatment

Systemic antibiotics are required to treat deep or generalised infection. Antibacterial shampoos or topical application of creams or ointments may be sufficient for the management of surface and superficial infections. Glucocorticoids should not be used in the management of deep pyoderma.

Demodex

Cause: *Demodex canis* (dogs) or *Demodex cati* (cats). Small cigar-shaped mites found in normal skin but causing no problems. In adults demodex infection is usually the result of immuno-suppression, e.g. diabetes mellitus or FIV in cats.

Signs: localised cases in young animals have non-pruritic alopecia. In cats adult disease may cause localised hair loss and scaling. In dogs severe cases may have generalised bacterial skin infection and systemic illness.

Diagnosis: skin scraping and identification of mites.

Treatment: in dogs amitraz baths or systemic treatment with ivermectin or milbemycin can be effective in refractory cases. There are no licensed products for use in cats.

Sarcoptes

Cause: *Sarcoptes scabiei, Notoedres cati.* These are obligate parasites that can only live on the host and infections are often caught from foxes.

Signs: pruritic skin disease particularly of ear margins, elbows and paws. Severe cases can make the animal systemically unwell.

Diagnosis: skin scrapes – may require multiple scrapes for identification of mites.

Treatment: in dogs weekly topical treatment with aludex, amitraz or Vet-Kem sponge-on. Selamectin or ivermectin 200 µg/kg s.c. repeated after 2 weeks may be useful in cats. All in-contact animals should be treated.

Cheyletiella

Cause: *Cheyletiella yasguri.*

Signs: pruritic skin disease with dandruff, disease in in-contact pets and humans. Infection may be asymptomatic.

Diagnosis: visual identification of mites on skin, on adhesive tape or in skin scrapings.

Treatment: sensitive to many parasiticides, e.g. ivermectin injections and selenium shampoos twice weekly, but need to treat all animals in household and the environment.

Lice

Cause: there are two types of lice found on dogs – biting (*Trichodectes canis*) and sucking (*Linognathus setosus*). The cat only has one type of louse, *Felicola subrostratus.*

Signs: pruritic skin disease and small itchy bites in pets, contact animals and humans.

Diagnosis: visual identification of lice in coat or on adhesive tape samples, or eggs seen attached to hair shafts.

Treatment: easily killed by any parasiticide active against fleas. Brushes and combs should also be treated to prevent spread.

Fleas

Cause: *Ctenocephalides canis* and *Ct. felis*. Signs are usually the result of an allergic reaction to flea saliva.

Signs: pruritic skin disease and hair loss, particularly over tail base. Allergic animals may have generalised pruritic disease whilst in-contact animals may be unaffected.

Diagnosis: visual identification of fleas or flea dirt found in coat.

Treatment: antiparasitic sprays, shampoos, spot-ons or internal treatment.

Harvest mites

Cause: *Neotrombicula autumnalis* (small orange spider-like mites). These are free-living mites with only the larval form being parasitic.

Signs: irritation usually confined to feet and legs, particularly in autumn.

Diagnosis: visualisation of mites between toes, on legs, head and ears.

Treatment: fipronil sprays or manual removal.

Ringworm

Cause: fungal infection of skin and hair – *Microsporum canis, Trichophyton mentagrophytes.*

Signs: may be no lesions or a range of alopecia and pruritus. Human contacts may be affected.

Diagnosis: examination of coat in UV light (Woods lamp), identification of spores on hair-shaft, fungal culture.

Treatment: oral antifungal treatment (griseofulvin), clipping and removal of infected hair.

Atopy

Cause: allergy to inhaled allergens (pollens, dust, fleas).

Signs: pruritic skin disease, initially seasonal but often develops to be present all year round. Typically first seen in animals around 1–2 years and gets progressively more severe with age.

Diagnosis: seasonal nature of disease, ELISA test, intradermal skin test.

Treatment: avoidance of allergen if possible, desensitising vaccination, reduction of pruritus with antihistamines, essential fatty acids and shampoo therapy, suppression of immune response with glucocorticoids.

Malassezia

Cause: an opportunist yeast *Malassezia pachydermatitis.*

Signs: severe pruritus of face, feet, skin folds.

Diagnosis: identification of yeast in adhesive tape samples.

Treatment: twice weekly topical treatment with selenium, enilconazole or chlorhexidine, oral antifungal drugs if very severe or shampooing ineffective.

Ear mites

Cause: infection with *Otodectes cyanotis* which may be transmitted from cat to dog.

Signs: otitis externa, head shaking, scratching, black waxy discharge from ears.

Diagnosis: identification of mites under microscopic examination of smear of ear discharge.

Treatment: many ear drops are effective (even those not containing a parasiticide); may be difficult to treat cats effectively and selamectin spot-on may be useful. All in-contact pets should be treated (even those that are asymptomatic).

DRUGS COMMONLY USED IN THE MANAGEMENT OF SKIN DISEASE

Antibiotics

Antibiotic selection should be based on culture and sensitivity results. Drugs which are able to penetrate the skin should be given and these must be given at a sufficient dose rate. To prevent antibiotic resistance developing treatment should be continued for a minimum of 2–3 weeks and for at least a week after all lesions have resolved. In cases of deep pyoderma treatment may last for 6 months or more.

Glucocorticoids

These are often misused in practice for the management of pruritic skin disease. Glucocorticoids should only be used when a diagnosis has been made *and* an indication for their use has been demonstrated. In allergic skin disease glucocorticoids may be required to control pruritus but should be used at the minimum effective dose and preferably no more frequently than every other day.

Antihistamines

In allergic disease mast cells release histamine which causes inflammation and irritation. These agents act by stabilising mast cells in the skin so that histamine is not released. The drugs are used to control pruritus and may be used alone or in combination with glucocorticoids.

Essential fatty acids (evening primrose oil)

These drugs have anti-inflammatory effects in some patients with pruritic skin disease. They can be used at the same time as glucocorticoids to reduce the steroid dose required.

Antifungal agents

The most commonly used drugs are griseofulvin tablets (for ringworm), ketoconazole tablets or enilconazole which can be applied topically.

Parasiticides

These may be applied externally (as washes or sprays) or administered systemically (as tablets or injections). It is important to identify the parasite accurately in order to prescribe the correct treatment and administration regime.

Formulations

Shampoos

Bathing is a very useful management strategy in almost all forms of skin disease. Bathing removes grease and dead skin layers and special shampoos can be used to manage skin conditions. Regular shampooing may start with a frequency of 2–3 times a week and gradually reduce as necessary. Frequent shampooing may cause drying of the skin and application of a humectant or moisturiser may help to counteract this.

Ointments

These are greasy preparations and are not usually used in pets.

Lotions

These are liquid preparations with the active ingredient dissolved or held in suspension. This formulation is useful to distribute a drug over a large area.

Creams

Creams can be made with a water-soluble or oily base. They are easier to apply than ointments.

THE EAR (Table 3.12)

ANATOMY AND PHYSIOLOGY

The ear is divided into:

- external ear canal
- middle ear
- inner ear.

Table 3.12	Important questions to ask the owner of a dog with ear disease
Question	Reason for question and interpretation of answer
How long has the problem been present?	Chronic ear disease is often associated with a conformational problem, e.g. narrowing of the ear canal or the presence of a primary untreated condition, e.g. neoplasia or allergic skin disease
Did head shaking come on acutely?	Acute head shaking and distress may suggest that a foreign body is present in the ear
Is the pinna involved?	Involvement of the pinna as well as the ear canal suggests the ear disease may be an extension of a skin problem
Has the animal previously had bouts of ear disease? If so are problems associated with a particular time of year?	Repeated bouts of ear disease, particularly if affecting the same ear each time, may indicate a problem with that ear, e.g. mass or polyp. Repeated bilateral problems may be associated with conformational or allergic disease. Food allergies are likely to be present all year round whereas problems associated with atopy may initially be most severe in the summer
Is the disease affecting one or both ears?	Problems affecting both ears are more likely to be due to generalised skin disease, e.g. atopy
Is the animal systemically unwell?	Severe bacterial infections may penetrate skin and cause systemic illness. Neoplasia or severe infection may invade inner ear and tympanic bulla causing neurological signs
Are any in-contact animals affected?	Parasitic ear disease, e.g. ear mites, can cause disease in in-contact animals. In this kind of disease treatment of all in-contact animals is important. Cats may be asymptomatic carriers and repeatedly infect dogs in the household

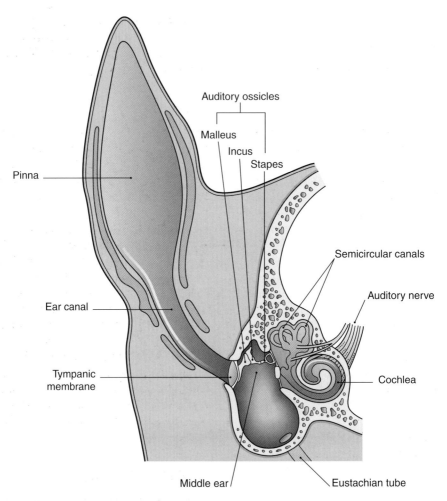

Figure 3.6 Schematic section through the left ear. (Reproduced with permission from Cunningham 1992.)

The external ear is the pinna and the ear canal. The ear canal has a vertical component which makes a right-angled turn into the horizontal canal. The ear canal is lined with modified skin. In most animals it is relatively hairless. The skin within the ear has a large number of sebaceous glands which secrete ear wax. The horizontal canal runs to the tympanic membrane (ear drum) which separates the external and middle ear. The middle ear is located within the tympanic bulla and comprises the three ossicles – its primary function is hearing. A branch of the facial nerve and the sympathetic nerve supply to the head run through the bulla and may be damaged by inflammation in the middle ear resulting in facial paralysis or Horner's syndrome, respectively. The inner ear is connected to the pharynx via the eustachian tube. The inner ear comprises the three semicircular canals (concerned with balance) and the cochlea (part of the auditory system). There are two nerves supplying the inner ear (the vestibulo-cochlear and the auditory nerve) (Fig. 3.6).

PATHOPHYSIOLOGY
Otitis externa

Once the natural flora within the ear canal are disturbed ear disease is likely to progress.

Cause

Underlying causes include:

- allergic skin disease (with breakdown of protective barrier)
- trauma due to foreign body in ear canal, e.g. grass awn
- poor air circulation in canal due to narrowed ear canal, hair within ear canal or floppy ear pinnae
- masses or tumour within the ear canal, e.g. nasopharyngeal polyps in cats
- primary infection with pathogenic bacteria or fungi
- parasites, e.g. ear mites *(Otodectes cyanotis).*

Signs

Irritation of the ear canal can be extremely distressing. Head shaking and ear scratching are commonly reported and there may be pain associated with the ear canal. Whatever the cause of the ear disease secondary infection is common and many of these infections produce a foul-smelling discharge. Acute cases may have reddening of the ear canal and excessive production of waxy secretions. As ear disease becomes chronic the ear canal lining becomes thickened and the canal narrows. Coloured discharges are common.

Diagnostic tests

Clinical examination is usually sufficient to provide the diagnosis. Full examination of the ear requires otoscopic examination of the tympanic membrane and horizontal canal. In most animals with severe ear diseases the canal is too painful to allow a detailed examination without sedation/analgesia or general anaesthetic. Further investigation is aimed at identifying the underlying cause. Examination of stained smears of material taken from the ear canal is often very useful. Bacteria can be seen and may be classified as rods or cocci which can give a clue as to their type and hence appropriate antibiotic therapy. Ear swabs should also be taken for culture and sensitivity examination. Yeast infections *(Malassezia)* are also

common and there is argument as to whether these are primary pathogens or whether their presence in large amounts indicates that other pathology is present.

Treatment

In all cases of ear disease the underlying cause should be addressed if possible. Otitis externa is frequently an extension of generalised skin disease into the ear canal and local treatment of the ear canal alone will not resolve the problem in the long term.

Most ear diseases require topical therapy at some stage. Ear drops are commonly prescribed but treatment is rarely performed well. Always demonstrate to owners the correct way to apply medication to ensure effective treatment is given from the start. In order for the drops to be effective they must come into contact with the ear canal lining. This will not happen if there is a lot of waxy debris or old ear drops within the canal. Before each application of drops the canal should be cleansed with ear cleaning solution to flush out all old debris. The canal is then dried to remove cleaning solution before application of drops.

Application of ear drops

- Ear disease can be very painful so it is important to restrain the patient well to avoid injury – difficult dogs may need to be muzzled.
- It is extremely difficult for one person to hold the animal *and* apply drops, so ask someone else to hold the animal.
- Clean the ear canal using a wax-dissolving solution, taking particular care to remove any old medication.
- Make sure you do not poke anything into the ear canal; try to flood the canal with fluid to float debris out.
- Dry canal thoroughly.
- Sit the animal in a comfortable position against a wall so that it cannot move away from you and preferably with its back in a corner so that it cannot move backwards.

- Lift the ear pinna (if necessary) and tilt the head so that the ear into which you will apply drops is uppermost.
- Holding the dropper above the opening of the ear canal, add the required number of drops.
- Do not touch the applicator on to the surface of the ear (if you do, clean it thoroughly afterwards to avoid carrying infection to the other ear).
- Allow the drops to run into the ear canal whilst keeping the animal restrained.
- Gentle massage of the vertical canal below the pinna will help distribution of drops.
- Keep the animal's head restrained so that it cannot shake and eliminate all the drops.
- Repeat with the other ear if necessary.

Remember that the active ingredients in ear drops are rapidly absorbed through the ear lining into the body and this can cause problems in some patients. Long-term administration of steroid ear drops can cause signs of Cushing's disease or result in a diabetic patient requiring increased insulin dose.

The administration of oral medications, e.g. antibiotics or anti-inflammatory agents, may also be required.

Many cases of ear disease require surgical intervention. This may be to remove an underlying cause, e.g. polyp, but in most cases it is to alter the anatomical conformation of the ear canal. Techniques such as lateral wall resection and vertical canal ablation are used to improve air circulation to the ear and provide better exposure of tissue for topical treatment. Total ear canal ablation (TECA) removes all external ear canal tissue and allows access to the tympanic bullae.

Prevention of trauma

Self-trauma is a prime perpetuating factor in ear disease. Head shaking is almost impossible to prevent but the use of appropriate anti-inflammatory drugs and analgesics may reduce this (many ear drops contain these agents). The use of an Elizabethan collar and bandaging of the hind paw can help to reduce the trauma induced by scratching the ear with a hind foot. Following surgery the ear is often bandaged to protect the surgical site and prevent interference with sutures – whilst this does provide protection the bandage should be removed as soon as practical since good air circulation will promote healing.

Head shaking may cause trauma to the ear pinna resulting in blood vessel rupture and haemorrhage within the cartilage layers. This forms a haematoma within the pinna. The haematoma can become an irritating focus and drainage is required in most cases.

Otitis media

Cause: usually an extension of chronic otitis externa into the middle ear. Occasionally infection may enter up the Eustachian canal.

Signs: typically vestibular disease with head tilt and ataxia. May be head shaking and signs of pain depending on cause.

Diagnosis: signs and radiography of bullae.

Treatment: systemic antibiotics and treatment of underlying cause. Severe cases may require drainage of the bulla (**bulla osteotomy**).

Otitis interna

Cause: tumour, inflammation or infection in tympanic bullae, can be an extension of otitis externa and media.

Signs: head tilt and balance disturbance, Horner's syndrome and facial nerve paralysis may be present due to damage to the nerves running through the bullae.

Diagnosis: otoscopic examination. Radiography of tympanic bullae may show bony changes or fluid within bullae. Magnetic resonance imaging (MRI) and computed tomographic (CT) scans may provide more detailed information.

Treatment: broad-spectrum antibiotics and surgical opening and bulla osteotomy may be necessary.

Deafness

Cause: disease of the detection apparatus in the ear (organ of Corti) or the auditory conduction system. Often a hereditary condition associated with white coat colour. Deafness can develop later in life and may be associated with degenerative changes due to chronic ear infection or the use of ototoxic drugs. Occasionally animals will be deaf because of wax and debris plugging the ear canal.

Signs: deafness in one ear can be very difficult to detect without using specialised tests. The presence of total deafness is much easier to detect due to lack of response to sound.

Diagnosis: specialist equipment to measure the electrical signals caused by detection of sound in the ear (brain stem auditory evoked potentials).

Treatment: no treatment for congenital disease and by the time of diagnosis most acquired disorders are irreversible. Removal of wax plugs may improve hearing.

DRUGS COMMONLY USED IN THE TREATMENT OF EAR DISEASE

There are many different formulations for the topical treatment of ear disease. Solutions or lotions are preferred for exudative conditions, oily formulations or ointments for dry conditions. Many preparations contain solvents, e.g. propylene glycol to dissolve wax.

Miticides

Permethrin and other miticides are available in ear drops. Some ear drops which have proven effect against ear mites actually do not contain any agent which is known to kill mites.

Antibiotics

Ideally the choice of antibiotic should be based on culture and sensitivity examination but this is rarely done as a first-line investigation of ear infection in general practice. However, smears of ear discharge can be stained and examined for the presence of rod or cocci bacteria which can help in selection of appropriate antibiotics.

Anti-inflammatory drugs

Glucocorticoids are used to reduce scarring. Systemic treatment may be needed in some cases.

Remember that steroids are absorbed through the skin and Cushingoid signs can develop with long term treatment. Other anti-inflammatory drugs include salicylic acid (which may be applied topically) or systemic NSAIDs.

Local anaesthetics

Ear disease is very painful and many preparations for treatment of infection contain local anaesthetics to control discomfort and reduce the risk of self-trauma.

ENDOCRINE SYSTEM

ENDOCRINE PANCREAS – ANATOMY AND PHYSIOLOGY

The pancreas is a V-shaped organ lying along the dorsal surface of the stomach and beside the duodenum. The **exocrine** cells of the pancreas produce digestive enzymes. The pancreas also produces **endocrine** secretions (hormones) that are released into the blood and affect the whole of the body.

Insulin is produced by the beta cells in areas of the pancreas called the **islets of Langerhans.** Insulin from all species looks very similar. Canine insulin is identical to porcine insulin and feline insulin is very similar to bovine insulin.

In the normal animal insulin is released when blood glucose is high. Insulin attaches to special receptors on muscle and fat cells and acts like a key in a lock – opening the door for glucose to enter the cells. Some tissues, e.g. the brain, do not require insulin in order to use glucose.

PATHOPHYSIOLOGY

Diabetic animals do not make enough insulin or their insulin does not work effectively and so glucose cannot get into cells. Glucose levels in the blood rise but the cells are starved of energy. Once blood glucose concentrations rise above a certain point more glucose passes through the kidney than can be recovered and glucose appears in the urine. This creates osmotic diuresis with excess water loss and the animal drinks more.

The cells have to find other sources of energy and switch from using glucose to burning fat. Metabolism of fat produces ketones and these build up in the blood. If blood levels get very high ketones may appear in the urine. High levels of ketones in the blood can be very dangerous.

SPECIFIC DISEASES

Diabetes mellitus (sugar diabetes)

There are two types of diabetes mellitus: insulin deficiency and relative insulin deficiency (insulin resistance).

Diabetic cats often have insulin resistance whereas dogs usually have true insulin deficiency, i.e. insulin-dependent diabetes mellitus (IDDM).

Cause

Diabetes mellitus is caused by a relative or absolute deficiency of insulin.

Signs

Diabetic dogs are often polydipsic and polyphagic and may be obese and losing weight. Cats with insulin resistance are typically normal weight or obese with a normal appetite and clinically well. Cats may become transiently diabetic at times of stress or concurrent illness, recovering for a time only to relapse later. There are often no significant findings but animals may have a big liver. Dogs may develop cataracts.

Diagnostic tests

In most dogs diagnosis is simple. Glucose in the urine *and* hyperglycaemia usually mean the dog is diabetic. Diagnosis in cats can be more tricky – hyperglycaemia is a common finding in sick cats. Stress (even as a result of struggling during blood sampling) may cause hyperglycaemia and occasionally this may cause glycosuria. Checking for glycosuria on urine samples collected from cats at home is one way of confirming that the glycosuria is real. Alternatively, a blood sample

to measure serum **fructosamine** can help as this tells us about the blood glucose concentrations during the previous few weeks.

Treatment

Often it is the veterinary nurse who plays a key role in the long-term management of diabetic patients.

The keys to successful management of a diabetic patient are:

- to treat any underlying diseases
- to treat any complications associated with diabetes mellitus
- to establish and maintain a normal bodyweight
- to provide a regulated lifestyle for the patient (food, exercise, insulin).

In most cases once a diabetic patient is stabilised there should be no need to change the routine unless circumstances change. Any changes to a routine should be continued for a minimum of 3 days to allow the patient to adjust before assessing the response. One of the common reasons for problems in stabilising diabetic patients is insulin doses being altered too frequently. All diabetic bitches should be spayed as soon as they are stabilised. This is because insulin requirements can change at different stages in the hormone cycle.

Dietary considerations

Diabetic diets must be consistent as insulin requirements are directly affected by food type and amount. Feeding a diet high in complex carbohydrates (starch) means that the liver takes longer to break down the food so glucose release is more controlled. Fresh water must always be available. Increased fibre content helps to control glycaemia. Calculate dietary requirements on the basis of the calorific requirements for the ideal weight of the patient. Obese, diabetic patients should be dieted by feeding two thirds of the dietary requirements for their ideal weight. Aim for a gradual return to normal body weight over several months.

Insulin

Most diabetic patients can be stabilised at home provided they are well and have a dedicated owner. Almost all diabetic dogs require insulin injections. A protocol for timing of insulin injection, feeding and monitoring should be explained to the owner. Owners are often initially very concerned about injecting their pets and need a lot of support. Traditionally animals have received daily insulin injections but often better control can be achieved by giving injections twice daily.

Some diabetic cats can be managed by a combination of dietary control and oral drugs which reduce blood glucose concentrations. The most commonly used of these is glipizide.

Monitoring

Urine glucose levels give an indication of how well blood glucose is controlled but it is not advisable for owners to alter insulin doses on the basis of urine glucose readings alone.

Complications

The most common problem in managing a diabetic is poor stabilisation. Often this is related to owner problems:

- improper handling or storage of insulin
- inadequate mixing of insulin prior to administration
- poor injection technique.

It is therefore important to question owners carefully and examine their injection technique if animals are difficult to stabilise. Blood samples taken at intervals throughout the day can be plotted to produce a **blood glucose curve.** From interpretation of the blood glucose curve it may be possible to understand why the animal is not well controlled.

Other stabilisation problems are as follows:

- Glucose concentrations never drop sufficiently low (Fig. 3.7). Increasing the dose of insulin should overcome this. If a patient requires more than 2.2 units insulin/kg to control blood

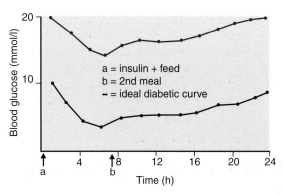

Figure 3.7   Inadequate insulin dose.

glucose it is likely that there is something working against insulin's effects. Increasing the dose of insulin further should eventually overcome the insulin resistance and control the diabetes (but it is important to find out what is causing the insulin antagonism).

- If blood glucose concentrations drop rapidly in response to insulin but rise again before the next insulin dose the insulin is not lasting as long as it should (Fig. 3.8). Switching to twice daily injections may resolve the problem, or use a longer-acting insulin preparation.

- If insulin doses are too high blood glucose concentrations may fall dangerously low (Fig. 3.9). This causes release of hormones which work against insulin. Blood glucose starts to rise but now the effects of insulin are beginning to wear off and blood glucose concentrations overshoot the acceptable level. Halving the dose of insulin should prevent the hypoglycaemia and then, if necessary, doses can be increased over time to control the diabetes.

- The major complication associated with treatment of diabetes mellitus is hypoglycaemia. You must be able to recognise this (confusion, ill at ease, hunger) and explain to owners how to deal with this crisis by feeding or providing sugar.

- Poorly controlled diabetic dogs may develop cataracts and other problems such as retinopathy and peripheral neuropathy. Complications associated with hyperglycaemia are less common in cats. Severe hyperglycaemia can progress to coma if untreated.

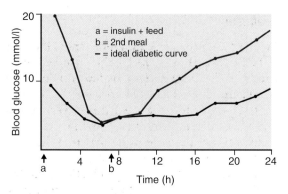

Figure 3.8 Inadequate duration of insulin action.

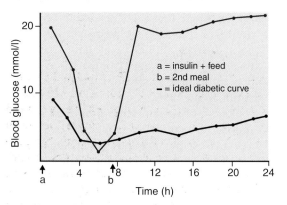

Figure 3.9 Overdose – Somogyi overswing.

Diabetic ketoacidosis

Cause

Insulin antagonism is commonly seen with conditions which increase hormones acting against insulin:

- infection (increases cortisol and glucagons)
- CHF (increases adrenaline (epinephrine) and glucagons)
- fever (increases cortisol, adrenaline (epinephrine) and growth hormone).

When an animal is starved it uses fat stores for fuel and this increases ketone production. It is very important not to withhold insulin if a diabetic patient fails to eat; if no insulin is given ketonaemia may develop rapidly. The recommendation is to administer 50% of the normal insulin dose to a diabetic patient who refuses food.

Dehydration is common in diabetic patients due to fluid loss in urine. As blood volume reduces there is less blood flow to the kidney making it harder for the patient to filter excess glucose or ketones.

Signs

Ketoacidotic patients are usually depressed/comatose, with a history of inappetence and vomiting (and often a past history of polydipsia and possible polyphagia).

Diagnostic tests

Laboratory tests show glucose and ketones in urine and often changes to blood electrolyte concentrations.

Treatment

This is a life-threatening condition requiring urgent attention and patients should be admitted for close monitoring.

Soluble insulin, either i.m. or i.v., in conjunction with intensive fluid therapy (physiological saline) is required. Blood glucose levels must be monitored regularly (ideally at least every hour).

Once a ketoacidotic patient has been stabilised, stopped vomiting and started eating, long-term management can be started as for any other diabetic patient.

Protocol for diabetic stabilisation

- Select starting dose of insulin which is usually 0.5–1.0 unit/kg (lower end of dose range for larger dogs).
- This is administered at a set time each day or divided into two equal doses and given at 12 hour intervals.
- In the initial stages the owner should bring the pet to the surgery for injection or the animal should be admitted to hospital.
- Select diet and calculate daily food requirement.
  — Once daily insulin: divide food intake, one third to be given with insulin and two thirds to be given 8 hours later.

— Twice daily insulin: divide food into two equal meals, one given with each insulin injection.
- Continue on this regime for 3 days monitoring urine glucose levels.
- After 3 days if results consistently show:
  — urine glucose more than 2% – increase insulin by 0.1 units/kg
  — urine glucose 0.1–1% – keep insulin dose the same
  — urine glucose negative – decrease insulin by 0.1 units/kg.
- Monitor urine glucose for a further 3 days before adjusting insulin dose unless complications arise.
- Alternatively perform a 24-hour blood glucose curve with 2-hourly blood glucose measurements to establish pattern of blood glucose throughout the day.

Insulinoma

Cause

An insulinoma is a tumour of the insulin-secreting (beta) cells of the pancreas. Most tumours are tiny and are only recognised as a result of the metabolic changes they cause. Insulinomas secrete insulin which reduces blood glucose.

Signs

Hypoglycaemia causes collapse, weakness and seizures. Clinical signs are worse after fasting and can be relieved by feeding.

Diagnostic tests

Persistently low blood glucose occurs with high insulin concentrations.

An intravenous glucose tolerance test helps to confirm a diagnosis. In patients with insulinoma blood glucose concentrations never reach normal peak concentrations and rapidly drop to sub-normal values. The tumour is usually too small to be seen on radiographs but may be seen on ultrasonographic examination of the pancreas. Patients with insulinoma should be screened for tumour spread (metastases) before surgery.

Treatment

Surgical resection of the tumour (removal of part of the pancreas containing the tumour) may relieve the clinical signs for a period of time (a few months up to 18 months). However, the tumour invariably spreads and as metastatic disease starts to produce insulin, clinical signs recur.

Medical management may control the signs if surgery fails or is not appropriate.

Diazoxide reduces insulin production from the insulin-secreting cells. Prednisolone is frequently given as glucocorticoids antagonise the effects of insulin resulting in increased blood glucose concentrations.

Dietary considerations

Frequent small meals of high carbohydrate (low simple sugar) content will help to even out release of glucose from the diet throughout the day. Avoid giving food with a high sugar content (even in a hypoglycaemic crisis) as this can stimulate additional insulin release from the tumour and, whilst alleviating the signs immediately, will result in rapid recurrence of hypoglycaemia. The long-term prognosis for patients with insulinoma is poor.

Special circumstances

Immediately after surgery the patient requires close monitoring and may need intensive nursing care. Acute pancreatitis is a common result of handling the pancreas during surgery and it should be assumed that all postoperative insulinoma patients have pancreatitis unless proven otherwise.

Patients can become transiently diabetic, requiring insulin injections for a period of time.

ADRENAL GLANDS – ANATOMY AND PHYSIOLOGY

There are two adrenal glands, one located on either side of the body just cranial to each kidney, and these produce cortisol (a glucocorticoid hormone). Cortisol production is controlled by another hormone, adrenocorticotrophic hormone (ACTH), which is produced by the pituitary gland in the brain. In times of stress the pituitary gland produces more ACTH which, in turn, stimulates the adrenal glands to make more cortisol.

SPECIFIC DISEASES

Hyperadrenocorticism (HAC), Cushing's syndrome

This is a very common endocrine disease in the dog but is rare in the cat.

Cause

There are three forms of hyperadrenocorticism, pituitary- and adrenal-dependent disease and iatrogenic:

- In adrenal-dependent disease a tumour of the adrenal gland produces cortisol without stimulation by ACTH.
- Pituitary-dependent disease is caused by a pituitary tumour releasing excess ACTH which stimulates both adrenal glands to grow (hypertrophy).
- Iatrogenic disease is the result of veterinary administration of glucocorticoids, e.g. prednisolone tablets.

Signs

Clinically the syndrome appears the same whatever the underlying cause:

- weight gain
- polydipsia/polyuria
- polyphagia
- alopecia.

Urinary tract infections (UTI) are common in dogs with HAC and diabetes mellitus because the immune system is suppressed by high steroid levels – UTI may also be difficult to detect because the normal changes in urine, i.e. increased red blood cells (RBCs) and white blood cells (WBCs), may not occur.

Diagnostic tests

The most common biochemical abnormality is increased **alkaline phosphatase** (ALP) concentration which occurs as a result of a combination of bile duct obstruction due to swelling of hepatic cells and release of a particular type **(isoenzyme)** of ALP. There are a number of tests used to diagnose HAC but none of these is 100% reliable. Ultrasonographic examination of adrenal glands can be useful for recognition of adrenal tumours (usually unilateral) or enlargement of both adrenal glands, which suggests pituitary disease.

Treatment

The standard treatment was a form of chemotherapy (mitotane), which destroys cortisol-producing cells in the adrenal gland.

A more recently licensed product is trilostane. This acts by blocking the production of cortisol by the adrenal glands. The medication is less toxic than mitotane and has fewer side effects. If treatment is stopped signs of disease will usually come back within a few weeks to months.

Monitoring for signs of recurrence of disease is done by repeating ACTH stimulation tests at regular intervals (every 3–6 months) or by monitoring for return of clinical signs.

Cats often respond poorly to drug treatment which may be toxic to them. They are usually treated by surgical removal of both adrenal glands.

Hypoadrenocorticism, Addison's disease

Cause

This is primarily a disease of dogs. In this disease the adrenal glands fail to produce adequate cortisol and mineralocorticoids.

Signs

Often chronic, vague and with a waxing and waning course. Animals may continue for several years with non-specific signs of illness before a crisis develops.

Diagnostic tests

Blood screens show high potassium and low sodium. Many blood screens do not include these electrolytes as a routine examination. Mild anaemia is common. An ACTH stimulation test is required for definitive diagnosis. Cortisol levels will be low and fail to rise after ACTH administration.

Treatment

Medical management is relatively straightforward in stable patients. Daily supplementation with the hormones that are lacking mineralocorticoids (Florinef) and glucocorticoids (prednisolone) usually corrects the deficit within a few weeks.

Special circumstances

If a patient is presented in a crisis then intensive nursing care is important. Fluid therapy is essential but this must be high in sodium and low in potassium, i.e. physiological saline. Soluble glucocorticoids (dexamethasone) are given i.v. and patients' serum electrolyte concentrations must be monitored closely. With good nursing care this is a very rewarding disease to treat. Once the crisis is resolved most patients lead a normal life on continued oral hormone supplementation.

THYROID GLAND – ANATOMY AND PHYSIOLOGY

The thyroid gland sits in the ventral neck just below the larynx. An inactive form of hormone is produced by the gland and this is converted to the active form in the tissues where it is used. Thyroid hormone controls metabolic rate and has effects on many tissues.

SPECIFIC DISEASES
Hypothyroidism

Cause

In dogs disease is caused by an immune-mediated destruction of thyroid tissue (**immune-mediated thyroiditis**) or idiopathic atrophy of the thyroid gland.

Signs

Typically a disease of middle-aged medium-sized bitches – rare in cats. Typical signs:

- skin disease
- lethargy and weight gain.

Owners frequently misinterpret the changes associated with the disease as signs of old age.

Diagnostic tests

Although there are a variety of laboratory tests that can be used to monitor thyroid gland function, none is 100% reliable and diagnosis of hypothyroidism can be quite difficult.
Routine blood screens should be taken for:

- mild non-regenerative anaemia (thyroid hormones are required for stimulation of bone marrow to produce new red blood cells)
- high cholesterol (metabolism of food is abnormal in animals with low thyroid hormone concentrations)
- raised liver enzymes, particularly ALP indicating bile duct obstruction (which may be due to abnormal fat metabolism causing fat deposition within the liver cells, and swelling obstructing normal bile flow in the bile ducts).

Circulating hormone concentrations can be measured but other tests are better for assessing thyroid function. There are many specific tests for thyroid function and the best method of diagnosis is to perform as many tests as possible and interpret the results together.

Treatment

Treatment is simple and usually very effective. Natural hormone deficiencies are replaced by twice daily oral supplementation with a synthetic hormone, levothyroxine (Soloxine). Most animals show clinical improvement within 7 days and all signs should resolve after several months on treatment. Treatment must continue lifelong or signs will rapidly return.

Monitoring

Thyroid hormone concentrations are monitored regularly to ensure that these remain in the normal range.

Hyperthyroidism

Cause

This is the most common endocrine disease in cats and is seen in older animals (usually 12 years and upwards). Most cases appear to be caused by a benign tumour of the thyroid gland.

Signs

Hyperthyroid cats can often be spotted by their appearance (thin, restless, aggressive with a dull, often matted, coat). A typical history is of a ravenous appetite and weight loss, often associated with vomiting or diarrhoea. Many cases are misdiagnosed as malignant neoplasia, or chronic kidney failure. In most cases a **goitre** (palpable enlargement of the thyroid glands) is present.

Tachycardia is caused by thyroid hormone stimulation of heart rate. The increased work can result in hypertrophic cardiomyopathy with all the associated complications, i.e. hypertension, poor cardiac output and the potential to develop thromboemboli.

Diagnostic tests

Routine blood screens should be taken for:

- mildly increased packed cell volume (PCV) (stimulation of bone marrow production of red cells by thyroid hormones)
- increased liver enzymes (mild hypoxic damage to liver tissue or a direct toxic effect of the hormones)
- mild hyperglycaemia (probably due to stress).

Measurement of serum thyroxine concentration usually provides a definitive diagnosis.

The presence of HCM is easily confirmed by radiographic and ultrasonographic examination of the heart.

Treatment

Removal of the affected thyroid gland is the treatment of choice. This can be done surgically or by the s.c. injection of radioactive iodine.

Before surgery the cat should be stabilised medically to increase anaesthetic survival. Carbimazole blocks the production of thyroid hormones.

Propranolol is often given to slow the heart rate. Aspirin may also be prescribed to reduce the risk of thromboembolic disease.

Medical management is normally maintained for around 2–3 weeks before surgery.

Treatment of hyperthyroidism is very rewarding as owners notice a rapid and dramatic improvement in their pet's condition soon after treatment is completed.

Special circumstances

Damage to the parathyroid glands during thyroidectomy may result in hypoparathyroidism and hypocalcaemia. Muscle twitching and seizures may be seen (usually within 48 hours of surgery, although they can develop after 1–5 days). Blood calcium is low. The diagnosis can be confirmed by the finding of low parathyroid hormone and low blood calcium concentrations. This condition is life-threatening and must be treated urgently; i.v. calcium will correct the acute crisis. Oral therapy with calcium supplementation should be started as soon as possible. In addition, vitamin D must be given orally because this is necessary for calcium to be taken up from the intestine. In many cats there is only transient damage to the parathyroid glands (disrupted blood supply at surgery) and calcium supplementation can be tapered over 3–4 weeks with regular monitoring of blood calcium.

PARATHYROID GLANDS – ANATOMY AND PHYSIOLOGY

The parathyroid glands are tiny glands lying in close contact with the thyroid glands. They produce parathyroid hormone (PTH) which is responsible for controlling serum calcium concentrations. Diseases of the parathyroid glands are rare.

SPECIFIC DISEASES
Hyperparathyroidism

Cause

This is caused by a tumour of the parathyroid glands. The tumour produces excess PTH causing increased uptake of calcium from the diet and release of calcium from bones, which, along with reduced calcium excretion, results in hyper-calcaemia. Unfortunately because the glands are so tiny the tumour can be difficult to detect and is usually recognised when the side effects of hypercalcaemia are seen.

Signs

Patients are usually presented with polydipsia/ polyuria and may already have irreversible kidney damage due to deposition of calcium within the kidneys.

Diagnostic tests

Diagnosis is based on the measurement of raised blood calcium, or preferably blood ionised calcium (the physiologically active form of calcium) *and* raised PTH concentrations in a single blood sample.

Treatment

Hypercalcaemia must be controlled as soon as possible to reduce the amount of renal damage caused. Surgical resection of the parathyroid glands is required and is usually effective. If both parathyroid glands are removed then permanent calcium and vitamin D supplementation will be required to prevent hypocalcaemia.

PITUITARY GLAND – ANATOMY AND PHYSIOLOGY

The pituitary gland is located on the ventral surface of the brain.

SPECIFIC DISEASES
Diabetes insipidus

Cause

There are two forms of diabetes insipidus (DI):

- **nephrogenic** (inability of the renal tubules to respond to antidiuretic hormone (ADH))
- **central** (insufficient production of ADH from the pituitary gland caused by damage to the pituitary or a tumour).

Signs

In both forms of the disease the animal is unable to concentrate urine so vast quantities are produced and, as a result of fluid loss, the animal becomes polydipsic (up to 10 l daily in a medium-sized dog). Animals with DI are generally healthy in all other respects.

Diagnostic tests

Routine screening tests to rule out other causes of polyuria/polydipsia. In animals with DI all parameters on routine blood screens should be normal, although there may be evidence of dehydration (mildly elevated PCV and plasma protein). Urine specific gravity will be low (often <1.003).

The water deprivation test is used to diagnose DI. It is very important that the contraindications to a water deprivation test are observed. The test must *not* be performed if:

- the patient has high blood urea (indicating possible kidney dysfunction)
- the patient has high blood calcium concentrations
- there are signs of any other disease which may explain the clinical signs (this disease must be investigated first)
- the patient cannot be monitored adequately for the entire period of the test.

This test is often performed inadequately in practice – in order for it to have any value a strict protocol must be adhered to.

If, at the end of the period of water deprivation, the animal has failed to produce concentrated urine despite losing 5% of its bodyweight a diagnosis of DI is made.

Treatment

Animals with central DI can be treated by supplementation with synthetic ADH (desmopressin, DDAVP). This is usually administered as nasal drops or drops into the conjunctival sac from where it is easily absorbed.

DRUGS COMMONLY USED IN THE MANAGEMENT OF ENDOCRINE DISEASE

Insulin

Most insulin used in pets is natural insulin produced by pigs. Insulin must be given by injection because it is a protein which would be digested if given by mouth.

Diazoxide

This is given by tablet and is used to treat hypoglycaemia. It inhibits insulin release, promotes glucose production from glycogen and reduces the uptake of glucose into cells thereby increasing levels in the blood.

Mitotane

This is a cytotoxic drug which selectively destroys the cortisol-producing cells of the adrenal gland. An overdose of mitotane can destroy the whole adrenal gland resulting in deficiency of glucocorticoids and mineralocorticoids.

Mineralocorticoid

These hormones, e.g. aldosterone, are produced by the adrenal glands and are concerned with the control of salt and water retention by the kidneys. They are important for maintenance of blood pressure. Supplementation of these hormones may be required if insufficient amounts are produced naturally.

Glucocorticoid

A hormone from the adrenal gland, e.g. cortisol, which acts to raise glucose levels. They are commonly used as anti-inflammatory agents. Supplementation is needed in animals whose adrenal glands are unable to produce sufficient amounts of hormone.

Levothyroxine (thyroxine)

This is a synthetic form of thyroid hormone (T_4). The hormone is distributed in the bloodstream and converted to the active form in the tissues where it will be used.

Carbimazole (Neo-Mercazole)

This drug blocks a step in the production of thyroid hormone. It is used in the management of hyperthyroidism – usually to stabilise the patient before surgery. Side effects are rare but may be seen with long-term treatment.

Beta blockers (propranolol)

These drugs slow heart rate and are particularly useful in cats with HCM.

Desmopressin

A synthetic form of ADH used in the treatment of diabetes insipidus. It has a longer duration of action than ADH and is usually given as eye drops 1–3 times daily (depending on the response).

HAEMOPOIETIC SYSTEM AND COAGULATION (Table 3.13)

NORMAL HAEMATOPOIESIS

In the normal adult animal production of most blood cells occurs within the bone marrow. The marrow contains many stem cells which are capable of producing different types of blood cells. When an RBC stem cell is stimulated it starts to divide to produce many cells which then

Table 3.13 Important questions to ask the owner of a bleeding animal

Question	Reason for question and interpretation of answer
Is the animal bleeding from more than one site, e.g. haematuria, blood in faeces/melaena?	Bleeding from more than one site makes it likely that the animal has a generalised haemostatic problem rather than a primary wound
Is the blood clotting?	If blood clots are forming then coagulation is probably OK. It is more likely that the haemorrhage is the result of a platelet or vascular disease or severe injury
Is there any bleeding around gums or bruising on skin?	Platelet deficiency is often associated with gingival bleeding, petechial haemorrhages or epistaxis
Have any swellings been noticed in the recent past?	Swellings may be due to bleeding into the tissues or under the skin. Owners may not be concerned about these and, because they see no evidence of blood loss, they fail to see the connection with the current bleeding problem

mature through a number of stages to produce the mature erythrocyte (RBC). There are many things which can stimulate the production of more RBCs but production is mainly controlled by **erythropoietin**, a hormone produced by the kidney. It takes about 7 days for an RBC to develop in the marrow and under normal conditions they last for about 110–120 days in the circulation in the dog. The RBC lifespan is shorter in the cat (only 69–79 days). If large numbers of RBCs have to be produced rapidly the marrow production may be supplemented by production of RBCs in other organs such as the liver and spleen. Platelets are formed from megakaryocytes in bone marrow and are not true cells but fragments of other cells. The mechanism for production of neutrophils and other white blood cells is very similar, with the exception of lymphocytes. Lymphocytes are also produced in the marrow but immature cells move in large numbers to lymphoid tissue for development.

NORMAL HAEMOSTASIS

Haemostasis is the mechanism which prevents excessive blood loss from damaged vessels; there are two phases: primary and secondary.

In **primary haemostasis**, a damaged blood vessel contracts to reduce the amount of blood loss and platelets start to stick to the sides of the hole in the vessel and release thromboplastin.

Secondary haemostasis is the formation of a blood clot to prevent further blood loss. The blood clot is formed by the interaction of many clotting factors (Fig. 3.10). The clotting factors are all produced in the liver except for factor VIII (also known as von Willebrand's factor) which is made in the lining of the blood vessels themselves. Finally the blood clot is broken down and removed by a process called fibrinolysis.

PATHOPHYSIOLOGY
Anaemia

Anaemia is defined as a lower than normal concentration of RBCs and this may be caused by:

1. excessive loss of red cells (haemorrhage)
2. excessive destruction of red cells (haemolysis)
3. inadequate production of red cells (Box 3.10).

Haemorrhage may occur as a result of a wound such as a cut or a non-healing lesion, e.g. ulcerated tumour or gastrointestinal ulcer. It may also be the result of a failure of the normal haemostatic mechanisms. Failure of haemostasis will allow even the small wounds encountered on a regular basis in everyday life to bleed significantly, e.g. animals with clotting defects may develop large bruises from being handled. Loss of blood cells due to haemorrhage may be visible externally if there is an obvious wound. However,

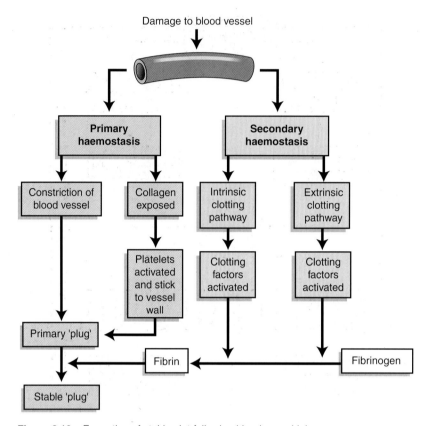

Figure 3.10 Formation of stable clot following blood vessel injury.

Box 3.10 Causes of anaemia

Haemorrhage	Haemolysis	Non-regenerative
Severe trauma (road traffic accident, internal organ rupture) Clotting disorder Neoplasia Haemorrhagic gastroenteritis Severe ectoparasite infection	Immune-mediated *Haemobartonella*	Bone marrow hypoplasia Iron deficiency Renal disease Leukaemia/ lymphosarcoma Lead poisoning

significant volumes of blood can be lost with no external signs of bleeding (see Figs 3.11, 3.12):

• Haemorrhage into body cavity, e.g. pleural space, or peritoneal cavity.

• Blood loss into GI tract or urinary tract which may be present at a low level for a long period and result in significant blood loss. If blood loss occurs over a long period of time the body may initially replace red cells as fast as they are lost, but as stores of iron (required to make haemoglobin) become depleted, further red cell production may stop.

Destruction of red cells (haemolysis) can occur within the blood vessels themselves (**intravascular haemolysis**), or damaged blood cells may be removed from the circulation as they pass through organs like the liver and spleen and be destroyed there (**extravascular haemolysis**). The most common reason for red cell destruction is activation of the immune response against red cells. This may occur as a result of a change in the appearance of the cells so that they are no longer recognised by the immune system, e.g. they have foreign proteins on their surface. This occurs in

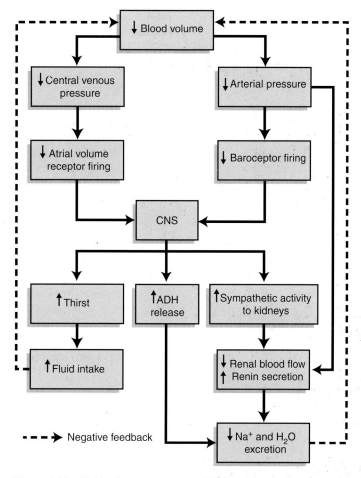

Figure 3.11   Fluid volume replacement following haemorrhage. (Reproduced with permission from Cunningham 1997.)

Haemobartonella infections in cats where proteins from the parasite within the cell appear on the surface. In dogs it is not uncommon for an idiopathic immune-mediated destruction of RBCs to occur. In this disease the immune system genuinely becomes overactive and starts to destroy normal RBCs.

Red cell production most commonly fails as a result of damage to the bone marrow. This can be caused by a tumour in the bone marrow, e.g. lymphosarcoma, or drugs such as oestrogen which can kill all the stem cells within the marrow. Leukaemias, causing excessive production of a single type of WBC in the bone marrow, may take up so much room with the production of white cells that red cell precursors are squeezed out.

SPECIFIC DISEASES

Coagulopathies (disorders of haemostasis)

These can be divided into two groups: congenital and acquired.

Congenital coagulopathies

Von Willebrand's disease

Cause: This is the most common congenital haemostatic disease. It is an inherited disease which can affect both sexes.

Signs: Severity of the disease varies from mild (with virtually no signs) to severe (with neonatal death).

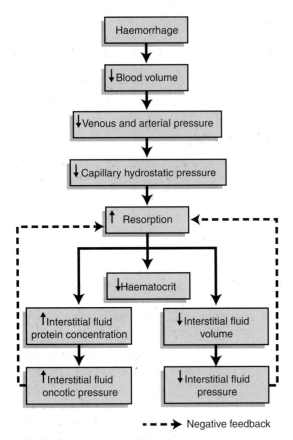

Figure 3.12 Capillary fluid shifts following haemorrhage. (Reproduced with permission from Cunningham 1997.)

Diagnosis: Mild forms of the disease may often be detected at the time of routine surgery when affected animals bleed more than expected. The disease is more common in certain breeds, e.g. Dobermann Pinschers, Scottish Terriers and Golden Retrievers, and it may be wise to check that clotting function is normal in these breeds before undertaking routine surgery. Von Willebrand factor levels can be measured and relatives of affected individuals should be tested to see if they are carriers.

Treatment: There is no specific treatment but once a diagnosis has been reached special precautions can be taken to reduce the risk of bleeding. In some cases fresh blood transfusion may be required to stop bleeding after surgery or an injury.

ACQUIRED DISORDERS OF HAEMOSTASIS

Anticoagulant rodenticide poisoning

Cause

The most common acquired coagulopathy is caused by ingestion of anticoagulant rat baits (containing warfarin or warfarin-like compounds). These poisons cause a reduction in vitamin K (which plays an essential part in the coagulation cascade).

Signs

Clinical signs are not seen until all body stores of vitamin K have been used up, which may not be for several days after ingestion of poison. Once vitamin K stores have been used up spontaneous bleeding (or severe haemorrhage in response to minor injury) results. Bleeding into the respiratory system (the trachea, lungs or pleural space) is common and can cause severe respiratory distress.

Diagnosis

Usually suspected on basis of clinical signs and potential exposure to poison. Clotting times are prolonged.

Treatment

The condition can be corrected by supplementation of vitamin K until the effects of the poison wear off (which may be up to 3–4 months in some cases). In the early stages of the condition, before the vitamin K has had time to take effect, it is vital to handle the patient with extreme care to prevent haemorrhage and bruising.

Liver disease

Coagulopathies can also be acquired as a result of severe liver dysfunction (usually cirrhosis) resulting in an inability to synthesise clotting factors. Some neoplastic diseases, especially haemangiosarcoma, can result in a condition called disseminated intravascular coagulation (DIC) where numerous tiny clots form in the blood. The formation of these clots uses up all the clotting factors and results in an acquired coagulopathy.

Anaemia

Cause

There are many causes of anaemia (see Box 3.10).

Signs

Anaemia reduces the oxygen-carrying capacity of the blood. As well as pale mucous membranes it may result in dyspnoea and exercise intolerance. If blood is being lost then signs may be due to hypotension as well as a lack of red cells. Collapse and fainting are not uncommon in this instance.

Diagnostic tests

Collection of a blood sample for haematological examination is essential. Crude estimation of severity can be obtained from PCV and measurement of RBC size (mean corpuscular volume or MCV) and density (mean corpuscular haemoglobin concentration or MCHC) can be used. Other investigations are directed at identifying the underlying cause of disease. Reticulocyte count and assessment of nucleated RBC numbers indicate the numbers of immature cells in the circulation and help to decide how regenerative the anaemia is.

Treatment

If a lot of blood has been lost then intravenous fluid replacement is indicated to support blood pressure. Ideally this should be in the form of blood or plasma but colloid solutions can also be used.

Blood transfusion to replace RBCs is not needed unless the animal is showing severe clinical signs. The severity of the anaemia at this time will depend on a number of factors, in particular how rapidly the PCV has dropped. It is unusual to see clinical signs as a result of anaemia alone in an animal with a PCV above 0.12 1/l. If the PCV drops below 0.10 1/l (or severe clinical signs are seen earlier) then a blood transfusion is probably necessary. If the patient has been haemorrhaging then whole blood is the best choice, however if anaemia is the result of red cell destruction or failure of RBC production then red cells only should be given if possible.

TRANSFUSION

The limiting factor to blood transfusion in practice is often the availability of a suitable donor animal. Blood donors should ideally be:

- clinically healthy
- fully vaccinated
- normal bodyweight
- *Haemobartonella* negative
- with PCV at top end of normal range
- of suitable temperament
- FeLV and FIV negative (cats)
- blood-type compatible with recipient (cats).

The donor is sedated and restrained comfortably. The jugular vein must be used for blood collection in order that sufficient volumes can be collected. Up to 10% of blood volume can be collected (or 20% if replacement fluids are given i.v.). The vein is prepared aseptically. Blood can be collected into a standard blood collection bag, or in smaller patients into a 50 ml syringe containing 7 ml of anticoagulant (acid citrate dextrose or citrate phosphate dextrose (CPD)). As blood is collected it should be mixed immediately with the anticoagulant. Repeated collections can be made from the same donor after 4–6 weeks provided PCV has returned to normal.

Fresh blood can be stored in a fridge for several weeks and will still be useful for replacing RBCs. However, clotting factors are only present in high concentrations in fresh plasma so this should be separated and frozen as soon as possible if not required for immediate use.

Remember that anaemia is not a diagnosis – it is merely a symptom of another disease. It is very important that the underlying cause is recognised and treated and that management of the anaemia is employed to keep the patient alive while appropriate diagnosis and treatment can be implemented.

DRUGS COMMONLY USED IN THE MANAGEMENT OF HAEMATOLOGICAL AND CLOTTING DISORDERS

Vitamin K$_1$ (phytomenadione)

Used in the management of clotting disorders associated with vitamin K$_1$ deficiency, e.g. anticoagulant rodenticide poisoning. It can be given subcutaneously but care should be taken in administration of injections in animals with bleeding tendencies as traumatic injection can result in haematoma formation. Intravenous administration of vitamin K$_1$ has been associated with anaphylactic reaction.

Bone marrow stimulants

These are used in anaemia caused by suppression of bone marrow function. Anabolic steroids have effects which should stimulate marrow production of RBC. The most effective anabolic steroid for this purpose is decadurabolin but nandrolone is often used. Epoietin is also available and whilst very effective in some cases of anaemia associated with chronic renal failure it is extremely expensive.

Anticoagulants

Heparin and warfarin have anticoagulant effects and can be used if the clotting system is overactive, e.g. DIC. Heparin acts by inhibiting factor XII activation but does not change the concentrations of clotting factors. Warfarin acts by antagonising the action of vitamin K.

CENTRAL NERVOUS SYSTEM
(Table 3.14)

SEIZURES

Advice to owners

Telephone advice

Owners may phone the veterinary practice whilst their pet is having a fit. Reassure the owner that

their pet is unconscious and not in pain – they should avoid handling it as they could be injured. They should be advised:

- to ensure the animal cannot injure itself, e.g. by falling downstairs
- to time the seizure accurately using a watch
- if the seizure stops within 5 minutes allow the animal to recover quietly at home
- if this is the first fit and no further seizures occur the next routine appointment should be made for the animal to have a veterinary examination.

If the fit lasts longer than 5 minutes the animal should be brought to the surgery if possible, or the vet should attend the animal immediately.

PATHOPHYSIOLOGY

The term **seizure** (convulsion or fit) is used to describe altered electrical activity in the brain. Seizures are a symptom of disease, not a diagnosis. For a seizure to start a small electrical discharge must be generated in the brain. This may be the result of damage to the cells in one area or changes in the fluid bathing the brain. Occasionally lack of oxygen (low oxygen in the blood or anaemia) or glucose to the brain cells can cause damage to them. Once an electrical discharge has started it spreads rapidly from cell to cell and usually involves the whole brain very rapidly. If the whole brain is involved the seizure is termed **generalised seizure.** Activation of the brain cells sends signals down the nerves to the muscles in the body causing them all to start contracting and this causes the signs of the seizure. Signs of seizure can be divided into three phases:

- **preictal** (the period before the seizure when some animals appear to sense that something is about to happen – in humans this is called the 'aura')
- **ictal** (the seizure itself)
- **postictal** (the period after the seizure before the animal returns to normal).

Sometimes only a small area of the brain is affected and this can result in a **partial seizure**

Table 3.14   Important questions to ask the owner of a seizuring animal

Question	Reason for question and interpretation of answer
How old is the animal?	Epilepsy most commonly starts between the ages of 1 and 3 years. Animals younger than 1 year are more likely to have congenital or infectious diseases. In older animals metabolic disease or tumours may be more likely
Is this the first fit?	If the patient has previously been diagnosed as epileptic occasional seizures are to be expected
If not the first fit, when was the last one?	Single seizures are rarely a cause for serious concern and the patient should be examined at the next routine surgery. If seizures are recurring frequently, are prolonged, or the animal is not recovering fully between seizures the patient should be assessed immediately
Do the attacks usually happen at a certain time of day? Or are they related to exercise or feeding?	Epileptic seizures tend to occur when the patient is relaxed (often in the transition between sleep and consciousness). Seizures associated with feeding (either after eating or after fasting) are more likely to be due to a metabolic cause. Seizures associated with exercise or excitement may be caused by cardiovascular disease
Is the animal well otherwise: any weight loss, anorexia or other signs?	Epilepsy is rarely associated with clinical signs of disease. Brain tumours and metabolic disease are more likely to be associated with other changes
Are all the fits the same?	Seizures from a single focus in the brain will all follow the same pattern. If the pattern of each seizure varies then multiple areas of the brain are affected – this makes epilepsy a less likely diagnosis
What are the fits like? Is the animal conscious (able to respond to owner)? What does the animal do during a fit? How long does a fit last? What does the animal do after a fit?	It is important to record the nature of each seizure so that any trends of progression or increasing duration can be monitored
Are the fits getting more frequent or lasting longer?	More frequent and prolonged seizures mean that the seizures are not being controlled and may indicate progression of the underlying disease, e.g. a growing brain tumour, or inadequate therapy
Is the animal completely normal between fits?	If the animal is completely normal between seizures it is less likely (but not impossible) that it has a severe underlying pathology such as a metabolic disease or brain tumour
Is there any history of trauma (recently, or in the past)?	Damage to the brain can cause seizures at the time of injury due to brain swelling and cell damage. Seizures may also start months or years after trauma as a result of scar tissue formation within the brain
Has there been potential access to poisons or drugs?	Many toxins can cause seizures and sudden onset of severe generalised seizures (particularly status epilepticus) should make you think of poisoning as a potential cause

(this is very rare in dogs but may be seen in cats). The signs of this will vary depending on which cells are affected. When faced with a seizuring animal there are two aims: to control the seizure and to establish the cause.

Cause

Seizures may be caused by disease inside the brain (intracranial) or diseases elsewhere in the body which affect the brain (extracranial). Some common causes of seizure are shown in Box 3.11. Epilepsy is a series of seizures in animals with no obvious disease – the seizures are caused by metabolic changes within the brain cells.

Signs

It is rare to find an obvious cause of seizures on clinical examination but vital signs should be monitored. Heart rate, temperature and respiration rate are all likely to be increased in an animal

Box 3.11   Causes of seizures

Intracranial disease	Extracranial disease
Trauma	Metabolic disease
Infectious disease	Hypoglycaemia
Brain tumour	Hypocalcaemia
Heatstroke	Hepatic encephalopathy
Hydrocephalus	Anaemia
Brain inflammation	Anoxia
Vascular disease	Poisoning
Idiopathic	

immediately after (or during) a seizure due to the physical exertion. Changes in these signs may also indicate a problem that has caused the fit. An irregular heart rate or pulse may be very significant. Always try to record details of clinical examination at the time of a seizure and then repeat the examination after the patient has fully recovered and compare the results.

Investigation

When presented with a seizuring animal the first step must always be to control the seizure. Once this has been done steps should be taken to investigate the underlying cause.

Obtaining a detailed history from the owner is important; you are trying to establish if the fit is likely to be due to a metabolic problem (e.g. hypoglycaemia), hypoxic episode (e.g. heart disease) or is truly epileptiform.

Diagnostic tests

Blood samples should be taken from the animal as close to the time of the seizure as possible. Some changes in the blood may only be present at the time of the seizure and the results of tests on samples from the animal between seizures may be completely normal. Tests should be done to check electrolyte concentrations (calcium, sodium, potassium), glucose, bile salts (to check liver function), RBC levels (for anaemia) and WBCs (for evidence of infection).

It may be necessary to take some cerebrospinal fluid (CSF) from around the brain to test for

infection or inflammation. This is called a CSF tap and involves anaesthetising the animal and putting a needle into the spinal canal at the back of the neck and drawing off a small amount of the fluid. This procedure is not without risk and is often only done as a last resort in general practice. There is a particular risk when performing this procedure in a patient with increased pressure in the cranium, e.g. a brain tumour. Sudden release of pressure by withdrawing CSF can cause fatal herniation of the brainstem through the foramen magnum.

Radiographs are rarely helpful but may aid diagnosis of some diseases, e.g. the finding of a small liver may suggest liver dysfunction and hepatic encephalopathy. Skull radiographs are almost never useful.

Other tests used to look for damage to the brain or congenital abnormalities, such as hydrocephalus, would be MRI and CT.

If anoxia is suspected to be the cause of the seizure then full examination of the cardiovascular and respiratory systems with radiographs, ultrasound and ECG is needed.

Treatment

If a cause of the seizures can be identified, successful management of this condition may be enough to control seizures. If no cause can be found then symptomatic control of the seizures with anticonvulsant drugs (as for epilepsy) is required. If the seizures continue to progress despite anticonvulsant treatment then investigations should be repeated to see if any abnormalities appear on the tests.

SPECIFIC DISEASES
Epilepsy

Cause

True epilepsy is a condition in which multiple seizures occur due to a metabolic disorder in the brain cells. It is relatively common in dogs and also occurs in cats. In some breeds of dogs (especially the German Shepherd dog) it is inherited.

Signs

Affected animals are usually between 1 and 5 years old. During a typical seizure the animal becomes unconscious, falls on to its side and makes running movements with its legs. Some animals may cry out and occasionally will defecate. Most attacks last between 3 and 5 minutes but patients may have behavioural changes before the seizure starts and can appear to be dazed for up to 24 hours afterwards. Recurrent seizures occur at intervals which vary between animals and occasionally an animal will have only one seizure during its lifetime.

Diagnostic tests

The history is important in suspecting epilepsy as a diagnosis but the condition can only be diagnosed by ruling out other causes of seizure. Tests may include blood samples, CSF tap, and radiographs of thorax and abdomen to rule out other diseases. Skull radiographs are rarely helpful but other imaging techniques such as MRI and CT may be needed to evaluate the brain for signs of disease or damage.

Treatment

Seizure control relies on oral anticonvulsant medication. The most common drugs used in the treatment of epilepsy are barbiturates, e.g. phenobarbital (commonly used in dogs) or diazepam (for use in cats). Once an animal starts on medication this must be given regularly for life; stopping anticonvulsant medication suddenly may itself cause seizures. Most animals with epilepsy can be controlled with medication so that they can live relatively normal lives.

Special circumstances

If an animal does not regain consciousness after 5 minutes or starts to seizure again immediately after a seizure it is said to be in **status epilepticus.** This is a serious condition because if a seizure lasts more than 5 minutes brain damage can occur. Emergency treatment must be started to keep the animal alive and then to control the seizure.

Intravenous anticonvulsant drugs are normally needed in these cases. In some animals with severe seizures it may be necessary to induce anaesthesia to stop the seizure and if so it is vital to monitor the patient in the same way as any other anaesthetised patient – paying particular care to maintaining a patent airway. If patients have to be anaesthetised for long periods then general nursing care is important, e.g. turning patient to prevent sores, providing fluid therapy and ensuring urinary function is maintained (with the placement of an indwelling urinary catheter if necessary).

DRUGS USED IN THE MANAGEMENT OF SEIZURES

Barbiturates

Phenobarbital and pentobarbitone are anticonvulsants used in the management of severe recurring seizures or status epilepticus. These drugs act by reducing the sensitivity of the brain cells so that it is harder for a seizure to get going. Phenobarbital is relatively short acting and is usually used early in the course of treatment and may be used as first-line oral medication in the dog and cat.

In status epilepticus pentobarbitone may be used intravenously for its prolonged action. This may induce anaesthesia necessitating endotracheal intubation and respiratory support as necessary. Barbiturates are metabolised in the liver and usually cause raised liver enzymes on blood screens. Bile salt measurements are required to monitor liver function and it is important to check this as the drugs can cause toxic damage to the liver.

Primidone (Mysoline) is metabolised in the liver primarily to phenobarbital and most of its effects are due to phenobarbital levels in the blood.

Diazepam (Valium)

Diazepam can be used as a first line in the oral control of seizures in the cat. In the dog, however, it has a shorter duration of action and is only effective when given by intravenous injection or per rectum (suppository). It is used in dogs to control status epilepticus.

Potassium bromide

This drug depresses the central nervous system, making seizures less likely. It is normally dissolved in water and given as an oral solution (on food). It is used in conjunction with phenobarbital and is particularly useful for control of clusters of seizures. It takes a long time (often several months) for the full effects of the drug to be seen. Side effects are uncommon. Because it is not metabolised in the liver it is a good drug to use in patients with liver disease.

ONCOLOGY (Table 3.15)

PATHOPHYSIOLOGY

A tumour is an uncontrolled proliferation of a single cell type. Most develop from a single abnormal cell which continues to divide free from the normal inhibitory mechanisms. When a tumour first develops the cells are dividing rapidly and the mass grows quickly. As the mass increases in size, cell division slows due to the difficulty of supplying an adequate blood supply to the increasingly large cell population. The behaviour of a tumour depends largely on the cell type from which it grew. In basic terms the behaviour of a tumour is classified as benign or malignant.

Cause

Benign

Benign tumours tend to be relatively slow growing and do not readily spread to distant sites (metastasise). Common examples of benign tumours are:

- adenoma
- fibroma
- lipoma
- melanoma
- papilloma.

Table 3.15 Important questions to ask the owner of an animal with a mass	
Question	Reason for question and interpretation of answer
When was the mass first noticed?	Masses which have been present for long periods may require less urgent attention. However, it is important to achieve an identification of every mass in order to provide the most appropriate treatment (even if this is to do nothing). Owners may fail to notice a mass until they come across it by chance, e.g. when grooming their pet
Has it changed since first noticed?	Masses which remain static for a long period are unlikely to change suddenly. Masses which do suddenly become irritating or ulcerate should be treated aggressively
Is the animal irritated by the mass?	Some masses are irritating because of their location, e.g. masses on the eyelid may rub on the cornea once they get to a certain size. Other masses become ulcerated and sore because of substances they produce, e.g. mast cell tumours releasing histamine. Irritating masses should be removed – not only on welfare grounds but because irritation may well be a sign of malignancy
Is the animal losing weight?	Many tumours cause cachexia and unexplained weight loss may be the first sign of serious neoplastic disease
Is the animal in good health otherwise?	Many tumours produce substances which make animals unwell. Signs of ill health may be due to anaemia, hypercalcaemia or toxic factors. Systemic infection may be present in animals with compromised immune systems, e.g. tumours invading bone marrow and affecting white blood cell production. Non-neoplastic masses may be associated with ill health, e.g. abscess and systemic infection or haematoma associated with anaemia

Malignant

Malignant tumours may be locally invasive or spread through the lymphatic or blood system to lymph nodes and distant sites. These tumours are more likely to cause systemic signs of ill health. Examples of these are:

- carcinoma (squamous cell carcinoma)
- sarcoma (lymphosarcoma, haemangiosarcoma).

Signs

There are a number of different presentations for neoplasia:

- visible mass noticed by owner
- physical effects of the tumour, e.g. a large abdominal mass causing abdominal distension or a thoracic mass causing coughing
- effects of mass, e.g. rupture of splenic tumour causing haemorrhage and collapse
- distant effects of neoplasia (paraneoplastic syndrome), e.g. polydipsia associated with hypercalcaemia in dogs with anal gland adenocarcinomas.

Full examination of the whole patient is essential when investigating a suspected tumour. Detection of distant metastasis is important and palpation of local drainage lymph nodes for signs of enlargement may give the first indication of tumour spread.

The mass itself should be thoroughly evaluated. Measurements of dimensions should be recorded along with details of mobility (can the mass be lifted clear of surrounding tissue or does it seem attached?) and characteristics, e.g. soft, firm, ulcerated, painful, etc.

Diagnostic tests

There are three important steps in the investigation of any mass:

1. Establish what the mass is.
2. Identify if it is localised or has spread elsewhere.

3. Rule out underlying disease or pre-existing conditions which might complicate management.

In most cases the mass should be identified before resection (rather than removing it and then sending the sample for histological diagnosis). Presurgical identification allows appropriate treatment planning and gives the surgeon information about the invasiveness and malignancy of the mass so that adequate surgical margins can be taken.

Fine needle aspiration

Needle aspiration is the removal of a few cells from a tumour for cytological staining and examination. This technique is simple and cheap to perform. A needle is inserted into the mass and then removed, attached to a syringe full of air, and the air is blown out through the needle over a microscope slide. This forces a bleb of cells on to the slide and these can then be smeared. Surface masses can be aspirated easily although ultrasound guidance may be required to collect samples from internal organs. This can provide a rapid and accurate diagnosis in tumours which shed cells easily. Some types of tumour do not readily give up cells and it may be impossible to collect a diagnostic sample by this method.

Core biopsy

This technique provides a small sample of cells for histological examination. A Tru-cut needle or biopsy 'gun' simplifies the technique. Basically, a large-bore needle is pushed into the mass cutting a core of tissues. This tissue must be preserved in formalin and sent for histological examination which can delay diagnosis. However, the sample can be rolled on a slide before fixing and some cells may be shed which can be examined cytologically.

Incisional biopsy

This involves taking a small sample of the mass as a surgical procedure. This technique is occasionally necessary in the examination of masses in inaccessible areas where radical surgery would be necessary for complete surgical excision, e.g. nasal tumours. In most cases a less invasive technique or complete surgical excision would be preferable.

Excisional biopsy

This technique is commonly used in practice in the management of small skin lumps. Whilst this does, in many cases, provide the owner with a single surgical, curative treatment when benign skin nodules are removed, the practice is rather sloppy. In cases of more malignant tumours a second, more radical surgery is required and the delay between first surgery and follow-up treatment may allow the tumour to spread locally or metastasise. It is good practice to aspirate every mass before undertaking surgery.

Other investigations

Examination of haematology screens and bone marrow samples is necessary for classification of leukaemias and to see how severely the bone marrow is affected. Blood screens may be useful in the evaluation of patients with other forms of tumour to identify systemic effects of the tumour, e.g. liver damage or production of substances causing hypercalcaemia. Additional laboratory investigations are used to assess the general health of the patient, to establish its ability to tolerate the planned treatment. Liver and kidney function may be important if anaesthesia is anticipated for radiotherapy or surgery. Many chemotherapeutic drugs can also be nephrotoxic or require hepatic metabolism. Haematological investigation is important if chemotherapy is planned as many of the agents have a suppressive effect on bone marrow.

Screening radiographs of thorax and abdomen are indicated in most cases to evaluate the extent of any internal tumour and to rule out the presence of distant metastases (particularly in lung fields). It is important to take at least two thoracic projections (left and right laterals or lateral and dorsoventral projections) to be sure of seeing metastases if they are present.

Ultrasonographic examination of tumours within internal organs may be useful but often MRI or CT will provide better detail if surgical treatment is being planned.

Treatment

There are three options for treatment:

- surgical removal
- radiotherapy
- chemotherapy.

Principles of surgery

The selection of treatment depends upon the tumour type and the health of the patient. If complete surgical resection is possible then this is the best option in almost all cases. Total surgical removal should result in complete cure. However, in many cases it is not possible to remove the whole tumour because it is too extensive, exists in multiple sites, or involves a vital organ which cannot be removed.

Principles of chemotherapy

Chemotherapy is the use of drugs which kill cells (**cytotoxic drugs**). Some tumour cells have a natural resistance to the effects of some drugs and others are able to develop resistance to these drugs with time. This is the reason why it is important to identify the tumour type so that the most effective treatment can be selected.

Most cytotoxic drugs act against cells when they are dividing, so rapidly dividing cells are most affected by these agents. Normal cells are also affected by cytotoxic drugs and rapidly dividing cells in the gastrointestinal tract and bone marrow are most at risk from these agents. Side effects of drugs are most commonly seen in these organs, i.e. diarrhoea or low WBC count due to bone marrow suppression. Cytotoxic drugs are most likely to be effective if used when cells are rapidly dividing – this occurs early in the course of the disease (usually before the mass is big enough to see) but also immediately after surgical resection of the primary mass.

Cytoxic drugs are usually given according to a set protocol. This includes a high dose of drugs in the first instance (**induction period**) and then a sustained lower level (**maintenance dose**). Drug therapy is usually given on a regular, intermittent basis so that normal cells have a chance to recover between treatments. Drug doses are calculated, not by bodyweight, but by body surface area (BSA). There is a conversion table which allows you to look up the BSA in m^2 if you know the weight of the patient.

In most animals we are aiming for a good, normal quality of life during treatment and so potential side effects are minimised by keeping drug doses low. Clinical cure is rarely attempted.

Cytotoxic drugs are a serious health hazard and should be handled only by properly trained staff using appropriate equipment, e.g. fume cupboards and protective clothing. They must never be used by pregnant women, or those who might become pregnant, as they can damage the foetus.

Principles of radiotherapy

Radiotherapy is the therapeutic use of radiation. High doses of radiation damage DNA in cells. This affects rapidly dividing cells more quickly than cells with a slow turnover, hence many tumours are susceptible to radiation. Lymphosarcoma and squamous cell carcinoma are particularly radiosensitive. Radiation treatment is usually given in multiple small doses (**fractions**) at regular intervals spread over a number of weeks. At any moment only a proportion of the cells in a tumour are actively dividing and hence susceptible to the effects of radiation. Radiation treatment at that time will kill those susceptible cells but over the next few hours or days other cells start to divide, and after a single dose of radiation the tumour would rapidly start to regrow. Fractionated doses give more chances to attack different groups of tumour cells. This also means that normal tissue affected by the radiation has time to recover between doses and so side effects of treatment are minimised. A course of radiotherapy requires that the patient be anaesthetised on a number of occasions and so it is important to ensure the patient is in a suitable condition to withstand this. Radiotherapy is often used as a follow-up treatment to surgical resection of a tumour. Following surgery the few remaining cells will start to divide rapidly and therefore be susceptible to radiotherapy.

Radiotherapy requires expensive equipment and specialist expertise and is only available at a few specialist centres.

Some tumours are much more sensitive to radiotherapy than others and particular types of chemotherapy are useful in particular disease. In many cases a combination of therapies is the best option, e.g. surgery followed by radiation or chemotherapy.

SPECIFIC DISEASES

Lymphosarcoma

Cause: neoplastic disease of the lymphatic system.

Signs: enlargement of multiple lymph nodes, occasional single mass in lymph node or skin.

Diagnosis: fine needle aspiration of enlarged lymph node for cytological examination usually provides diagnosis although in a few cases biopsy is required.

Treatment: although the tumour is very radiosensitive the generalised nature of the disease usually makes this form of therapy impossible. Chemotherapy can be effective in providing remission for up to 1–2 years, in some cases.

Osteosarcoma

Cause: malignant tumour of bone.

Signs: lameness, pain or swelling typically affecting specific sites, e.g. proximal humerus in giant-breed dogs.

Diagnosis: radiographic changes in affected sites with concurrent new bone proliferation and bone destruction. Fracture may occur at site of lesion. Radiographic screens for pulmonary metastasis before treatment are important.

Treatment: radical surgery is required (usually amputation of affected limb) but almost invariably metastases will still appear around 1 year later. Additional chemotherapy can prolong survival times.

DRUGS COMMONLY USED IN THE TREATMENT OF NEOPLASTIC DISEASE

Cyclophosphamide

This is one of the most commonly used cytotoxic drugs, especially for the treatment of lymphosarcoma. It is normally given orally (usually on an every-other-day basis) but can be given intravenously. Side effects are not usually severe but bone marrow suppression can occur. However, accurate dosing in small dogs and cats is difficult because of the large tablet size. Tablets should not be broken (due to the risk to people handling the drug), so it is hard to get small doses. This problem is usually overcome by administering larger doses on a less frequent basis, e.g. weekly. At high doses gastrointestinal signs (vomiting and diarrhoea) are likely. The most serious complication associated with this drug is haemorrhagic cystitis. If this develops during treatment the drug should be stopped immediately and a different form of chemotherapy prescribed.

Doxorubicin

Mostly used in the management of lymphosarcoma but can be used to treat osteosarcoma and soft tissue sarcomas, e.g. haemangiosarcoma. It is given intravenously and perivascular injection *must* be avoided as it is very irritant. May be nephrotoxic in the cat. Marrow suppression occurs after injection, with a drop in WBC count (which recovers after 3 weeks). Gastrointestinal and acute allergic reactions can be seen. To prevent anaphylactic reactions an antihistamine premed is often given. The drug has a cardiotoxic effect which builds up over a number of doses so cardiac ultrasound should be monitored on a regular basis in animals receiving treatment. The total dose of drug given in a course of treatment should not be more than 240 mg per m^2.

Vincristine

Often used for the treatment of leukaemia and lymphosarcoma. This is a useful drug as it causes relatively little bone marrow suppression and so can be used in combination with other drugs. It is administered intravenously and is irritant perivascularly so an intravenous catheter should be placed before injection.

POISONING (Table 3.16)

ADVICE TO OWNERS

Telephone advice

Instructions given to the owner in cases of suspected or known poisoning are important:

Table 3.16	Important questions to ask the owner of an animal with suspected poisoning
Question	Reason for question and interpretation of answer
What signs are being shown?	Clear documentation of the signs gives a baseline from which to judge whether the patient is getting better or worse. Taking a good history may indicate another cause of the signs (apart from poisoning)
Are the signs getting worse?	Urgent attention is required if the symptoms are progressing
Has the animal had any access to possible poisons? If so: What poison? When did the exposure occur? How much was eaten/drunk?	It can be very difficult to identify the source of a poisoning from the signs alone. If owners can identify a potential source of the poisoning ask them to bring this with them. Knowledge of the cause of the poisoning may allow likely signs to be predicted and potential antidotes to be obtained. Knowing how much was eaten or drunk will give some idea of the likely severity of symptoms and the timing of exposure may affect treatment offered, i.e. if recent ingestion then it may be practical to promote vomiting
Is the animal on any medication?	Overdose of some medications can be toxic or cause signs associated with poisoning. Patients already receiving anticonvulsants may be likely to develop severe seizures if medication is stopped suddenly

- Protect the animal and remove it from the source of the intoxication.
- Take care of people exposed to the animal as disorientated or frightened animals may become aggressive and people may be at risk from contamination with noxious substances by handling the animal.
- In cases of topical exposure the worst of the contamination may be washed off to reduce further absorption. Protective clothing must be worn and water only should be used.
- Animals should be allowed to drink water which may act as a diluent for ingested poisons. If the animal is convulsing or unconscious no attempt should be made to administer anything by mouth.

Do not advise the owner to make the animal vomit.

PATHOPHYSIOLOGY
Cause

A poison is defined as any substance which in small amounts can cause sickness or death. Poisons are usually categorised in broad groups:

- insecticides
- rodenticides
- human/veterinary medicines
- herbicides
- plant poisons.

Signs

Poisoning should be suspected in any animal which suddenly develops severe clinical signs, especially status epilepticus. If the clinical signs do not match those anticipated with the suspected poisoning it is important to treat the signs that occur.

Diagnosis

It is rare to make a definitive diagnosis in a case of suspected poisoning but it may be necessary to collect samples for later analysis in case of legal disputes. Blood samples are often required for monitoring the condition of sick patients.

Treatment

A patient must be stabilised before any other treatments are instigated. Proceed as follows:

- If the animal is unconscious, respiratory and cardiovascular function should be assessed and support provided if necessary. Unconscious animals should be intubated with a cuffed endotracheal tube and manually ventilated if respiration is depressed. If blood loss is severe blood transfusions may be given. Fluid loss can be corrected with plasma expanders or Hartmann's solution.
- Seizures should be controlled with anticonvulsants, e.g. diazepam or anaesthetics. Avoid treating the excitement associated with alphachloralose toxicity if possible as animals subsequently become depressed and sedation will exacerbate this effect. Depressed or unconscious patients must be closely monitored and appropriate support of vital functions given as necessary.
- Core body temperature may be elevated or depressed and any variances from normal should be regulated by the use of cold water or alcohol baths or external heating devices, respectively. Many poisons result in slow metabolism and hypothermia. Active warming with heat pads, warm i.v. fluids or baths is often needed. Shocked animals should be closely monitored as peripheral vasodilation can cause a fatal reduction of blood pressure. Some poisonings cause hyperthermia and if temperature rises above 105°F cooling is necessary to prevent tissue damage. Alcohol cooling is the safest method as it is difficult to reduce body temperature too low. Ice bags or cold water baths may also be used but careful monitoring is required to prevent overchilling.

Minimising toxin absorption gives the patient the best chance of recovery.

Topical exposure

Toxic or irritant substances on the coat should be removed by clipping or bathing. It may be necessary to use a solvent, e.g. vegetable oil, to remove tar or oil. Avoid using detergents and soaps as they may dissolve some substances and allow them to pass through the skin.

Ingested poisons

Initial treatment is aimed at removing as much of the poison as possible from the GI tract before it is absorbed. If an irritant has been ingested more damage to the oesophagus may be caused by removal, so the poison in the GI tract should be diluted and, if possible, absorption reduced by binding to an inert substance.

Emesis

Vomiting can be induced if it is less than 2 hours since poison was ingested. Some substances, e.g. chocolate and aspirin, stay longer in the stomach and emesis may be useful for up to 6 hours after ingestion. Vomiting should never be induced if the animal:

- is already vomiting
- is depressed or unconscious
- has no gag reflex
- has ingested a caustic or petroleum-based substance.

Techniques

- 'Syrup of ipecac' (ipecacuanha emetic draught) causes vomiting within 15 minutes and can be repeated after 20 minutes if no vomiting occurs. However, this is only effective in half of all patients and if the animal fails to vomit gastric lavage must then be performed to remove the syrup which may be poisonous itself.
- Apomorphine injections can result in prolonged vomiting.
- The effectiveness and safety of table salt, washing soda, xylazine and hydrogen peroxide is questionable.

Gastric lavage

This is a useful technique if it is less than 2 hours since ingestion of the poison when it is likely that the poison will still be in the stomach. It can be performed in an unconscious animal, otherwise it requires light anaesthesia.

Technique

- To prevent the aspiration of stomach contents into the lungs a cuffed endotracheal tube is required and the head should be lowered with respect to the stomach.
- A tube is passed down the oesophagus into the stomach and 5–10 ml/kg warm water washed in and sucked out using a 50 ml syringe.
- This process is repeated 10–15 times, until the lavage fluid is returning clear.
- An adsorbent can be added to the final lavage fluid and left in the stomach for 10 minutes before washing out to assist in removal of the toxin.

Adsorbents

The most commonly used adsorbent is activated charcoal. A slurry of 1 g charcoal to 5–10 ml water is administered at 2–8 g/kg by stomach tube using a funnel. Alternatively the adsorbent can be administered 3–4 times daily for 3–4 days after intoxication. Cathartics, e.g. sodium hydroxide, are sometimes used along with adsorbents.

Diuresis

Diuresis helps in elimination of many toxins but should not be used in patients with:

- shock
- reduced renal function
- heart disease.

Intravenous fluids given at 2–3 times maintenance rate will increase the glomerular filtration rate and flush out soluble toxins. Urine output must be measured and if renal output is inadequate peritoneal dialysis may be necessary. Diuretic drugs should only be used to promote toxin elimination if intravenous fluid therapy is given and urine output is more than 0.1 ml/kg per minute. In acute renal failure diuretics may be used to stimulate urine output when it is low.

If the toxin has been identified it may be possible to administer an antidote. In general these must be given as soon as possible after poisoning to be effective. However, there are few specific antidotes and even if there is one it may not be readily available in the practice. All patients require symptomatic treatment whether or not an antidote is given. Antidotes should only be used if the poisoning is severe as many have severe side effects.

SPECIFIC POISONS
Coumarins (warfarin)

Cause: ingestion of rat poison – repeated small doses are more toxic than single large doses. Cats may be poisoned by eating poisoned rodents.

Signs: not present for 1–2 days following ingestion of poison. These relate to haemorrhage and include depression and weakness as a result of blood loss. Other signs relate to the site of bleeding, e.g. dyspnoea and coughing, as a result of haemorrhage into the respiratory tract. Prolonged bleeding from minor wounds, e.g. venepuncture sites, is common.

Diagnosis: usually suspected from history and signs. Whole blood clotting time (WBCT), one stage prothrombin time (OSPT) and activated partial thromboplastin time (APTT) are all increased. Treatment usually has to be given on suspicion of diagnosis but enquiries should be made to identify the particular type of coumarin that the patient has had access to, as this will have an influence on the duration of treatment required.

Treatment: trauma must be avoided – cage rest and minimal handling are important aspects of management. In severe cases whole blood administration and oxygen therapy may be required. Vitamin K_1 supplementation is needed until the patient is able to make its own clotting factors again. The duration of replacement therapy depends upon the type of coumarin ingested – clotting times should be checked after treatment has been stopped and therapy continued if necessary.

Metaldehyde

Cause: found in some forms of slug pellets. These seem to be very palatable to dogs although poisoning in cats is rare.

Signs: mainly neurological signs – hyperaesthesia, convulsions, tremors and incoordination. These may progress to opisthotonus, nystagmus and tachycardia.

Diagnosis: based on signs and often known ingestion of slug pellets.

Treatment: emesis or gastric lavage recommended in early stage. Liquid paraffin may help to reduce further absorption. If seizures are severe anticonvulsants can be given.

Ethylene glycol

Cause: found in antifreeze which appears palatable to small animals and they will often drink it voluntarily. There may be a history of recent car radiator drainage.

Signs: occur within 1 hour of ingestion, and are due to kidney damage and acute renal failure. Vomiting, ataxia/weakness, dehydration, polydipsia and polyuria with milder cases developing oliguric renal failure and more severe toxicoses progressing to central nervous system depression, convulsions or coma.

Diagnosis: serum levels peak at 3 hours and urinary excretion is evident at 6 hours.

Treatment: the initial aim is to prevent absorption and metabolism by the use of emetics and cathartics. Supportive care requires correction of fluid balance and metabolic acidosis. Once the patient is rehydrated continue intravenous fluids until all toxin is eliminated.

DRUGS COMMONLY USED IN THE MANAGEMENT OF POISONED ANIMALS
Activated charcoal

This is an absorbent compound which traps toxins in the gut and prevents them from being absorbed into the bloodstream.

Anticonvulsants

Seizuring is a common sign associated with poisoning. Phenobarbital or pentobarbitone is used in the management of severe recurring seizures or status epilepticus. These drugs act by reducing the sensitivity of the brain cells so that it is harder for a seizure to get going. Phenobarbital is relatively short acting and is usually used early in the course of treatment. In status epilepticus pentobarbitone may be used intravenously for its prolonged action. This may induce anaesthesia necessitating endotracheal intubation and respiratory support as necessary.

Diazepam has a relatively short duration of action and is given by intravenous injection or per rectum (suppository). It is used in dogs to control status epilepticus.

Emetics

Apomorphine is an opioid agent given by injection and is an extremely effective emetic. Ipecac syrup is given orally and is available in many practices. A few crystals of washing soda placed on the back of the tongue can be an effective method of emesis. Hydrogen peroxide is a relatively unreliable emetic.

Diuretics

Loop diuretics (e.g. furosemide (frusemide)) are effective and osmotic diuretics, e.g. mannitol, can also be used. They are most effective in the elimination of toxins that are renally excreted in an unchanged form. If diuresis is being induced the patient should be catheterised so that urine production can be monitored and fluid balance must be maintained by administration of appropriate intravenous fluids.

NUTRITION

It is beyond the scope of this chapter to discuss the nutritional requirements of the healthy animal. Specific nutritional requirements in the management of specific medical conditions are given in the treatment sections of each disease section.

It is very important to consider the nutritional needs of any sick patient as they are likely to be very different from the healthy animal. In most diseases calorie requirements are increased but appetite may be suppressed. Initially metabolism slows to conserve energy resources but subsequently metabolism is accelerated to repair injuries. A relatively minor trauma can increase metabolic requirements by 10%. In the face of increased caloric requirements breakdown of body tissues occurs:

- Fat is broken down to fatty acids.
- Protein is metabolised to amino acids and glucose.

Stressed animals have more difficulty utilising carbohydrates and preference is given to fat metabolism. Malnutrition during illness can result in delayed recovery (poor wound healing and reduced immune function), and loss of body tissues (muscle wastage and weakness).

Sickness increases nutritional requirements in a number of ways.

Attention should be paid to ensuring all sick patients eat adequately. Techniques to encourage eating include offering highly palatable, strong-smelling, warmed food and frequent feeding of small meals. Convalescent diets are usually concentrated feeds which have a high fat content and contain high levels of high biological value protein. These diets should be used with caution in many medical conditions in which there are specific nutritional requirements. In some cases assisted feeding by the placement of naso-oesophageal or oesophagostomy, pharyngostomy or gastrostomy feeding tubes may be necessary. Syringe feeding is not recommended as there is a risk of aspiration of food material into the respiratory tract. Provided that there is a functional gastrointestinal tract enteral nutrition is the most practical and beneficial form of providing nutrition. Parenteral feeding, i.e. intravenous feeding, is very expensive and requires high levels of monitoring.

Assisted feeding should be considered in patients where:

- There are poor body reserves at the start of disease (malnourished animals).

- There is a substantial loss of bodyweight during disease.
- Oral intake is reduced for more than 3 days.

Appetite stimulants, e.g. intravenous diazepam and B vitamins, can be useful for encouraging feeding in inappetant cats.

PART

2

Musculoskeletal system

Stephen J Baines

INTRODUCTION

Although musculoskeletal system disease is generally considered to be a surgical topic, the reality is that medical management is appropriate for many disorders affecting the musculoskeletal system. In addition, in those cases requiring surgical management, medical therapy is likely to play an important part in the pre- and postoperative management of the case. This section will review the musculoskeletal system in health and disease, with a bias towards medical disorders and their therapy. However, some basic knowledge of surgical management needs to be included in order to understand the rationale for medical therapy.

ANATOMY AND PHYSIOLOGY OF THE MUSCULOSKELETAL SYSTEM

Bones

The functions of bones are to:

- provide strength to the skeleton
- provide support to the soft tissues
- act as levers for muscles and tendons
- provide protection for vital organs
- act as a reservoir of calcium and phosphate.

The structure of a typical long bone is shown in Figure 3.13. The bone consists of:

- diaphysis
- epiphysis
- physis
- metaphysis
- medullary cavity
- periosteum

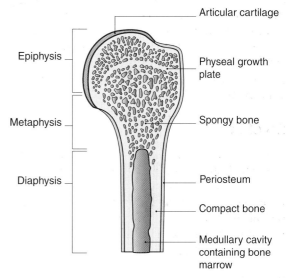

Figure 3.13 Anatomic features of a typical long bone. (From *Pre-Veterinary Nursing Textbook* by Masters and Bowden (2001). Reprinted by permission of Elsevier Science.)

- endosteum
- articular cartilage.

The diaphysis comprises an outer cylinder of cortical bone surrounding the central medullary cavity. In skeletally immature animals, increase in bone length occurs by growth at the physis (growth plate), which separates the epiphysis from the metaphysis. Once maturity is reached, the physis closes and the metaphysis and epiphysis unite to form a single metaphysis. The epiphyses arise from separate centres of ossification and have an articular surface covered by hyaline cartilage. The remainder of the long bone is covered by periosteum and the inner surfaces of the diaphysis are covered by endosteum.

Bone is composed of:

- organic matrix
- mineral
- bone cells.

The organic matrix consists primarily of proteoglycans and collagen and comprises approximately one third of the bone tissue. The mineral, which makes up most of the remaining two thirds, consists of calcium phosphate in the form of hydroxyapatite. The cells include osteoblasts, osteocytes and osteoclasts, and these cells regulate the structure and mineral composition of the bone.

Osteoblasts are bone-forming cells which are found on the surface of cortices or trabeculae on which matrix is being formed. Osteocytes are osteoblasts that have become trapped in this developing matrix. Osteoclasts are large, multinucleated cells involved in bone removal. Removal of bone by osteoclasts and deposition of bone by osteoblasts allow the growth and remodelling of bone to occur.

Bone matrix exists as either compact cortical bone or spongy cancellous bone. Cortical bone is found primarily in the diaphyses of the long bones and cancellous bone is found at the metaphyses. In the formation of bone, either embryologically or during healing with the formation of a callus, bone tissue is first formed as woven bone, with random orientation of the collagen fibres and is then remodelled into lamellar bone, with collagen fibres arranged in an organised, parallel fashion.

Joints

Joints are classified according to the amount of movement possible:

- synarthroses: immovable joints, e.g. the sutures in the skull
- amphiarthroses: partially movable joints, e.g. the pubic symphysis
- diarthroses: freely movable joints, e.g. hip joint.

Diarthrodial joints are the most important type from the point of view of musculoskeletal system disease and are further classified according to the type of movement they permit:

- enarthrosis or ball and socket joint, allowing movement in all planes, e.g. hip
- condylarthrosis or condyloid joint, allowing movement in flexion, extension, abduction and adduction, but no rotation, e.g. carpus
- sellar or saddle-shaped joints, allowing movement in flexion, extension, abduction and adduction, and slight rotation, e.g. interphalangeal joint
- ginglymus or hinged joint, allowing movement in flexion and extension only, e.g. elbow
- trochoid or pivot joint, allowing rotatory movement only, e.g. atlanto-axial joint
- arthrosis or plain joint, allowing only a slight degree of gliding between adjacent bones, e.g. between individual carpal and tarsal bones.

The structure of a typical diarthrodial joint is illustrated in Figure 3.14 and comprises:

- articular cartilage
- synovial fluid
- synovial membrane
- fibrous joint capsule
- ligaments.

Hyaline articular cartilage covers the articular surfaces of joints and lies immediately above the subchondral bone. Its function is to provide a smooth surface for articulation, to protect the ends of the bones from concussive injury and to provide a growth zone for the epiphysis in skeletally immature animals.

Articular cartilage consists of chondrocytes embedded in a matrix composed of proteoglycan aggregates, collagen and other fibres and water. The proteoglycan aggregates consist of a number of proteoglycans bound non-covalently to a hyaluronic acid core (Fig. 3.15). The basic structure of the proteoglycan is a monomer subunit composed of glycosaminoglycans (GAGs) attached covalently to a central protein core. GAGs are long, unbranched carbohydrates made up of repeating disaccharide units. The predominant GAGs of articular cartilage are chondroitin sulphate and keratan sulphate.

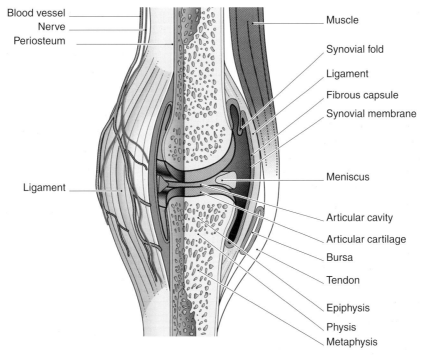

Figure 3.14 Anatomic features of a typical diarthrodial joint.

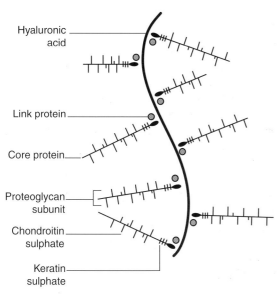

Figure 3.15 Schematic representation of the proteoglycan aggregate of articular cartilage.

Synovial fluid is a dialysate of plasma, to which mucopolysaccharide is added. This mucopoly-saccharide is responsible for the viscosity of the fluid. Synovial fluid provides lubrication within the joint and provides nutrition for intra-articular structures, such as articular cartilage, ligaments and menisci.

The synovial membrane lines the fibrous joint capsule and intra-articular ligaments. It constitutes a barrier between the blood and the synovial fluid and maintains the intrasynovial environment by producing mucopolysaccharide and clearing debris by phagocytosis.

The fibrous joint capsule is attached to the bones forming the joint and forms the external borders of the joint. Together with the synovial membrane, the joint capsule keeps the synovial fluid within the joint and, in conjunction with ligaments, muscles and tendons, limits the movement of the adjacent bones. These ligaments may be thickenings within the joint capsule itself, or may be distinct intra- or extra-articular structures. Defects in the joint capsule allow intra-articular tendons to leave the joint and allow the synovial membrane to form a bursa beneath a tendon.

Menisci are intra-articular fibrocartilaginous structures which facilitate joint lubrication, act as shock-absorbers and improve joint congruity.

Muscle and tendon

Striated muscle, as found in the musculoskeletal system, is composed of numerous long muscle cells or sarcomeres arranged into long muscle fibres (Fig. 3.16). Individual muscle fibres are surrounded by the endomysium and are bound together in bundles or fascicles. Individual fascicles are separated by the perimysium and groups of fascicles form the muscle, which is covered by a fascial layer, the epimysium.

Tendons are extensions of the muscle at each end and attach the muscle to bone at its origin and insertion. Tendons are composed of long spiralling bundles of collagen fibres arranged in parallel rows which are embedded in ground substance and extracellular fluid. The collagen fibres and tenocytes are surrounded by the endotenon and the entire tendon is surrounded by the epitenon. The free-gliding motion of the tendon is provided by the outer sheath or paratenon, which separates tendons from each other and may form a synovial sheath at areas of local pressure. Tendons act to facilitate and transmit forces developed by muscles across joints. Retinacular bands may alter the pull of the tendon as it crosses the joint. Tendons have a greater elasticity than ligaments, which may protect muscles and tendons from the sudden application of force.

Ligaments

Ligaments are composed of longitudinally oriented bundles of collagen fibres. Ligaments provide stability to joints and serve to guide joint motion.

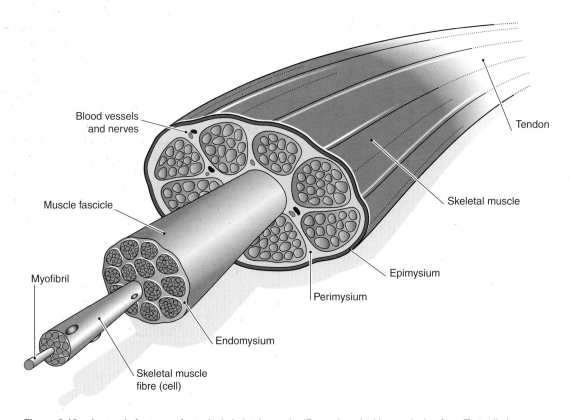

Figure 3.16 Anatomic features of a typical skeletal muscle. (Reproduced with permission from Tartaglia.)

This structure gives them much greater tensile strength in tension than in shear or torsion. However, ligaments are relatively inelastic, compared to tendons, and, if the tensile load exceeds the ligament's elasticity, the collagen fibres become permanently damaged.

DIAGNOSIS

The diagnosis of disorders of the musculoskeletal system is based primarily on the clinical examination of the patient. Ancillary diagnostic aids may be used to confirm a clinical diagnosis or to document the severity of the disease. However, over-reliance on additional diagnostic tests should be discouraged, since there may be discordance between the findings. For instance, some animals have severely disabling osteoarthritis (OA) with minimal changes on radiographs and others will have marked radiographic changes, but do not display lameness.

History and presenting complaint

The owner's primary complaint should be clearly identified. The nature of the onset and duration of the problem are recorded. It should be identified whether the condition is static or progressive and continuous or intermittent. Association with rest or exercise, and the ground surface should be determined. Alteration in the animal's willingness to exercise and change in temperament are noted.

The animal's signalment, previous medical history and proposed or current use of the animal (e.g. breeding, showing, racing or working) are noted. Knowledge of the health and medical history of the parents and siblings may be useful if hereditary disease is suspected.

Examination

Physical examination

The aim of the physical examination is to identify the general health of the animal and to identify any concurrent or underlying medical disorders. The suitability of the patient for sedation or anaesthesia and surgery also needs to be assessed.

Orthopaedic examination

The aim of the examination is to identify the patient's primary problem and to assess its clinical severity. A thorough examination of the entire musculoskeletal system is performed to rule out any concurrent orthopaedic disease, particularly in the contralateral limb. A screening neurological examination is often performed to rule out neurological disease as the cause of the disorder. The clinical findings are gathered from observation, palpation, manipulation and gait analysis.

The general body condition and condition of the coat and hair are assessed. The animal's general disposition (friendly, nervous or aggressive) and the likelihood of the owner being able to handle the animal during the examination are assessed. The conformation of the trunk is assessed for abnormalities (lordosis, kyphosis and scoliosis). The limbs are evaluated for angular deviations (valgus or varus), flexural deformities (hyperextension or hyperflexion) and rotational deformities (toe-in or toe-out). The animal's behaviour at rest may yield important information. Animals with a hindlimb lameness may tend to sit and those with a forelimb lameness may lie down. Resting limb while standing, shifting of weight between the limbs and apprehension or multiple attempts to sit or stand may be apparent.

The animal's gait is evaluated before examining the limbs to avoid exacerbating problems by performing manipulations which might induce pain or discomfort. The animal is observed as it walks on the lead away from and towards the examiner. The procedure is then repeated at the trot. Faster gaits may be required to evaluate some disorders and a period of off-lead exercise may be useful. Certain manoeuvres may be required to exacerbate subtle lamenesses, such as moving the animal in tight circles and encouraging the animal to climb kerbs or stairs.

Gait abnormalities which may be seen include:

- short stride length
- abnormal joint movement
- dragging of toenails
- limb circumduction during protraction
- hypermetria

- stumbling
- general weakness
- ataxia
- criss-crossing of legs
- abnormal sounds (clicks, snaps)
- head bob (head elevates when lame leg hits the ground).

The aim of palpation is to detect general abnormalities of the musculoskeletal system and the entire animal should be palpated. With the animal standing symmetrically, the contralateral limbs are examined simultaneously. The animal is examined for the presence of swellings affecting bone or soft tissues, muscle atrophy, focal areas of heat or pain and wounds. The general conformation of the animal, symmetry of the major bony landmarks and equality of weight-bearing between the two paired limbs are also evaluated.

A systematic examination of each limb should be performed. The limbs should be examined with the animal lying in lateral recumbency, although the forelimbs may be examined with the animal sitting, and the hindlimbs with the animal standing. The limbs should be evaluated from the toes proximally. The abnormal limb should be examined last and any manoeuvres which might cause pain should be performed last. This allows the animal to relax during the examination and allows the clinician to learn the animal's response to manipulation. Comparison with the contralateral limb is useful in determining the clinical significance of any finding, although it must be remembered that bilateral disease is common.

The joints are examined for effusion, peri-articular swelling, range of motion, instability, crepitus and pain. The limbs are examined for swelling, muscle atrophy, malalignment of bony landmarks, wounds and focal areas of pain.

Additional procedures may be performed if indicated following the results of the orthopaedic examination. These include tests of hip joint laxity (Barden's hip lift test, Ortolani test) and tests of cranio-caudal instability in the stifle joint due to cranial cruciate ligament rupture (cranial drawer sign, tibial compression test). These manoeuvres may induce pain and are better performed with the animal sedated or anaesthetised, e.g. during radiography.

Neurological examination

A screening neurological examination is performed to rule out neurological diseases as the cause of the disorder. Tests of sensory function (paw position, reflex stepping and sway tests) and motor function (wheelbarrowing, extensor postural thrust, hemistanding and hemiwalking) are performed. Each limb is evaluated for muscle tone, muscle atrophy, spinal myotactic reflexes, presence of cutaneous sensation and deep pain perception. If any abnormalities are identified, or if there is a high index of suspicion for neurological disease, a full and complete neurological examination is performed.

Imaging

Following the clinical examination, one or more imaging procedures are generally used to help reach a specific diagnosis and to assess the stage of the disease. The results of these procedures are interpreted in the light of the clinical findings.

Radiography

Radiography is the most commonly used diagnostic aid. Radiographs should be used to evaluate clinical findings rather than as a survey to identify any abnormality.

Two orthogonal radiographs are generally required. On occasion, additional oblique or sky-line views may be required, e.g. when investigating complex joints such as the carpus or hock.

Stressed radiographs are used to confirm abnormal joint laxity due to ligament damage. Stress is applied to the joints using ties, sandbags or foam wedges. Abnormal angulation of the bones and a change in the joint space will be identified in the unstable joint.

Contrast radiography (arthrography) is performed by the injection of a water-soluble iodine-containing positive contrast agent into the joint, following arthrocentesis. Arthrography is used to delineate the surface of articular cartilage, to identify the position and integrity of the joint capsule and to identify the presence of other intra-articular structures, e.g. joint mice. This technique is commonly used in the shoulder joint to identify cartilage lesions in osteochondrosis and to image the tendon and sheath of the biceps brachii muscle.

Ultrasound

Ultrasonography is used to examine the soft tissues. It may be employed to examine tendons, tendon sheaths, e.g. the biceps tendon, and certain large joints, e.g. the stifle. However, the high echogenicity of bone limits its routine use.

Scintigraphy

Scintigraphy is performed by evaluating the uptake of a radiopharmaceutical by various tissues, following its intravenous injection. The commonly used isotope is ^{99m}Technetium diphosphonate, which is incorporated into the hydroxyapatite crystals of bone. Uptake is dependent on local blood flow and metabolic activity of the tissues. The soft tissues and bone are evaluated at different times post-injection. Scintigraphy allows the anatomic location of areas of inflammation or bone turnover to be identified, but does not reveal anything about their significance or aetiology. As such it is a useful screening test for occult lameness or the detection of metastases, but does not allow a definitive diagnosis to be made.

Computed tomography

CT is a cross-sectional imaging technique based on X-ray absorption. The X-ray beam is passed through the patient at various angles and the data are collected and analysed to give a cross-sectional image. These images allow visualisation of anatomic structures without the superimposition found in standard radiographs. CT is superior to MRI for the visualisation of osseous structures, e.g. fragmented medial coronoid process in the elbow joint.

Magnetic resonance imaging

MRI is a cross-sectional imaging system which uses radiofrequency rather than X-ray photons to produce the images. The patient is placed in a strong magnetic field which aligns the magnetic vectors of the atoms in the body. Radiofrequency waves are then passed through the body to deflect the magnetic vectors. Depending on the characteristics of the atoms in a given tissue, the vectors return to alignment with the magnetic field at different rates and emit radiofrequency waves which are detected by a receiving coil. This information is relayed to a computer which generates a cross-sectional image. A major advantage of MRI is the ability to differentiate soft tissue structures, which allows visualisation of cartilage, ligaments, tendons and subchondral bone.

Diagnostic aids

Following the clinical examination and appropriate imaging procedures, ancillary diagnostic aids are often required to reach or confirm a diagnosis. The results of these tests are then interpreted in the light of the clinical findings.

Non-invasive diagnostic aids

Routine blood screens may detect underlying or unrecognised medical disorders which need treatment. Measurement of a few basic parameters, e.g. PCV, plasma protein, may be required as part of a pre-anaesthetic work-up.

A complete blood count may reveal an inflammatory leucogram in animals with wounds or inflammatory disorders (e.g. polyarthropathies). Anaemia may be due to blood loss in trauma cases, or anaemia of chronic disease.

Animals with polyarthropathies may show elevations in alanine aminotransferase, aspartate aminotransferase, and alkaline phosphatase. Animals with destructive lesions of bone may also show elevation in alkaline phosphatase. Globulin levels may be elevated because of increased production and albumin may be decreased in animals with protein-losing nephropathy or enteropathy associated with immune-mediated polyarthritis. Elevations in creatine kinase levels may be seen in animals with myopathies.

Proteinuria may be seen in animals with glomerulonephropathy associated with immune-mediated polyarthropathies. Collection and routine analysis of the urine is an important part of ensuring adequate renal function in the trauma patient.

Culture of body fluids or tissues is important in the diagnosis and management of infectious disorders of the musculoskeletal system, primarily septic arthritis, osteomyelitis and discospondylitis. Culture of synovial fluid or synovial membrane may be used to differentiate infectious from non-infectious arthritis. Improved results may be obtained if the sample is submitted into blood culture medium rather than a bacteriology swab or a plain tube. If a sample of the lesion cannot be retrieved, then culture of a urine sample or blood sample may identify the organism if a haematogenous aetiology is suspected. Culture of the surgical wound may be performed immediately before closure if wound contamination is considered likely, e.g. cases of open fractures, and in complex procedures where infection would be disastrous, e.g. total hip replacement.

Serologic tests may be used in the diagnosis of polyarthropathies. These include rheumatoid factor (elevated in rheumatoid arthritis) and antinuclear antibody (elevated in systemic lupus erythematosus (SLE)). Antibodies directed against erythrocytes, leucocytes or platelets may be identified in patients with multisystemic polyarthritis. The measurement of antibody against specific pathogens may also be used, e.g. *Toxoplasma*, *Neospora* and *Borrelia*.

Invasive diagnostic aids

Although well-used in equine lameness, nerve blocks are not used routinely in small animal orthopaedics. The aim is to identify the location of the source of pain by causing resolution of the lameness following the injection of local anaesthetic. The main uses are local (individual nerves) or regional (ring block) anaesthesia of the digits and intra-articular blocks. If the technique

cannot be performed in the conscious animal, a long-acting local anaesthetic (e.g. bupivicaine) is administered during a short-acting general anaesthetic (e.g. propofol) to ensure the local analgesia is still present following recovery.

Electromyography (EMG) examines the action potentials in small numbers of muscle fibres. Spontaneous activity in muscles is abnormal and indicates either denervation of the muscle, because of a lesion in the lower motor neurone supplying the muscle, or the presence of a myopathy. The major use of this technique is to differentiate denervation (where the EMG is abnormal) and disuse (where the EMG is normal) in animals with lameness and muscle atrophy. Nerve conduction velocity (NCV) studies will allow the speed of conduction within peripheral nerves to be examined in animals where a peripheral neuropathy is suspected.

Synovial fluid analysis is a valuable aid to establishing a diagnosis in joint disease. Most patients will require sedation or general anaesthesia. The hair is clipped from around the joints and the skin is prepared aseptically. Synovial fluid is aspirated with a 21 or 23 gauge needle attached to a 2 ml or 5 ml syringe. Very little fluid is recovered from a normal joint. Normal synovial fluid is clear, colourless or pale yellow and viscous. Gross abnormalities seen in joint disease include increase in volume, reduction in viscosity, turbidity and change in colour.

A direct smear is made of the joint fluid and if enough is collected, fluid is placed into ethylenediaminetetraacetic acid (EDTA). The cell count, cell type and morphology are assessed. This should allow the differentiation of inflammatory and degenerative arthropathies, and the separation of infectious from non-infectious joint diseases. The results of synovial fluid analysis in different joint diseases are illustrated in Table 3.17.

Tissue biopsy may be required to achieve a definitive diagnosis, particularly in animals with myopathies or focal bone lesions. Synovial membrane biopsies are usually taken at arthrotomy, although a tissue sample may be recovered arthroscopically or percutaneously with a needle. Muscle biopsies are performed by removing an ellipse of tissue following an open surgical approach to the

Table 3.17 Synovial fluid analysis in canine joint diseases

Parameter	Normal joint	Osteoarthritis	Immune-mediated arthritis	Septic arthritis
Colour	Clear/pale yellow	Yellow	Yellow, +/− blood tinged	Yellow, +/− blood tinged
Clarity	Transparent	Transparent	Transparent or opaque	Opaque
Viscosity	Very high	High	Low or very low	Very low
Mucin clot	Good	Good–fair	Fair–poor	Poor
Spontaneous clot	None	+/−	Often	Often
Leucocytes (mm^3)	<1000	1000–5000	>5000	>5000
Neutrophils	<5%	<10%	10–95%	>90%
Mononuclear cells	>95%	>90%	5–90%	<10%
Protein (g/dl)	2.0–2.5	2.0–3.0	2.5–5.0	>4.0

muscle. The sample is allowed to rest on a piece of card or may be pinned to a piece of cork prior to fixation, to prevent muscle contracture. Bone core biopsies are taken percutaneously with a needle, e.g. Jamshidi type.

A rigid arthroscope is introduced into the joint to allow the direct visualisation of the joint and the intra-articular structures, and permit sampling of tissue within the joint. Arthroscopy is a less invasive procedure than arthrotomy and may be used to collect synovial membrane biopsies. However, because of the size of the arthroscopes, arthroscopy is limited to the larger joints of large-breed dogs. Disadvantages include the expense of the equipment and the necessity to learn a difficult and demanding technique.

Some joint diseases may only be confirmed following an open surgical approach to the joint. Although surgery is more invasive than arthroscopy, this approach may also allow treatment of the lesion.

TREATMENT OF MUSCULOSKELETAL DISEASE

Disorders of the musculoskeletal system may be treated surgically or non-surgically. Non-surgical therapy may be further divided into medical therapy, which is dependent on the administration of drugs, and conservative therapy, which consists primarily of changes to the patient's lifestyle. The therapies considered as non-surgical treatment also have a role to play in the post-operative care and rehabilitation of the surgical patient. Non-surgical therapy may also include the use of bandages and slings to support or limit the use of the affected part.

Many disorders may be treated in a number of different ways and the most appropriate therapy may depend on the nature and severity of the disease, the nature of the animal and its intended use and the owner's wishes. For instance, the majority of fractures are treated surgically, but animals with chronic joint disease are treated non-surgically initially, with surgical management performed if this treatment is not successful.

Non-surgical management – the aims

The success of non-surgical management often depends on the expectations of the owner and clinician. If it is expected that one off-the-shelf treatment regime will work for all animals or will always work for a single individual, and that all diseases will always be cured, then the clinician will be disappointed. If non-surgical management is used with an understanding of the disease process and with reasonable expectations, it may be successful. The clinical signs and underlying pathological changes may change during the dog's life and therapy may have to be adjusted to account for this variability.

Reasonable expectations of the non-surgical management of musculoskeletal disease are relieving pain, maintaining joint function and allowing normal activity. Expectations that are often stated but may not be achieved are minimising damage to articular cartilage, promoting articular cartilage repair and minimising the development and progression of osteoarthritis. Unreasonable expectations are achieving a cure of chronic conditions such as osteoarthritis and the prevention of progression of chronic diseases.

Conservative management

Exercise

Restricted exercise This has traditionally been a mainstay of therapy in patients with joint disease, particularly osteoarthritis, and patients learn to live with the limitations of the disease. The rationale for limited exercise is that exercise places stress on the abnormal, thickened and inflamed peri-articular tissues, causing the release of inflammatory mediators, which results in acute exacerbation of pain. By limiting exercise, inflammation is minimised and the joint will not be painful. In addition, exercise may lead to additional mechanical trauma to the joint, potentially accelerating the disease process. However, severe exercise restriction may result in exercise intolerance, loss of muscle mass and tone, decreased range of motion, exacerbation of cartilage destruction and social maladjustment.

Controlled exercise This has the benefit that muscle strength and cardiovascular fitness will be maintained, without causing joint inflammation, stiffness and pain. Joint movement is important in maintaining cartilage nutrition, and adequate development of the peri-articular soft tissues is important in the stabilisation of the lax joint. The correct amount of exercise is that which the animal can tolerate without exacerbating signs of stiffness or lameness and may have to be identified by trial and error.

Cage rest This may be appropriate as the sole method of treatment of minimally displaced or well-splinted fractures, e.g. certain pelvic fractures. It is also used post-operatively for certain fractures to prevent disruption of the repair by weight-bearing. The treatment of young puppies with joint laxity by severe exercise restriction by limiting them to a small cage, e.g. of $1\,m^3$ size, has been reported. Placing a puppy in a small area forces it to sit, thereby maintaining an abduction–flexion position. This method of treat-

ment has been shown to prevent the development of hip dysplasia (HD) in genetically predisposed dogs. However, these dogs did not develop well socially and this method of treatment is not recommended.

Many animals present initially with a bout of lameness or gait abnormality brought on by an acute flare-up or increase in severity of osteoarthritis. For the first 7–10 days, these animals should be restricted to lead exercise only, for short walks of 5 minutes' duration, 3–4 times daily. Simple passive range of motion physiotherapy exercises may be of benefit, particularly before a walk. Care should be taken to provide comfortable bedding. Over the next 3–5 weeks, the amount of lead exercise may be slowly increased. As the first line of treatment, no off-lead exercise should be allowed for 4–6 weeks. It must be emphasised that free access to a garden off the lead is not allowed.

After this initial period, lead exercise of increasing duration and a gradual return to off-lead exercise should be instituted, as detailed below. The main reason for the apparent failure of conservative management to improve clinical signs is a failure to adhere to these recommendations.

The aim of long-term management is to find a level of exercise with which the dog can cope, which does not exacerbate clinical signs. Exercise should be the same each day and moderate in intensity. Periods of inactivity (e.g. during the week) followed by excessive exercise (e.g. at the weekend) are to be avoided. Common sense should dictate the amount of exercise, ensuring adequate periods of rest in between. Lead exercise at a controlled pace is least likely to be detrimental. Off-lead exercise or playing with toys or other dogs is more likely to exacerbate the disease. A non-weightbearing exercise such as swimming is beneficial and yields the positive benefits of exercise while placing minimal stresses on the joint.

Weight control

Prevention of obesity is recommended to decrease the stresses placed on joints and peri-articular tissue. Obesity is a major risk factor in the development of osteoarthritis in humans and weight loss leads to relief of pain and increased ability to exercise. In dogs, dietary restriction and weight loss can reduce the incidence of HD and the development of OA.

The key to weight loss is to reduce calorie intake to less than caloric expenditure. A key first step is being able to quantify exactly how much food the animal normally eats and, ideally, the caloric density of that food. It should be borne in mind that if dietary management is instituted at the same time as exercise restriction, then caloric expenditure will also decrease. A target weight should be set. In addition, a target body shape should be set: the ribs should be easily palpable and the dog should have a definite indentation cranial to the wing of the ilium, i.e. a waistline.

A simple and achievable target for weight loss is to aim to reduce the animal's weight by 15% over 3 months. A simple formula exists to identify the proposed caloric intake of a dog with a target weight in mind:

diet calories = 60–70% of the calorie requirement for the target weight

The caloric requirement for a particular weight is given by:

calories (kCal/day) = (30 × weight (kg)) + 70

The most common reasons for failure are:

- owner or animal non-compliance
- poor estimation of bodyweight
- poor estimation of calorie requirements and calorific density of food
- defence of body fat, by reducing energy use and increasing hunger.

Environment and nursing care

Variation in the severity of arthritis with a change in the environmental temperature is well-recognised and keeping the animal in a warm environment may help alleviate the pain associated with OA. Providing a well-padded and warm bed within easy access will also make the animal more comfortable and help alleviate the pain of OA. Minimising contact with other dogs so that vigorous playing does not occur may be required during periods of acute exacerbation. Maintenance of a low-stress environment is important in the management of systemic diseases such as the polyarthropathies. Hand feeding and encouragement to eat may be required for anorexic animals.

Physiotherapy

The benefit of physiotherapy in the rehabilitation of canine patients is largely overlooked. The rational application of physical therapeutic modalities has the potential to improve the long-term outcome of animals with orthopaedic disease, including those managed both surgically and non-surgically. Physiotherapy is the treatment of diseases and injuries with physical agents such as heat, cold, water, sound, electricity, massage and exercise. The objectives are to promote healing and an early return to function and to prevent complications occurring from disuse of the affected area.

Positive benefits of physiotherapy include:

- increase in blood and lymphatic flow
- early resolution of inflammation
- prevention or minimisation of muscle atrophy
- prevention of peri-articular contraction
- positive psychological effects for patients and owners.

Veterinary rehabilitation protocols are based primarily on those proven to be of use in human medicine.

Passive range of motion exercise This is used whenever a patient has lack of motor control or is unwilling to use the limb because of pain. The objective of this therapy is to move the limb gently through a comfortable range of motion which requires no effort on the part of the patient.

Aims of passive range of motion exercise include:

- maintenance of normal range of motion in the joints
- prevention of soft tissue contracture
- improvement in blood and lymphatic circulation
- stimulation of sensory awareness

• reduction in the detrimental effect of immobility on articular cartilage.

These exercises should be performed slowly with the muscles relaxed. The therapy involves moving the limb through an unrestricted, pain-free motion for 10–15 repetitions, two or three times a day. One modification is to move the joint up to and beyond a normal range of motion and then hold the joint at this end point for up to 5 minutes. The technique chosen depends on the patient's comfort level and at no time should the patient experience discomfort. Painful manipulation may lead to reflex inhibition of movement, limited limb use, soft tissue contracture and a delayed return to function. The judicious use of NSAIDs or the application of a hot pack before these exercises may allow more pain-free movement.

Massage The benefits of massage include:

• increased arterial and lymphatic flow
• stretching and breakdown of adhesions
• provision of muscle relaxation
• provision of analgesia.

An even rhythm should be used during massage. A slow rate of massage will improve the circulation, reduce oedema and provide relaxation. Increasing the rate, when using frictional massage, will loosen adhesions. Light pressure achieves relaxation and reduction in oedema and firmer pressure is of more use in frictional massage.

Two commonly employed techniques are effleurage (stroking movement) and petrissage (kneading and pressing the muscles). Effleurage is performed by running the hands gently over the limb, from distal to proximal. Light contact is maintained and movement of the skin over the soft tissues will aid breakdown of adhesions. Petrissage is performed by lifting and kneading the soft tissues and rhythmically squeezing the deeper muscles. Initially, small circles are made with the heel of the hand, with gradually increasing pressure. Massage therapy may be performed every 24 to 48 hours.

Local application of heat This has been used for the treatment of arthritis in humans for a long time, although the exact mechanism of action is not understood. Warmth may only contribute to an overall feeling of well-being and thus relaxation in the animal. The heat produced by stretching or moderate exercise ('warming up') does allow improvement in musculoskeletal function. The rationale for this is that collagen fibres will elongate with increased temperature, which allows the peri-articular tissues to stretch and provide a better range of motion.

After the acute inflammation has subsided (after 48–72 hours following an injury or surgery), application of local warmth (40–45°C) to an area before massage or passive range of motion exercises is beneficial. This can be done by applying hot packs, using bags of fluids or damp hand towels that have been placed in a microwave.

The benefits of local warmth include:

• increase in resorption of extravasated fluid and reduced level of oedema
• stimulation of local metabolism and increased local delivery of nutrients
• increase in compliance of soft tissues, reducing joint stiffness and pain.

Treatment sessions should last 10–20 minutes and should be performed two to three times a day. The temperature of the heat source should be 40–45°C. The temperature of the skin should be assessed every 2–3 minutes. If the skin is hot to the touch, then more insulating towels should be placed between the heat source and the patient.

Monitoring the outcome of conservative therapy

An objective measure of the outcome of conservative therapy is required if rational decisions regarding future therapy are to be made. This is particularly important where the apparent response to therapy is slow. Comparisons of objective measurements allow the identification of improvement with positive feedback for the owner and veterinary surgeon.

Baseline measurements should be taken before starting therapy and then should be repeated at regular intervals. Suitable measurements include:

• range of motion in the joint
• circumference of the affected leg or legs
• lameness score
• activity level

- weight
- relative body condition.

In addition, subjective measurements also have a part to play. An assessment of the dog's general demeanour, willingness to exercise and appetite will give important information as to the success of therapy and the patient's quality of life.

Medical management

Drugs of a number of different classes have been used for the management of musculoskeletal disease in humans and animals. Medical therapy is used primarily in the management of joint disease and the most important facet of drug therapy in this respect is pain control.

Non-steroidal anti-inflammatory drugs

Pain and inflammation are present in OA and therefore the use of NSAIDs has been the mainstay of therapy for humans and animals with OA.
Pain associated with OA may arise from:

- synovitis
- microfractures of subchondral bone
- irritation of periosteal nerve endings by osteophytes
- stretching of peri-articular soft tissues by joint effusion or bone deformity
- muscle strain.

NSAIDs work by inhibiting cyclo-oxygenase, which is responsible for the production of prostaglandins (PGs) from arachidonic acid. PGs are important in the inflammatory process and may augment pain perception. NSAIDs may also influence neutrophil chemotaxis and stabilise lysosomal membranes, thus preventing the release of enzymes involved in inflammation.
Although NSAIDs provide pain relief, it is clear that they do not reverse or impede the progression of OA. Damaged chondrocytes continue to produce proteolytic enzymes that degrade the cartilage matrix. In fact, there is some evidence to indicate that NSAIDs may actually accelerate the degenerative process. NSAIDs may decrease the proteoglycan content of cartilage, thus rendering

it more susceptible to mechanical damage. However, this evidence is not conclusive and is not a reason to withhold the use of these drugs in patients with OA.
A number of licensed drugs are available, including carprofen, meloxicam, ketoprofen and phenylbutazone. These drugs should be used judiciously, making a clinical judgement of the risks of therapy and the potential benefit to the patient. They should be used at the smallest dose that provides a beneficial effect and should be discontinued if the animal can exercise without them. Long-term therapy may be required, but this should not be assumed, and reducing the dose and weaning the dog off the drug should be attempted. Using these drugs solely to permit a high level of physical activity is counterproductive in the long term.
Side effects include gastrointestinal irritation and ulceration, renal and hepatic toxicity and blood dyscrasias. Many of the patients with OA are geriatric and may have pre-existing renal and hepatic disease, which may potentiate side effects. Withdrawal of the drug and reinstituting therapy at a lower dose or with a different drug may be required.

Corticosteroids

Corticosteroids may be used at anti-inflammatory doses for the management of osteoarthritis or at immunosuppressive doses for the management of immune-mediated joint disease. Corticosteroids act primarily by inhibiting phospholipase A_2, thus reducing the levels of PGs, leukotrienes and other inflammatory mediators. In addition, they may also inhibit the action of matrix metalloproteinases. At higher doses, they suppress the immune response.
Corticosteroids are very effective in the treatment of acute inflammation. Intra-articular administration of single doses of corticosteroids is occasionally used, e.g. in the treatment of bicipital tenosynovitis. There appears to be relatively little detrimental effect following single doses of corticosteroids. However, the chronic nature of OA means that long-term therapy is required. Chronic parenteral and intra-articular

therapy with corticosteroids has been shown to lead to cartilage matrix degradation and break-down. For this reason, they are not recommended for chronic use. Corticosteroids are generally used either as the last resort for the treatment of OA refractory to other medications or to control an acute exacerbation of clinical signs, using a low dose for a few days only. Corticosteroids are the mainstay of therapy in animals with immune-mediated joint disease and may be used alone or in conjunction with other drugs.

Joint fluid modifiers

Normal chondrocytes produce polysulphated glycosaminoglycans (PSGAGs) and hyaluronic acid (HA) to maintain or repair the joint. These agents have been used frequently to treat carti-lage injuries in the horse. However, these drugs have not been fully evaluated in dogs, although anecdotal reports suggest that they may be valuable in the management of OA.

PSGAGs The mechanism of action of PSGAGs (Adequan) is not completely understood. In OA, cartilage proteoglycans are depleted and have a reduced ability to bind to HA. Lack of this PSGAG–HA aggregation decreases the cushion-ing effect of cartilage and makes the cartilage more susceptible to biomechanical damage.

Reported benefits of PSGAGs include:

- inhibition of destructive proteases in synovial fluid
- stimulation of proteoglycan synthesis
- increases in HA synthesis
- minimisation of cartilage fibrillation and erosion.

The ideal dose of PSGAGs for dogs with chronic OA is unknown. Recommended doses include 1–5 mg/kg i.m. once or twice a week for 4–8 weeks, followed by maintenance therapy at intervals of 1–3 months as needed to control clinical signs. PSGAGs have also been adminis-tered intra-articularly at 0.6 mg/kg once weekly. However, great care should be taken to ensure aseptic technique is maintained since PSGAGs have been shown to potentiate joint infection. Side effects include abnormalities of haemostasis, consisting of prolongation of the activated partial thromboplastin time, prothrombin time, activated clotting time and bleeding time.

HA Hyaluronic acid (Hylartil) is the most abundant component of synovial fluid and acts as a lubricant for articular surfaces and as a source of nutrients for avascular cartilage.

Reported benefits of HA include:

- scavenging of oxygen radicals
- inhibition of access of inflammatory enzymes to articular cartilage
- modulation of the cellular inflammatory response
- inhibition of PSGAG release from cartilage
- reduction of structural changes in cartilage seen in arthritis.

To date, no controlled studies on the use of HA in the management of OA in small animals are available. HA is administered by intra-articular injection, although no published dose rate is available.

Pentosan polysulphate (Cartrophen) Using this drug may be worthwhile in some animals with OA, particularly those that have gait abnor-malities but do not show a great deal of pain. It is less effective in animals with severe OA.

Glucosamine is an amino-saccharide and is the precursor to the disaccharide unit of GAGs. Chondroitin sulphate is a long-chain polymer of repeating disaccharide units (galactosamine and glucuronic acid).

The reported benefits of glucosamine include:

- provision of the raw materials for synthesis of GAGs and HA
- provision of a regulatory stimulus for cartilage synthesis.

The reported benefits of chondroitin include:

- increased synthesis of GAGs
- inhibition of degradative enzymes in the joint.

Controlled trials in humans with OA using glucosamine and chondroitin sulphate have shown a positive effect, as have trials with dogs following cranial cruciate ligament rupture. Cosequin (Nutramax Laboratories) is a nutra-ceutical marketed as a chondroprotective agent.

It contains glucosamine, chondroitin sulphate and manganese ascorbate. Studies in experimental animals have shown that a combination of these three ingredients was more efficacious than any agent used singly. Side effects include reduced haematocrit, haemoglobin and leucocyte count.

Essential fatty acids (EFAs)

It is proposed that n-3 and n-6 polyunsaturated fatty acids may reduce the production of PGs and therefore reduce pain. A decreased incidence of synovitis was seen in human patients with rheumatoid arthritis following treatment with these EFAs. One study performed to examine the effects of EFAs on dermatological disease in dogs noted that the patients seemed to be less painful and stiff following this medication. However, controlled clinical trials investigating the efficacy of these agents in dogs with OA are not available.

Vitamin C (ascorbate)

Vitamin C has been recommended to prevent HD in young dogs. The rationale for the use of vitamin C is that ascorbate is necessary for the hydroxylation of proline to hydroxyproline, a major component of collagen. It is proposed that a puppy deficient in vitamin C might have weak collagen, which might contribute to hip laxity. However, there is no definite proof of its effect.

Antibiotics

Antibiotics are indicated for infectious diseases of the musculoskeletal system, primarily osteomyelitis and septic arthritis. As with any organ system, treatment should be based on the results of culture and sensitivity testing. However, empirical treatment may be used before these results are known, or if no organism is cultured, but there is evidence of an infectious process, e.g. bacteria and degenerate neutrophils seen on cytological examination.

A broad-spectrum, bactericidal drug should be used initially and suitable choices include cephalosporins (e.g. cefalexin), clavulanate-potentiated amoxicillin and fluoroquinolones (e.g. enrofloxacin). Many isolates are beta-lactamase-secreting bacteria and antibiotics inactivated by this enzyme, e.g. ampicillin, are not a suitable first choice.

Chemotherapeutic drugs

Chemotherapeutic drugs are indicated for some forms of immune-mediated polyarthritis and for post-operative chemotherapy for musculoskeletal neoplasia. For immune-mediated polyarthritis, the commonly used drugs include cyclophosphamide and azathioprine. Side effects include myelosuppression and haemorrhagic cystitis. In neoplastic disease, cisplatin and doxorubicin are most commonly indicated. Side effects include nephrotoxicity and cardiotoxicity respectively.

Chrysotherapy

Therapy with gold salts is not commonly used, but may be indicated for cases of rheumatoid arthritis. Sodium aurothiomalate may be given by intramuscular injection, or auranofin may be given orally. Side effects include renal impairment, pulmonary fibrosis, corneal ulceration and diarrhoea.

Bandages, casts and slings

External coaptation may be used in injuries affecting the musculoskeletal system. These may be applied as a first aid measure prior to definitive treatment (e.g. splinting of a long bone fracture prior to surgery); as the sole method of treatment (e.g. incomplete or minimally displaced, well interdigitating fractures); as an adjunct to closed reduction of a luxated joint (e.g. Ehmer sling following coxofemoral joint luxation); or as an adjunct to surgery (e.g. external support of a pancarpal arthrodesis with a cast).

Bandages are used to protect a wound, to provide some external support to the limb, which may limit movement and reduce pain, and to reduce swelling of the limb. A splint is a bandage into which a stiffer material has been incorporated, usually along only one aspect of the limb. These may be premade splints or moulded splints made from thermoplastic or fibreglass material. A cast is a complete cylinder of rigid material which provides external support. Slings allow some degree of immobilisation of the limb and prevent weight-bearing. The forelimb may be immobilised with a Velpeau sling and the hindlimb with an Ehmer sling. A carpal flexion bandage prevents weight-bearing, but allows movement of the elbow and shoulder.

Surgical management – the aims

There is no space to give a detailed description of the types of surgical therapy and their indications. However, some basic knowledge of the surgical orthopaedics is required if appropriate medical care is to be provided.

Surgical therapy for bone disorders

Fracture fixation is a major part of surgical orthopaedics. Fracture repair may be achieved by external coaptation with casts and splints, or by the use of implants. These consist primarily of external skeletal fixators, screws and plates, interlocking nails and intramedullary pins. Adjunctive fixation of smaller fragments with screws, K-wires and cerclage wire may also be performed. Amputation may be required with irreparable fractures and other diseases, e.g. bone tumours.

Angular limb deformities in the young, growing dog may be treated by osteotomies or ostectomies to remove the effect of tension in individual bones of a pair (e.g. the ulna following premature closure of its distal growth plate), periosteal transection (to reduce the tethering effect of the periosteum) and staples across the growth plate (to retard growth on that side of the bone). In the adult dog, angular limb deformities may be treated by osteotomies and fixation of the bones.

Surgical therapy for joint disorders

Lavage may be performed following arthrocentesis for infectious arthritis. Arthroscopy is primarily a diagnostic tool although some conditions may be treated arthroscopically, e.g. osteochondrosis of the humeral head. Arthrotomy allows debridement of articular cartilage, e.g. in osteochondrosis, and fixation of intra-articular fractures. Joints with abnormal angulation of the bearing surfaces may be treated by osteotomy and fixation of the adjacent bones to re-align the joint surfaces, e.g. triple pelvic osteotomy in patients with abnormal hip laxity, or osteotomy alone, e.g. proximal dynamic ulna osteotomy in patients with ununited anconeal process.

Arthrodesis may be used to treat intractably painful joints, e.g. the hock with chronic osteochondrosis, or to treat ligamentous injuries, e.g. hyperextension injuries of the carpus. The chronically painful joint may also be treated by excision arthroplasty or by total joint replacement, e.g. the hip. Arthrodesis and excision or replacement arthroplasty are salvage procedures which are reserved for animals in which appropriate non-surgical management is failing.

Surgical therapy for muscle disorders

Muscle tears and ruptures may be subject to evacuation of the haematoma, debridement of the damaged muscle and primary closure. The primary repair is augmented with tension sutures placed in the muscle sheath. Resection of muscles may be performed for pain relief, e.g. pectineus myotomy or myectomy in hip dysplasia. Tenotomy may be required to alleviate the signs associated with muscle contracture, e.g. infraspinatus contracture.

Surgical therapy for tendon disorders

Primary repair of lacerated tendons may be performed. A suture pattern such as the Bunnell, locking loop or 3-loop pulley suture should be used. Additional techniques are required to support the joint and remove tension from the repair during the period of healing. Various techniques have been described to achieve tendon lengthening or shortening, following muscle contracture or inappropriate management of tendon rupture. The tendon of a functioning muscle may be transposed to perform the function of a nonfunctioning muscle (e.g. transposition of a carpal flexor to the extensor aspect of the joint in radial paralysis) or to augment the repair of an adjacent tendon (e.g. the use of the peroneus brevis tendon to fill a defect in the common calcaneal tendon). Surgical repair or prosthetic replacement of the surrounding retinaculum or ligaments may be required for tendon displacement.

Surgical therapy for ligament disorders

Surgical treatment of a second-degree sprain may involve imbrication or plication of the ligament, followed by external support. Surgical treatment of third-degree sprains involves primary repair of the damaged ligament with or without augmentation of the ligament with prosthetic suture material passed around screws or bone anchors. Large avulsed fragments of bone may be reattached with a screw, a screw and spiked washer or a loop of cerclage wire or non-absorbable suture passed through a bone tunnel. Post-operative immobilisation of the joint may be achieved with external coaptation, external fixators, temporary lag screws or cerclage wire.

COMMON MUSCULOSKELETAL CONDITIONS

Diseases affecting bones

Congenital abnormalities

Congenital deformities are not common and may involve a transverse defect in the limb (amelia), a longitudinal defect (hemimelia), duplication of the limbs (polymelia), longitudinal splitting of the distal limbs (ectrodactyly), the presence of one or more extra digits (polydactyly) and the fusion of two or more digits (syndactyly). The clinical significance of these conditions depends on the type of deformity and the degree of weight-bearing that is possible.

Metabolic abnormalities

The parathyroid gland produces parathyroid hormone in response to a decrease in serum calcium concentration. Parathyroid hormone acts on the bone to increase calcium release, on the intestine to increase calcium absorption and on the kidneys to reduce calcium excretion. The absorption of calcium from the bone results in a weaker structure which causes lameness, folding fractures of the long bones and compression fractures of the vertebrae. In addition, resorption of alveolar bone may result in the loss of teeth and new woven bone may obliterate the nasal cavity and cause thickening of the maxilla and mandibles. Treatment is aimed at correcting any underlying disease, while restricting the animal to strict cage rest to prevent pathological fractures.

Primary hyperparathyroidism This condition occurs as a result of oversecretion of parathyroid hormone due to a functional disorder of the gland. This is generally an adenoma, although carcinomas have been reported. Surgical removal of the gland is indicated.

Nutritional secondary hyperparathyroidism This occurs due to chronic hypocalcaemia, resulting in the secretion of parathyroid hormone. The hypocalcaemia results from the inadequate intake of calcium, e.g. an all-meat diet, or from diets with an abnormal calcium:phosphate balance, from malabsorption syndromes or from the presence of calcium-binding compounds (e.g. phytates) in the diet. This condition is treated by correcting the diet and treating any underlying disease.

Renal secondary hyperparathyroidism Resulting from chronic renal failure and impaired excretion of phosphate, hyperphosphataemia produces a compensatory fall in serum calcium, which stimulates the parathyroid gland. Chronic renal failure may result from juvenile nephropathy, interstitial nephritis, glomerulonephropathy and pyelonephritis. Treatment is palliative, as the condition is associated with chronic, irreversible renal damage.

Vitamin D deficiency This is uncommon and is known as rickets in immature animals and osteomalacia in adult animals. Dogs are unable to synthesise vitamin D in their skin and are dependent on the diet to supply this vitamin. In the immature animal, this deficiency results in the loss of the normal arrangement of chondrocytes at the growth plate and a failure of mineralisation of the cartilaginous matrix. This results in thickened, irregular growth plates and enlarged metaphyses, with the development of soft bones, which may bow. In the adult animal, the signs are less marked, with lameness being the main feature. The condition is treated by correcting the diet by providing adequate levels of vitamin D and the correct ratio of calcium to phosphate (1.2–1.4:1).

Vitamin A deficiency This is more common in the cat than the dog, since cats are unable to convert carotene to retinol. It is caused by dietary deficiency of the vitamin in immature animals. Clinical signs include lameness with malformed, shortened long bones, narrowed growth plates and thin cortices. Feeding of a balanced diet (containing 5000 IU vitamin A/kg dry matter) with supplementary vitamin A (200 IU vitamin A/kg body weight) is indicated.

Hypervitaminosis A Also more common in cats than dogs, it is generally seen in cats fed on a high liver diet for many years. Excess vitamin A is toxic to chondrocytes and osteoblasts and causes cartilage destruction, osteopenia and accelerated bone remodelling. In the cat, exostosis formation often affects the vertebrae and the joints in the region of tendinous and ligamentous attachments. A balanced diet containing normal levels of vitamin A should be fed.

Endocrine

Hypopituitarism Congenital growth hormone deficiency (hypopituitarism) results in a smaller animal of normal proportions (proportionate dwarf). Affected animals are usually a normal size for the first 1–2 months of life, but then grow more slowly and are obviously much smaller than litter mates by 3–4 months. Retention of the secondary hairs and lack of primary hairs result in a soft, woolly coat. Most animals are presented for evaluation as the growth plates are closing and a significant response to growth hormone is unlikely. Most animals die by 4 years of age.

Hypothyroidism The signs of congenital hypothyroidism (cretinism) are similar to hypopituitarism since the lack of thyroxine prevents the developing bone from responding to growth hormone. There is a delay in the closure of the growth plates and in the appearance of the epiphyses, and the long bones are shortened. However, in contrast to hypopituitarism, the animal develops as a disproportionate dwarf with a large broad head, a thick, protruding tongue, a wide square trunk and short limbs. Treatment is by thyroid supplementation using L-thyroxine.

Hyperadrenocorticism This may result from Cushing's syndrome or from chronic administration of exogenous corticosteroids. Glucocorticoid excess reduces osteoid formation and interferes with its formation by increasing urinary excretion of calcium and interfering with the action of vitamin D. The result is osteoporosis of the skeleton and dystrophic calcification of the soft tissues, such as the skin, bronchi and renal pelvis.

Congenital or acquired hypogonadism This condition results in the delayed closure of growth plates and increased bone length. Thus castrated male cats are more likely to suffer physeal fractures following trauma compared to entire cats of the same age, who would be more likely to suffer long bone fractures.

Infectious diseases

Osteomyelitis is an inflammatory condition affecting the bone cortex and marrow cavity. Infectious osteomyelitis is primarily due to bacterial infection; fungal infection with *Aspergillus* and *Cryptococcus* has been reported in the UK, but is rare. The common bacteria isolated are staphylococci, streptococcci, coliforms, *Pseudomonas* spp. and *Proteus* spp. As with most infectious diseases, the severity of the condition depends on the number and virulence of the infecting organism and the effectiveness of the host response. The host response may be reduced by systemic factors, such as diabetes mellitus, hyperadrenocorticism or hypoproteinaemia. More importantly, the host resistance to infection may be reduced by local factors, such as the presence of blood clots, devitalised tissue, poor blood supply and the presence of implants and suture material, all of which may be seen post-operatively with poor surgical technique.

Infection may arise from open wounds, from the spread of bacteria from an adjacent septic focus or, rarely, from haematogenous spread. Open wounds include open fractures, puncture wounds affecting bones and iatrogenic contamination at surgery.

Treatment is based on long-term (4–6 weeks) administration of antibiotics, ideally following culture and sensitivity testing. In acute cases, the area should be debrided and surgical drainage should be established. In chronic cases, sequestra and foreign material should be removed and any fractures should be evaluated for stability and healing. If the fracture has healed, the implants are removed. If the fracture has not healed, but the implants are secure and stabilising the fracture, they are left in place. If the implants are loose, they are removed and rigid internal (bone plate) or external (external fixator) fixation is applied.

Acute osteomyelitis Infection generally arises from wounds involving the bone. The infection may spread along the marrow cavity or under the periosteum. Acute osteomyelitis is characterised by depression, anorexia and pyrexia, with lameness and pain on palpation of the affected area.

Chronic osteomyelitis may follow an acute episode, or may be insidious in onset. Systemic signs are much less common. Chronic infections often become walled off from the rest of the bone and may be seen as an area of cortical bone which has lost its blood supply and become sclerotic (sequestrum) surrounded by an area of osteolysis (involucrum) which may connect to the skin as a draining tract (cloaca).

Neoplastic diseases

Bone may be affected by tumours arising directly from bone, metastatic deposits from tumours elsewhere in the body, or tumours of the soft tissue which invade bone. The majority are primary tumours and of these approximately 98% are malignant. Osteosarcoma accounts for approximately 80–90% of the malignant tumours, with chondrosarcoma, fibrosarcoma and haemangiosarcoma comprising most of the remainder. Benign tumours include osteoma, chondroma and giant cell tumours. Metastatic tumours may arise from many tissues, but the usual primary tumours are carcinomas of the mammary glands, prostate, tonsils, pancreas and bronchi.

Primary malignant bone tumours are normally found in middle-aged to old large-breed dogs and have a predilection for the metaphyses of long bones. Presenting signs are lameness and swelling of the metaphysis. Metastatic tumours and tumours arising from the soft tissues can arise at any site, although they will cause similar clinical signs.

Since the majority of tumours are malignant, the prognosis is guarded to poor. Most animals will have metastasis at the time of presentation, although micrometastases may not be visible radiographically. Surgical options include amputation or, at some locations, excision (e.g. distal ulna) or limb-sparing surgery (e.g. distal radius). Chemotherapy (e.g. cisplatin with or without doxorubicin) will improve the survival time. Palliative treatment with radiotherapy or NSAIDs may be used if surgery is not an option.

Miscellaneous or unclassified diseases

Metaphyseal osteopathy A developmental disease of young, rapidly growing dogs of unknown aetiology, this occurs mainly in large- and giant-breed dogs and causes mild to marked lameness, which is usually self-limiting. Clinical signs include hot, swollen metaphyses, depression and pyrexia. Radiography reveals an irregular radiolucent band in the metaphysis, parallel to the physis, and adjacent sub-periosteal or extra-periosteal calcification. Treatment consists of appropriate analgesia and nursing care.

Panosteitis This is a condition of unknown aetiology, affecting the larger breeds of dog, particularly the German Shepherd dog. Clinical signs are usually seen between 5 and 18 months and consist of recurrent bouts of shifting lameness of variable severity. Systemic signs such as depression, anorexia and pyrexia may be seen in severely affected cases. Radiography may reveal ill-defined patches of soft-tissue opacity within the medullary cavity and thickening of the trabeculae and cortices. Treatment consists of analgesia, supportive care and exercise restriction during bouts of lameness.

Hypertrophic osteopathy This condition arises secondary to chronic diseases affecting the thorax and, less commonly, the abdomen or neck. These diseases are generally mass lesions, primarily tumours, affecting the lungs, abdominal organs, especially the bladder, and the oesophagus. The aetiology is unknown, but it is suggested that the primary disease affects the vagal or intercostal nerves, resulting in a neurovascular response. The clinical signs consist of bilaterally symmetric soft tissue swellings of the distal limbs, particularly affecting the metacarpus and metatarsus. Radiography reveals palisading periosteal new bone along the diaphyses of the phalanges and metacarpal and metatarsal bones. Treatment is aimed at treating the primary disease and successful treatment may result in resolution of the clinical signs. However, since many of the primary initiating diseases are malignant, treatment may not be possible or may be followed by recurrence.

Multiple cartilaginous exostoses This is a rare, benign condition of puppies, characterised by proliferation of new bone and cartilage at various sites. These projections grow with the developing skeleton and cease growth as maturity is reached. The bony proliferations may be asymptomatic, or may impinge on adjacent tissues. No treatment is required, unless clinical signs result from local pressure of the masses, in which case surgical excision is indicated.

Craniomandibular osteopathy This is a non-neoplastic proliferative disease which occurs primarily in young West Highland White, Scottish and Cairn terriers, although it is seen occasionally in larger breeds, such as the Dobermann and German Shepherd dog. The lesions consist of bilaterally symmetrical palisading periosteal new bone along the mandible and the petrous temporal bones. Puppies may be reluctant to eat and may drool saliva. The disease is generally self-limiting and treatment consists of analgesia and nursing care, with the provision of a highly palatable, energy-dense diet. The prognosis depends on the severity of the disease, particularly with respect to the degree of involvement of the temporo-mandibular joint.

Aseptic necrosis of the femoral head (Legg–Calvé–Perthes disease) This is a non-inflammatory, non-infectious disease which results in necrosis of the femoral head and neck. The aetiology is unknown, but ischaemia resulting from vascular compression or aberrant sex hormone activity has been suggested. The bone of the femoral head and neck becomes necrotic and deformed. Collapse of the subchondral bone results in cracking of the articular cartilage. The necrotic bone eventually fills in with new bone, but the resulting deformity causes joint incongruity and instability. This condition causes a painful lameness and results in the development of marked OA.

The condition is found in young, small-breed dogs and is bilateral in 12–15% of dogs. The clinical signs consist of a progressive hindlimb lameness, often with marked muscle atrophy. Radiography reveals focal lucencies within the femoral head and neck, an increased coxo-femoral joint space and periarticular osteophytes. Conservative management, consisting of rest, analgesia or the use of an Ehmer sling, has been described, but surgical excision of the femoral head and neck produces better, more consistent and more rapid results.

Bone cysts These are rare in dogs. They may involve one bone (monostotic) or multiple bones (polyostotic). They are fluid-filled and generally benign in nature, although if they weaken the structure of the bone, they may predispose to pathologic fractures. A biopsy is required to differentiate them from bone tumours. Small cysts do not require treatment, but symptomatic or large cysts may be curetted and packed with a cancellous bone graft to encourage healing.

Traumatic diseases

A fracture is a partial or complete break in the continuity of the bone or cartilage. A fracture is accompanied by varying degrees of injury to the surrounding soft tissues and compromise of locomotor function. Diagnosis is based on the history of trauma, clinical examination and radiography. Surgical management, consisting of open or closed reduction and internal or external fixation of the fracture is considered appropriate for the majority of fractures. External coaptation with a splint or cast may be used for minimally displaced or incomplete (greenstick) fractures and cage rest may be used for non-articular pelvic fractures which do not disrupt the weight-bearing axis, do not compromise the diameter of the pelvic canal and do not cause neurological deficits. A major consideration from a medical point of view is the identification of any factors which may have predisposed to the occurrence of the fracture, such as underlying diffuse bone disease, e.g. nutritional secondary hyperpara-thyroidism, or localised bone disease, e.g. cysts or tumours. Failure to recognise factors which might precipitate a pathological fracture may result in failure of the surgical repair.

Diseases affecting joints

Degenerative arthropathies

Traumatic arthritis 'Sprain' is caused by a single, acute injury to the joint. It may result in:

- stretching, tearing or laceration of joint capsule
- tearing, laceration or avulsion of ligaments
- intra-articular fracture of bone
- detachment of articular cartilage
- tearing or displacement of menisci.

Treatment depends on the severity of the case, and may include confinement and restricted exercise, external support of the joint, surgical exploration of the joint, repair or replacement of damaged joint capsule and ligaments and removal of torn menisci. Some animals will develop OA, particularly if trauma has induced instability. Chronic repeated trauma may also produce OA.

Intra-articular haemorrhage Haemophilia is a rare inherited defect in the production of clotting factors, which predisposes to bleeding episodes. Intra-articular haemorrhage will result in synovial inflammation, articular cartilage damage and joint capsule fibrosis.

Osteoarthritis This is the commonest form of joint disease affecting the dog. It may be regarded as the end-stage of many different joint disorders rather than a specific disease process.

OA may be defined as primary or idiopathic where there is no obvious initiating cause, and secondary, which is the commonest form, where the disease follows some other abnormality of the joint. Common causes of OA are joint laxity, e.g. hip dysplasia, ligamentous injury, e.g. cranial cruciate ligament rupture, osteochondrosis and intra-articular fractures.

OA results in a change in chondrocyte metabolism, with a change in composition and degeneration of the cartilage matrix. Superficial chondrocytes are lost and the cartilage becomes worn away. The subchondral bone may show sclerosis and cyst formation and peri-articular osteophytes develop. The synovial membrane and joint capsule become hyperplastic and hyper-trophic resulting in thickening of the joint. Synovial fluid may increase in volume.

There is no absolute cure for arthritis and the disease is a chronic progressive one. The main-stay of therapy is conservative and medical therapy as outlined above. Some diseases, e.g. OA secondary to cranial cruciate ligament rupture or articular osteochondrosis, may benefit from surgical correction of the underlying disorder.

Inflammatory arthropathies

Bacterial infective (septic) arthritis This condition is uncommon in small animals. It may arise from haematogenous spread of bacteria from other sites of infection (e.g. pyoderma, gingivitis, urinary tract infection), from puncture wounds affecting the joints, by extension from adjacent foci of infection e.g. abscesses or from iatrogenic contamination following arthrotomy.

Animals generally present acutely, with a hot, swollen, painful joint. Occasionally, animals may show a low-grade, gradual-onset lameness. Septic arthritis usually involves a single joint; multiple joint involvement is generally associated with haematogenous spread of bacteria from a distant septic focus, and is more common in young animals. Synovial fluid analysis allows a definitive diagnosis to be made and allows traumatic arthritis and immune-mediated arthritis to be ruled out.

Antibiotic therapy is the main treatment, although this is augmented in most cases by joint lavage, performed either with needles or catheters introduced percutaneously, by arthroscopy or by arthrotomy. Intra-articular antibiotic therapy may be provided using gentamicin-impregnated methyl methacrylate beads (Septopal), which allows a high local concentration of antibiotic while minimising the risks of systemic side effects.

Lyme disease This is caused by the tickborne spirochaete *Borrelia burgdorferi*. Recurrent episodes of lameness affecting one or more joints and pyrexia may be seen. Polyarthritis associated with infection by *Mycoplasma* and bacterial L-forms has also been recorded. Articular infections associated with fungi (e.g. *Coccidioides immitis*, *Cryptococcus neoformans*, *Blastomyces dermatitidis* and *Aspergillus terreus*), rickettsiae (e.g. *Ehrlichia*) and protozoa (*Leishmania*) have been reported, but are unlikely to be seen in the UK, except in imported animals. Viruses do not seem to cause joint infections, although a transient polyarthritis may occur following vaccination, which may be an immune-mediated response.

Inflammatory, non-infectious, immune-mediated arthritis In this group of chronic, progressive diseases which generally affect multiple joints, especially the more distal joints, e.g. carpus and tarsus, differentiation is made on the basis of the radiographic changes, e.g. erosive vs non-erosive, immunological tests (e.g. rheumatoid factor, anti-nuclear antibody) and presence of other systemic signs (e.g. glomerulonephritis in SLE). Synovial fluid is typically turbid and increased in volume, with an elevated nucleated cell count, consisting primarily of non-degenerate neutrophils.

Erosive arthritis is generally caused by rheumatoid arthritis, Felty's syndrome, periosteal proliferative arthritis and polyarthritis of greyhounds, as well as septic arthritis. The remainder of the polyarthritides are non-erosive.

The prognosis depends on the diagnosis and the severity of the disease. The principal aim of therapy is to provide symptomatic relief of the signs by suppression of the immune response and by control of inflammation. Some cases require continuous therapy, whilst in other cases therapy may be withdrawn. Prednisolone is the mainstay of therapy for the immune-mediated polyarthropathies, and many cases can be successfully managed with this drug alone. However, in refractory cases, multisystemic disease or erosive disease, more aggressive drug therapy may be required. Immune-mediated polyarthritis associated with infections, neoplasia, gastrointestinal disease and idiosyncratic drug reactions may resolve following removal of the inciting factor, but some of these cases also need prednisolone to control the inflammatory joint disease. Lifestyle management is an important adjunct to therapy. Particular care should be paid to maintaining a low-stress existence with exercise moderated to the dog's abilities.

Surgical management is rarely indicated, although synovectomy, arthrodesis and excision arthroplasty may be considered as potential salvage procedures. Repair of subluxation and ligamentous injuries may also be of benefit, but the surgical failure rates are higher than in normal animals because of the ongoing pathology and because of the deleterious effects of the medication on wound healing.

Rheumatoid arthritis This is a chronic, symmetric polyarthropathy, which results in erosive changes on radiography. Various other criteria must be fulfilled before a definitive diagnosis can be made. These include: stiffness after rest; pain in one or more joints; swelling of two or more joints over a 3-month period, generally with symmetric involvement of contralateral joints; subcutaneous nodules; abnormal synovial fluid; seropositivity for rheumatoid factor and characteristic histological appearance of the synovial membrane and the subcutaneous nodules. The prognosis is poor, with progressive erosion and destruction of the joints. Therapy may preserve the quality of life, but ultimately euthanasia will be necessary.

Felty's syndrome is rare and consists of rheumatoid arthritis with splenomegaly and neutropenia. Periosteal proliferative polyarthritis is occasionally seen in the dog, but is more common in the cat. Bony proliferation is seen around the joint at the attachments of ligaments and tendons. Polyarthritis of greyhounds is uncommon, and may be an infectious arthritis caused by *Mycoplasma spumans* rather than an immune-mediated disease.

Systemic lupus erythematosus SLE presents as a bilaterally symmetric, non-erosive polyarthritis. This is a multisystemic disease and other manifestations include pyrexia, immune-mediated haemolytic anaemia, leucopenia and thrombo-cytopenia, immune complex glomerulonephritis, dermatitis, polymyositis, meningitis, pleuritis and gastrointestinal disease. Diagnosis is based on the clinical signs, lack of erosive changes, demonstration of auto-antibodies to erythro-cytes, leucocytes or platelets in patients with reduced numbers of these cells and the presence of anti-nuclear antibody (ANA).

Canine idiopathic polyarthritis This is the most common form of immune-mediated polyarthro-pathy in the dog. A diagnosis is achieved by exclusion, and other causes of polyarthritis as well as infectious (e.g. Lyme disease) and septic arthritis need to be ruled out. Immune complex deposition may also result in additional signs, such as dermatitis, glomerulonephritis and uveitis. Four sub-types of disease are recognised. Type I, uncomplicated idiopathic arthritis, is the most common form and no underlying disease is detected. Type II disease (reactive arthritis) is associated with infections remote from the joint, type III (enteropathic arthritis) is associated with gastrointestinal disease and type IV is associated with neoplasia remote from the joints.

Immune-mediated polyarthritis may be seen as part of the polyarthritis/polymyositis and polyarthritis/meningitis syndromes. Non-erosive polyarthritis is also reported as a vaccination reaction, generally in the young animal follow-ing the primary vaccination course, and as an idiosyncratic drug reaction.

In human medicine, the accumulation of various crystals within the joints has been associated with arthritis (crystal-induced arthritis). Gout, the accumulation of urate crystals in the joint, and pseudogout, the accumulation of calcium pyrophosphate or calcium phosphate crystals, are rare in dogs. Calcium hydroxyapatite-like crystals have been seen in joint fluid from normal and abnormal joints and their significance is unclear.

Congenital arthropathies

Congenital luxation and subluxation of joints are seen occasionally. The main joints affected are the stifle, with medial or lateral luxation of the patella, the shoulder, with medial displacement of the humeral head, and the elbow, with lateral displacement of the head of the radius or the proximal ulna or both.

Treatment options include closed reduction, open reduction and open reduction with stabil-isation. If a diagnosis is made early, then reduction of the joint may allow the joint to develop normally. However, there is often a marked lack of joint congruity at diagnosis and it may be difficult to reduce the joint or maintain reduction once achieved. Mildly affected animals may tolerate the abnormality with minimal lameness. Arthrodesis of the joint or amputation may be required in severely affected animals.

Developmental joint disease

Osteochondrosis This is a disease process characterised by an abnormality in the orderly progression of fibrous tissue to cartilage and then to bone during the development of skeletal structures. The main manifestation is within the joint, where thickened areas of articular cartilage may form (osteochondrosis) which may fissure and form a flap (osteochondrosis dissecans). This disease tends to affect certain anatomic sites in the joint, e.g. the caudal humeral head and the medial humeral condyle. It may also affect primary centres of ossification (e.g. the radial carpal bone), secondary centres of ossification (e.g. the medial humeral epicondyle) and the cartilage of the growth plate (retained carti-laginous cores in the distal ulna).

Surgical debridement of the thickened carti-lage and the flap is indicated in most cases, although the outcome is better for the large joints such as the shoulder and stifle, than for the smaller and more congruent joints such as the elbow and hock.

Hip dysplasia A common cause of lameness in the dog, this is a multifactorial disease with a hereditary component. It is caused by abnormal coxofemoral joint laxity, which may progress to subluxation or complete luxation. This lack of joint congruity results in abnormal joint wear and the development of osteoarthritis. Clinical signs of hindlimb lameness are generally seen at 4–12 months old, although some dogs do not show signs until a few years old. Physical examination will confirm joint laxity in the young dog and radiographs reveal varying degrees of coxofemoral subluxation and secondary osteoarthritis.

Non-surgical management is used initially and the majority of animals will respond and be able to cope with the disorder. However, surgical management is indicated in those animals which do not respond and may consist of a triple pelvic osteotomy in the immature animal and excision arthroplasty or total hip replacement in the adult animal.

Elbow dysplasia This is the term given to a group of developmental disorders affecting the elbow joint. The underlying cause may be asynchronous development of the radius and ulna or failure of the semilunar notch of the ulna to develop. These abnormalities result in abnormal elbow joint congruity. This may manifest as ununited anconeal process of the ulna or fragmented medial coronoid process of the ulna. Osteochondrosis of the medial humeral condyle is also included in this group of disorders, as is ununited medial epicondyle of the humerus. These conditions will result in osteoarthritis of the joint. Surgical management is indicated if an early diagnosis is made, but if osteoarthritis is already present, non-surgical management is used.

Conformational abnormalities These may be congenital or acquired as a result of nutritional bone disease, fracture malunion or growth plate disorders. Conformational abnormalities include straight hocks, straight stifles, valgus or varus deformities of various joints and hyperextended or hyperflexed joints. Congenital conformational abnormalities should be recognised since they may predispose to other orthopaedic disorders. The underlying cause of acquired deformities should be identified and corrected if possible. Some conformational abnormalities are considered normal for the breed, e.g. chondrodystrophy in the Bulldog, Pekingese and Pug.

Metabolic arthropathies

Mucopolysaccharidosis This is a rare inherited metabolic disease, seen primarily in cats. Various forms are reported and common features include dwarfism, facial abnormalities, multifocal neurological defects, skeletal deformities and ocular disease.

Ehlers–Danlos syndrome A connective tissue disorder characterised by hyperelasticity of collagen in the skin, blood vessels and joints, this condition results in excessive laxity of the joints.

Neoplasia of joints

Tumours affecting the joints are uncommon. They may arise from tissues within the joint (e.g. synovial membrane and fat), from extra-articular tissue (e.g. bone, cartilage and fibrous tissue) and from metastatic spread from other tumours. The commonest primary tumour is synovial sarcoma. The tumours are generally malignant and treatment is by amputation of the digit if a single toe is affected, or the limb if more proximal joints are affected. Limb-sparing by excision and joint arthrodesis is a possibility for the rare benign lesions.

Diseases affecting muscles

Myopathies

Myopathies are relatively uncommon and may be broadly categorised as inherited, congenital non-inherited and acquired disorders.

Animals with myopathies of skeletal muscles of the limbs may present because of muscular weakness, stiffness, variation in muscle bulk, either hypertrophy or atrophy and muscle pain. Myopathies affecting muscles with a more restricted distribution may cause signs such as regurgitation if the pharyngeal or oesophageal muscles are affected, or pain on opening the mouth if the masticatory muscles are affected.

Hereditary myopathies These include myotonia and Labrador neuromyopathy.

Hereditary myotonia This has been described in the Chow and other breeds. This causes difficulty rising and marked stiffness, which reduces on exercise. The muscles are hypertrophic, but have normal tone. A myotonic dimple may be seen on muscle percussion. Diagnosis is based on EMG and muscle biopsy. The disease is a chronic progressive one, although the stiffness may be reduced by procainamide.

Labrador neuromyopathy This is caused by selective atrophy of type II muscle fibres. This results in stiffness, extension of the limbs, difficulty in holding the head erect and collapse. The signs worsen on exercise and improve with rest. Diagnosis is based on EMG and muscle biopsy. There is no treatment. After an initial progression, the signs usually stabilise, such that the animal can undertake short walks.

Acquired myopathies

Bacterial myositis This is uncommon. Acute myositis may accompany open fractures or puncture wounds affecting muscles. Chronic myositis may be associated with deep granulomas and draining sinuses, e.g. associated with a foreign body.

The parasites *Toxoplasma gondii* and *Neospora caninum* can cause acquired polymyositis, with hindlimb weakness as the primary sign (**protozoal myositis**). Neospora may also affect other organ systems including the central nervous system, and these signs may predominate. Diagnosis is based on clinical signs and serologic testing. The treatment of choice is clindamycin.

Idiopathic masticatory muscle myositis This is inflammation and destruction of the masticatory muscles which may be seen as an acute, subacute or chronic disease. The acute disease may cause pain and swelling of the muscles, resulting in reluctance to open the mouth. In the chronic form, gradual atrophy of the muscles is seen, which may be followed by fibrosis and an inability to open the mouth. Diagnosis is based on clinical signs and muscle biopsy. Treatment includes anti-inflammatory doses of corticosteroids and mechanical traction to open the jaws if there is restriction to opening of the mouth.

Idiopathic polymyositis This group of diseases is characterised by inflammation of the skeletal muscles. It may be associated with SLE and other immune-mediated joint diseases, dermatitis and neoplasia. Clinical signs include weakness and muscular pain, with a stiff gait. Treatment with corticosteroids is indicated.

Myasthenia gravis This disease may be seen as a congenital or acquired form. The disease is caused by a lack of receptors for the neurotransmitter acetylcholine in the neuromuscular junction. The major sign is premature fatigue that is relieved by rest. The administration of drugs which block the enzymatic destruction of acetylcholine at the neuromuscular junction allows this neurotransmitter to persist and for neuromuscular activity to occur. Administration of a short-acting drug with this function (edrophonium) forms the basis of a diagnostic test and a long-acting drug (pyridostigmine) is used for treatment.

Metabolic myopathies These result from some abnormality in muscle metabolism, which may affect only the muscles, or may have a more widespread tissue distribution. These disorders may be caused by abnormalities in the mitochondria or in the glycogen metabolic pathway. Muscular weakness may also accompany serum electrolyte abnormalities (hyperkalaemia or hypokalaemia) and hypoglycaemia.

Ischaemic myopathy This muscle inflammation and necrosis may result from interruption of the blood supply to the muscles, e.g. by thrombi or emboli, by casts or bandages that are placed too tightly or by intramuscular injections.

Many endocrine disorders may induce a secondary myopathy. The most well-documented are hyperadrenocorticism, hypoadrenocorticism and hypothyroidism.

Muscle disorders have been seen following chronic administration of corticosteroids.

Muscle atrophy

This is not a specific disease, but is one of the commonest clinical signs accompanying muscle disease.

Generalised muscle atrophy is seen in malnutrition or cachectic states, e.g. neoplasia, organ failure. Localised muscle atrophy may result from disuse or neurogenic disease. Disuse atrophy occurs in any muscle group after a period of relative or absolute inactivity and is generally seen in the limbs in association with orthopaedic disorders. Neurogenic atrophy results from the loss of motor innervation to the muscle. Neurogenic atrophy is more rapid and more marked than disuse atrophy, and may have a more localised distribution.

Traumatic injuries of muscle

Traumatic injuries of muscles and tendons are termed strains. Strains may be acute or chronic and single or multiple in nature. They may occur anywhere within the musculotendinous unit (muscle origin, muscle belly, musculotendinous junction, tendon body and tendon insertion) and may vary in severity from mild to complete rupture.

Mild injuries produce minimal changes in gait and may be overlooked in all animals apart from athletic individuals, where a decrease in performance may be noticed. Diagnosis may be made by deep palpation of the affected area. Conservative management, consisting of rest and confinement, will result in resolution of the problem.

Rupture of the musculotendinous unit causes a more marked lameness, with an inability actively to flex and extend the associated joint and bear weight. Surgical repair and external coaptation, if possible, are required to restore normal function. Spasm or contracture of the muscle may prevent spontaneous healing. If it does occur, spontaneous second intention healing results in disorganised scar tissue, which may not be strong enough to allow weight-bearing or may result in muscle contracture which will limit function.

Muscle ruptures are more common in athletic dogs and the rupture is due to the development of endogenous forces within the muscles during racing. Rupture of the long head of triceps and gracilis muscles is the most common. Healing may occur by second intention, but the resulting fibrosis may limit motion of the associated joint. Surgical exploration, evacuation of the haematoma and primary repair of the muscle, followed by 2–3 months of strict rest, offers the best results.

Muscle laceration may occur in conjunction with open wounds following trauma. The basic principles of wound management apply and the wound may be subject to primary closure, delayed primary closure or healing by second intention. Primary suture repair of the lacerated muscle is performed if the wound is closed.

A few distinct syndromes of muscle fibrosis and contracture are seen in small animals and produce chronic lameness, sometimes with characteristic gait abnormalities. Contracture of the infraspinatus muscle is seen primarily in working dogs and is thought to arise from chronic repetitive trauma to the muscle or tendon. Treatment is by sectioning the tendon of origin.

Contracture of the quadriceps muscle is generally seen in young animals associated with femoral fractures and their repair, although a congenital form has also been reported. Quadriceps contracture results in hyperextension of the stifle joint. Restoration of normal function is attempted by freeing adhesions between the muscle and the femur, encouraging use of the limb and maintaining a degree of stifle flexion with a dynamic transarticular external fixator.

Fibrotic myopathy has been described involving the supraspinatus, gracilis, quadriceps and semitendinosus muscles. The aetiology is unknown, but may include trauma, neuropathy, myopathy or a congenital predisposition. Surgical resection of the affected muscle is reported but the prognosis is guarded since the condition tends to recur at the surgical site. Myositis ossificans involves the localised or generalised calcification of skeletal muscles. It may be due to trauma, myositis or ossification of haematomas. Surgical excision may be curative.

Diseases affecting tendons

Tendon disorders are often accompanied by open wounds and conformational abnormalities (e.g. plantigrade stance with Achilles tendon disruption), which aids in diagnosis.

Laceration and rupture

These injuries involve complete or partial disruption of the substance of the tendon. The goal of therapy is to restore the continuity of the tendon by primary repair, followed by support of the repair by external coaptation, external fixation or temporary immobilisation of the joint with a lag screw. Tendon laceration is often accompanied by an open wound. The wound may be debrided and lavaged, followed by primary repair of the tendon and primary closure of the wound. Alternatively, the wound may be managed as an open wound and delayed primary repair performed.

Contracture

Muscle fibrosis and tendon contracture may result from a previous injury and may limit the function of the associated joint. Surgery is seldom indicated unless there is marked chronic lameness or conformational abnormality. The most common disorders are fibrotic myopathy of the semitendinosus and semimembranosus muscles, contracture of the flexor tendons of the carpus and contracture of the infraspinatus tendon. Surgical treatment comprises either sectioning of the tendon, thus sacrificing the function of the muscle, or lengthening the tendon, thus preserving the function of the muscle.

Displacement

The displacement of a tendon from its normal position, particularly as it crosses a joint, may result in limb dysfunction and chronic lameness. Tendon displacement usually results from trauma to supporting ligaments or other stabilising soft tissue structures. Examples include displacement of the tendon of origin of the biceps brachii over the shoulder, the tendon of origin of the long digital extensor muscle in the stifle and the superficial flexor tendon of the hindlimb over the hock. Surgical treatment involves repair of the tendon retinaculum or associated ligaments or detachment of the tendon from its origin and fixation (tenodesis) to the underlying bone.

Avulsion

Trauma to the musculotendinous unit may result in avulsion of the tendon of origin (e.g. long digital extensor and gastrocnemius) or insertion (e.g. common calcaneal tendon) from the bone. The avulsion may occur at the bone–tendon interface, or the tendon may remain intact, resulting in an avulsion fracture of the bone. Avulsed tendons are attached to the bone by passing suture material through a tunnel made in the bone. Avulsed bone fragments may be re-attached with a bone screw or suture material passed through a bone tunnel.

Diseases affecting ligaments

Damage to a ligament is termed a sprain. The tensile strength of ligaments varies with age. In the immature animal, an avulsion fracture is likely to occur, whereas in the mature animal, the ligament is likely to fail in the midsubstance. Sprain injuries are categorised into three classes:

- First-degree sprains involve the tearing of relatively few fibres with resulting haematoma and oedema formation and fibrin deposition. Healing occurs by invasion of the fibrin by fibroblasts and is relatively rapid with normal anatomy and function being restored.
- Second-degree sprains are characterised by damage to a larger number of collagen fibres, more extensive haematoma formation and a more marked functional defect, although the ligament remains grossly intact.
- Third-degree sprains are characterised by complete or partial disruption of the substance of the ligament or avulsion of the ligament from bone. Avulsion fractures of the origin or insertion of the ligament may also occur. Joint instability will be present and function is completely lost.

Treatment

The initial treatment of ligamentous injuries involves the basic principles of first aid, i.e. cold and immobilisation. After the initial injury, the affected area should have a cold temperature applied (e.g. cold water or melting ice) two or three times a day for 15–20 minutes. After 24–48 hours, the cold treatment is replaced by the application of heat via warm water, head pads or ultrasound. A soft bandage should be applied from the toes to above the affected area. More rigid external coaptation is required if joint instability is present.

For first-degree sprains, treatment consists of bandaging the limb and enforced rest for 7–10 days. This is followed by 7–10 days of lead-only exercise and then a gradual return to normal exercise. Second-degree sprains are treated by immobilisation of the joint and strict rest for 2–3 weeks. This is followed by 2–3 weeks in a soft bandage and lead-only exercise, followed by gradual return to normal activity. Surgical treatment of second- and third-degree sprains is indicated if joint instability is present. The post-operative management is similar to that for second-degree sprain.

REFERENCES

Cunningham JG 1992 Textbook of veterinary physiology. WB Saunders, Philadelphia, p 216

Cunningham JG 1997 Textbook of veterinary physiology, 2nd edn. WB Saunders, Philadelphia, pp 254, 255

Evans HE 1993 Miller's anatomy of the dog, 3rd edn. WB Saunders, Philadelphia

Masters J, Bowden C (eds) 2001 Pre-veterinary nursing textbook. Butterworth-Heinemann in association with BVNA, Oxford, p 19

Nelson RW, Couto CG 1992 Essentials of small animal internal medicine. Mosby, St Louis

Tartaglia L 2002 Veterinary physiology and applied anatomy. College of Animal Welfare, Oxford, p 84

Williams DL 2002 Veterinary ocular emergencies. Butterworth-Heinemann, Oxford, pp 14, 18

4

Medical diagnostics

*Jonathan Wray   Edward J. Hall
Alasdair Hotston Moore*

PART
1
Examination techniques

Jonathan Wray

ROUTINE PHYSICAL EXAMINATION AND HISTORY TAKING

INTRODUCTION

No diagnostic test comes close to matching a thoroughly taken history and diligently performed physical examination for the useful information generated as well as cost- and time-effectiveness.

The order in which a history is taken and physical examination performed is not so important as the need for it to be complete in every sense. Thus the adoption of a routine that is logical and suitable to the examiner will encourage a thorough job to be done with minimal risk of omission. The suggested plan for history taking and physical examination detailed below is certainly not the only way to perform it, merely the author's preferred method.

Principal obstacles to obtaining a full set of clinical data are:

1. Inadequate consultation time for a thorough history and physical examination.
2. Deviations from the adopted plan of history taking and physical examination leading to omissions.
3. Not keeping full and detailed records.
4. Overinterpretation or underinterpretation of findings due to preconceptions, assumptions

and 'conclusion jumping' on the part of the examiner.

HISTORY TAKING

It is usual for a history to be taken prior to physical examination being performed as not only does this allow the examination of the animal to be more directed towards the primary owner complaint, it also allows time for fractious animals to become 'acclimatised' to the examination room and examiner. Much of the relevant information may already be known to the examiner, recorded on the animal's records, or easily available if needed and time can be saved in newly presenting patients by the use of waiting-room questionnaires to record pertinent details and by follow-up telephone interviews if adequate time is unavailable during the consultation period.

A medical history should include:

1. Routine preventative, dietary and environmental history
   a. age, breed, sex and neutering/reproductive status (if not already known)
   b. vaccination and worming status
   c. dietary history (what fed, what amount, how often and any treats/scraps)
   d. environmental history
      i.   contact with other animals of the same species and their health and vaccination status (especially fighting behaviour in cats)
      ii. indoor vs outdoor lifestyle (especially cats) (where exercised)
      iii. predatory/scavenging behaviour
      vi. history of travel abroad
2. Description of previous medical problems and response to treatments given
3. Description of the current medical problem or problems
4. Further questioning of the owner regarding specifics of the problems described, response to any medications administered and determination of functional integrity of unmentioned body systems.

Emphasis should be placed upon trying to establish:

- what *the owner* perceives to be the most concerning problem
- what the duration, speed of onset and dynamics of the illness course are as perceived by the owner
- specifics of timing (e.g. relation of vomiting to time of eating), quantification of body fluid 'ins and outs', character of emissions, changes in health status/demeanour/appetite/bodyweight, etc.

The history should be concluded by the examiner asking more detailed questions of the owner to establish specifics of the condition and to attempt to differentiate between similarly presenting conditions (for instance attempting to differentiate between vomiting versus regurgitation of food). In several instances certain 'key questions' can quickly direct the examiner to the more pertinent problem. For example, asking about the presence or absence of abdominal heaving during episodes of sickness can usually reliably determine whether vomiting or regurgitation is occurring. Finally, any body systems for which information has not been volunteered should be asked about to establish normal functional integrity.

PHYSICAL EXAMINATION
Approach and technique

As with the history, the exact order in which a physical examination is performed is of secondary relevance to the need for it to be done thoroughly and for the examiner to adopt an established routine. It is equally important that all physical examination findings (*both abnormal and normal*) are recorded in a clearly understandable manner. Any areas which could not be satisfactorily examined should also be noted; these may be revisited later or, for example, repeated when the animal is sedated.

Normal values

Every effort should be made to ensure that the examiner is familiar with the normal ranges for physical parameters for all veterinary species to be examined along with an appreciation of the degree of possible inter- and intra-individual variation. There is no substitute for the repetitive examination of healthy animals of as many species and breeds as possible to establish this baseline of personal experience.

Initial observations

Frequently, invaluable information can be gained by observing the animal prior to 'hands on' physical examination and this observation at a distance can often be performed whilst a history is being taken. In particular, note should be made of body condition, coat quality, mental alertness and appropriateness of behaviour, body and head posture and gait.

Physical examination and recording

The author prefers to examine animals in a 'head to tail' direction though there are advocates for many different approaches, for example concentrating on examining one body system at a time. Again, this is very much a matter of personal choice and approach is largely irrelevant so long as the examiner finds his or her own most 'user-friendly' technique and adheres to it in such a way that a complete examination is always performed. All findings should be recorded and an aide-mémoire such as in Figure 4.1 can be invaluable. A schematic aide-memoire is shown in Figure 4.2.

DIAGNOSTIC APPROACH

Concept of the problem-based approach

The most successful diagnosticians are those who maintain an open mind and who base decisions on facts ('evidence-based' approach) rather than trying to fit a disease to a pattern of clinical signs ('pattern recognition' approach) which may lead to errors of omission.

Steps in formulating a diagnostic plan

Steps in formulating a problem-based diagnostic plan are outlined in Box 4.1.

The problem list comprises historical, physical examination and laboratory abnormalities that may aid the clinician in producing a differential diagnosis list. Some problems are more specific (i.e. have a shorter differential diagnosis list) than others and more weight should be placed on these more 'pivotal' findings. For example, if initial questioning, physical examination and previous laboratory findings establish the following problem list:

- lethargy
- inappetence
- lymphadenomegaly
- hypercalcaemia

then of these the last two, lymphadenomegaly and hypercalcaemia, are potentially much more useful and specific findings, since lethargy and inappetence are common to most ill animals.

A differential diagnostic list is essential to avoid omissions and again more weight should be placed on the more specific problems identified. A useful aid to establishing a thorough differential list is the use of the mnemonic DAMNIT-V which helps classify differential diagnoses according to aetiology (Box 4.2)

The type and extent of diagnostic procedures performed will, of course, depend on many practical factors such as the facilities, equipment and expertise available, the cost-constraints of the owner and the level of investigation required by the owner. The adage that 'common things occur commonly' should always be borne in mind.

NEUROLOGICAL AND OPHTHALMOLOGICAL EXAMINATION

INTRODUCTION

Any animal suspected of having neurological disease must receive a *full* neurological examination. Needless to say, a thorough history should be taken prior to the examination. Of particular importance is determining the speed of onset, duration and progression of the disease as this can offer invaluable clues.

PHYSICAL EXAMINATION

Body weight (kg)	Temperature	Pulse rate	Heart rate	Respiratory rate

		Normal	Abnormal	Describe abnormal
1. General	Body condition	☐	☐	_____
	Coat	☐	☐	_____
Inspection	Gait	☐	☐	_____
	Behaviour	☐	☐	_____
	Mental status	☐	☐	_____
2. Head and neck — Inspect	Face, head, nostrils, neck, eyes, ears	☐	☐	_____
	Conjunctival mucous membranes	☐	☐	_____
	Mandibular lymph nodes	☐	☐	_____
Palpate	Salivary glands	☐	☐	_____
	Larynx	☐	☐	_____
	Trachea to thoracic inlet	☐	☐	_____
3. Mouth	Lips	☐	☐	_____
Inspect, lift lips	Teeth & gingiva (outer surfaces)	☐	☐	_____
	Teeth & gingiva (inner surfaces)	☐	☐	_____
Open mouth	Tongue	☐	☐	_____
	Hard palate	☐	☐	_____
	Tonsils	☐	☐	_____
4. Forelimbs — Inspect and palpate	Prescapular lymph nodes area	☐	☐	_____
	Flex & extend joints	☐	☐	_____
	Nails, pads & dew claws	☐	☐	_____

PHYSICAL EXAMINATION

		Normal	Abnormal	Describe abnormal
5. Trunk	Character of respiratory movements and rate	☐	☐	_____
Inspect	Chest	☐	☐	_____
	Abdomen	☐	☐	_____
	Chest	☐	☐	_____
	Cranial abdomen	☐	☐	_____
Palpate	Midventral abdomen	☐	☐	_____
	Pelvic abdomen	☐	☐	_____
	Cardiac apex	☐	☐	_____
Auscultate	Cardiac base	☐	☐	_____
	Rate & rhythm	☐	☐	_____
	Lungs	☐	☐	_____
Inspect and palpate	Mammary glands	☐	☐	_____
	Testicles	☐	☐	_____
	Prepuce	☐	☐	_____
	Penis	☐	☐	_____
6. Hindlimbs	Popliteal lymph nodes	☐	☐	_____
	Extend & flex joints	☐	☐	_____
Inspect and palpate	Nails, pads & dew claws	☐	☐	_____
	Femoral pulse rate & character	☐	☐	_____
	Tailhead	☐	☐	_____
	Tail	☐	☐	_____
7. Perineum	Perineum	☐	☐	_____
Inspect	Anus	☐	☐	_____
	Vulva	☐	☐	_____
	Scrotum	☐	☐	_____

Figure 4.1 Physical examination chart. (University of Bristol.)

Aims of the neurological/ophthalmological examination

By the end of a neuro-ophthalmic examination the examiner should be able to answer the following questions:

- Does this animal have evidence of neurological disease?
- What is (are) the location(s) of the lesion(s)?
- How severe is the lesion and what are its dynamics of progression?
- What differential diagnoses/aetiologies are likely?
- What further investigation is required?
- What is the prognosis?

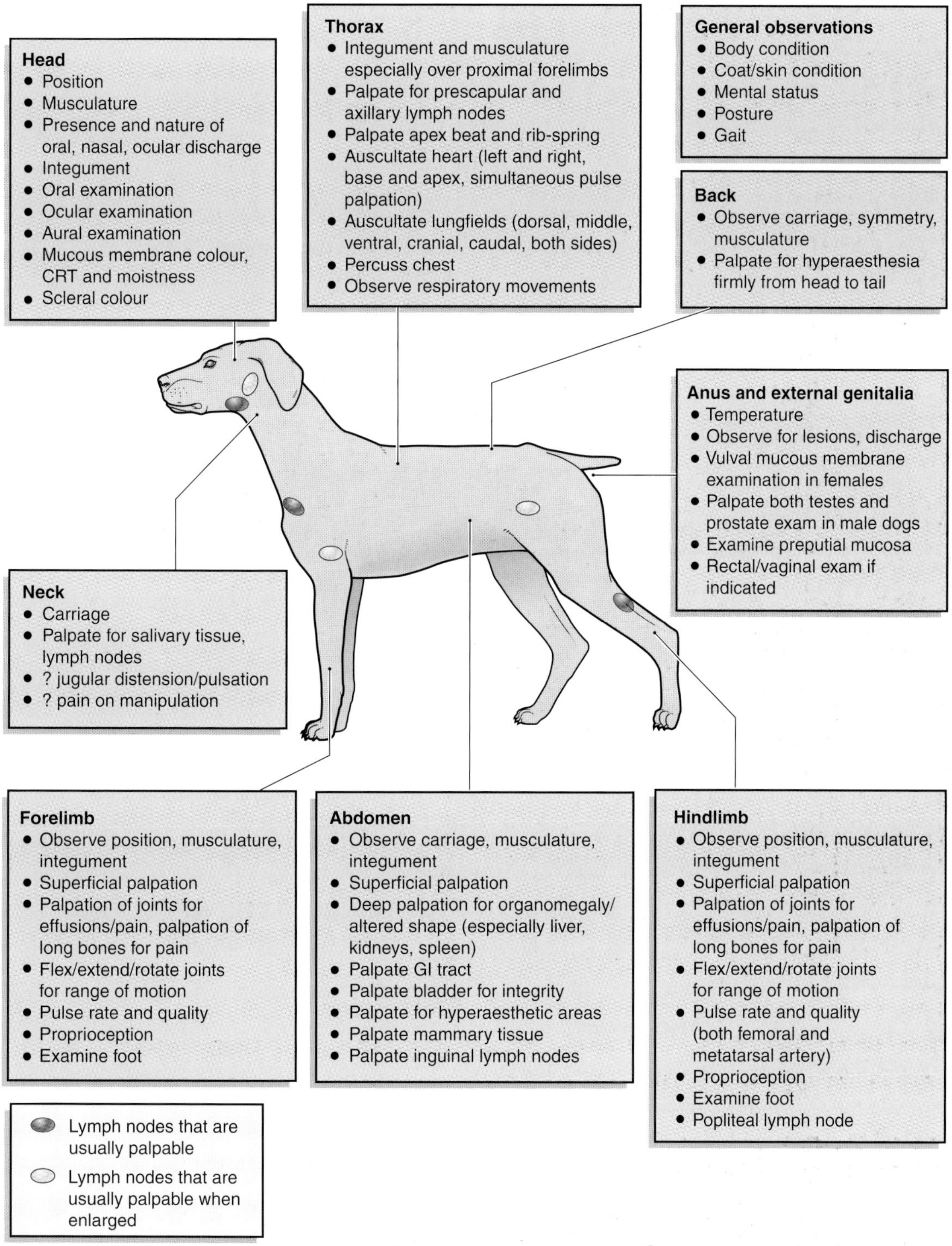

Head
- Position
- Musculature
- Presence and nature of oral, nasal, ocular discharge
- Integument
- Oral examination
- Ocular examination
- Aural examination
- Mucous membrane colour, CRT and moistness
- Scleral colour

Thorax
- Integument and musculature especially over proximal forelimbs
- Palpate for prescapular and axillary lymph nodes
- Palpate apex beat and rib-spring
- Auscultate heart (left and right, base and apex, simultaneous pulse palpation)
- Auscultate lungfields (dorsal, middle, ventral, cranial, caudal, both sides)
- Percuss chest
- Observe respiratory movements

General observations
- Body condition
- Coat/skin condition
- Mental status
- Posture
- Gait

Back
- Observe carriage, symmetry, musculature
- Palpate for hyperaesthesia firmly from head to tail

Anus and external genitalia
- Temperature
- Observe for lesions, discharge
- Vulval mucous membrane examination in females
- Palpate both testes and prostate exam in male dogs
- Examine preputial mucosa
- Rectal/vaginal exam if indicated

Neck
- Carriage
- Palpate for salivary tissue, lymph nodes
- ? jugular distension/pulsation
- ? pain on manipulation

Forelimb
- Observe position, musculature, integument
- Superficial palpation
- Palpation of joints for effusions/pain, palpation of long bones for pain
- Flex/extend/rotate joints for range of motion
- Pulse rate and quality
- Proprioception
- Examine foot

Abdomen
- Observe carriage, musculature, integument
- Superficial palpation
- Deep palpation for organomegaly/altered shape (especially liver, kidneys, spleen)
- Palpate GI tract
- Palpate bladder for integrity
- Palpate for hyperaesthetic areas
- Palpate mammary tissue
- Palpate inguinal lymph nodes

Hindlimb
- Observe position, musculature, integument
- Superficial palpation
- Palpation of joints for effusions/pain, palpation of long bones for pain
- Flex/extend/rotate joints for range of motion
- Pulse rate and quality (both femoral and metatarsal artery)
- Proprioception
- Examine foot
- Popliteal lymph node

- Lymph nodes that are usually palpable
- Lymph nodes that are usually palpable when enlarged

Figure 4.2 Schematic aide-mémoire for physical examination. CRT, capillary refill time; GI, gastrointestinal.

Method of neurological/ophthalmological examination

Materials needed

- Somewhere to walk and turn the animal that is free of distractions and personnel traffic.
- A quiet area that can be darkened.
- Pen-torch.
- Tendon hammer.
- Ophthalmoscope/magnifying hand lens.
- Mosquito forceps.

Other useful items of equipment can usually be improvised from practice stores and won't be listed.

Order of examination

This is probably not as essential as the need to perform a thorough and complete examination. A period of observation is, however, essential before performing 'hands on' tests and may reveal subtle changes that may be overlooked if the examiner is too focused on minutiae. Test of nociception should be left until last to maintain good examiner/patient relations and tests of deep pain sensation are unnecessary in the fully ambu-

latory animal. The author prefers the following order of examination:

1. general observations
   a. mental status
   b. posture
   c. movement
   d. muscle tone
2. ophthalmic examination
3. cranial nerve examination
4. postural reactions
5. spinal reflexes
6. nociception.

Recording

A standardised way of recording information is essential so that colleagues can easily and unambiguously access pertinent information and so that comparisons between examinations can be easily made. A neurological examination sheet (Fig. 4.3) fulfils these needs and acts as a useful aide-mémoire to prevent omission of important tests.

Unifocal vs multifocal lesions

Every attempt should be made to try and explain the neurological findings by a single lesion in one anatomical site. If this is not possible, the possibility of either a misleadingly inaccurate examination or of a multifocal lesion should be considered.

DIVISIONS OF THE NERVOUS SYSTEM AND INTRODUCTION TO TERMS USED

Definitions

The central nervous system (CNS) comprises the brain and the spinal cord. The peripheral nervous system (PNS) comprises the spinal segmental nerves (both sensory and motor) and autonomic nerves which lie outside the CNS. For the purposes of this chapter the nervous system may be functionally divided into autonomic (unconscious, homeostatic, regulatory) portions and somatic portions (usually concerned with more easily recognisable functions such as ambulation).

NEUROLOGICAL EXAMINATION SHEET

Animal details:

Date:

Examiner:

History:

Mental status:

Gait and posture:

Muscle tone:

Fundus:

Cranial nerves

I Olfaction

II Optic
Menace
Following
Obstacles

III Oculomotor
Direct PLR
Indirect PLR
Ventro-lateral
strabismus (±)

IV Trochlear
Lateral rotation (±)

V Trigeminal
Motor (mastication)
Sensory (mand, max, ophth)

VI Abducent
Medial strabismus (±)
Corneal reflex;
globe retraction

LEFT RIGHT

VII Facial
Facial muscles

VIII Vestibulocochlear
Cochlear
Vestibular (±)
Head (±)
Nystagmus (±)
- Spontaneous (±)
- Positional (±)
- Direction

IX Glossopharangeal and X Vagus
Swallowing/gag

XI Accessory
Trapezius muscles

XII Hypoglossal
Tongue muscles

LEFT RIGHT

Postural reactions

	LF	LH	RH	RF
Wheelbarrow	—	—	—	
Extensor thrust	—			—
Hemistand				
Hemiwalk				
Proprioception				
Hopping				
Placing				
Tactile				
Visual				
Righting				

Spinal reflexes

		L	R
Thoracic limb			
Biceps	C6 – C7		
Triceps	C7 – T2		
Ext. carpi radialis	C7 – T2		
Flexor	C6 – T2		
Crossed extensor			
Pelvic limb			
Patellar	L4 – L6		
Cranial tibial	L6 – S2		
Gastrocnemius	L6 – S2		
Flexor	L6 – S2		
Crossed extensor			
Others			
Anal	S1 – S3		
Panniculus	T3 – L1 & C8 – T2		

Nociception

	Superficial pain		Deep pain	
	L	R	L	R
Thoracic limb				
Pelvic limb				
Head				
Perineum				

Grading scale

0	Absent
1	Decreased
2	Normal
3	Exaggerated
4	Very exaggerated
X	Not examined
±	Present/Absent

Assessment/localisation:

Differential diagnoses (tick)

☐ Degenerative   ☐ Metabolic   ☐ Inflammatory   ☐ Cardiovascular
☐ Anomalous   ☐ Neoplastic   ☐ Immune-mediated   ☐ Orthopaedic
☐ Allergic   ☐ Nutritional   ☐ Traumatic
☐ Autoimmune   ☐ Infectious   ☐ Toxic

Figure 4.3 Neurological examination sheet. PLR, pupillary light response. (University of Bristol)

Functionally neurones may also be subdivided into **afferent** neurones (those conducting impulses towards the CNS) and **efferent** neurones (those conducting impulses from the CNS). Most afferent neurones are sensory in nature whilst most efferent neurones are motor in nature.

Upper motor neurones (UMNs) are collections of nervous tissue specialised to initiate and maintain normal movement and muscle activity. Lower motor neurones (LMNs) are connections between the CNS and effector muscle groups or organs and connect to UMNs in the ventral horns of grey matter of the spinal cord.

Divisions of the brain

Divisions of the brain are extremely confusing as many terms are used interchangeably and divisions are often described based on embryological, functional or anatomical boundaries. For the purposes of this chapter it is useful to think of the brain as comprising four functional divisions:

1. the **forebrain** comprising the cerebral cortex/basal nuclei (telencephalon) and the thalamus/hypothalamus (diencephalon)
2. the **brainstem** comprising the midbrain (mesencephalon), pons (metencephalon

with cerebellum) and medulla oblongata (myelencephalon)

3. the **cerebellum**
4. the **vestibular system** which comprises a peripheral portion within the bony labyrinth of the ear, and a central portion within the medulla and cerebellum.

Simplistically the forebrain is responsible for the processing and interpretation of sensory information, cogitation, behaviour and the initiation and coordination of motor activity. The brainstem is responsible for maintenance of arousal of the forebrain and is the 'junction box' for most cranial nerve functions; it is also a site through which most afferent and efferent nervous traffic has to pass. The cerebellum is essentially regulatory in nature and helps to 'fine tune' coordination and movement; in itself it does not tend to initiate any activity. The vestibular apparatus is concerned with balance. A summary of divisions is shown in Figure 4.4.

Divisions of the spinal cord

The spinal cord is best considered as a cylindrical body divided into a number of segments like a stack of coins. From each segment paired nerves arise from either side comprising generally sensory afferent nerves dorsally and motor efferent nerves ventrally. The sensory and motor neurones innervating the limbs emerge from two swellings (intumescences) within the cord referred to as the brachial plexus (or intumescence) and the lumbosacral plexus (or intumescence). These segments are referred to according to the paired nerve roots which emerge from them but do not correspond exactly to the bony verterbrae which they are most adjacent to. The spinal cord segments can be grouped together to form five distinct divisions (see Fig. 4.5).

Localisation of lesions using upper and lower motor neurone signs

Because of these anatomically distinct sections and the divisions between UMNs and LMNs careful examination can be used to determine the site of a lesion to one of six functional divisions

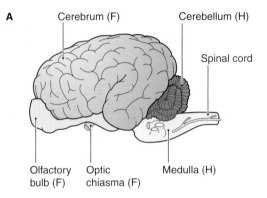

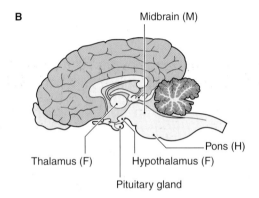

Figure 4.4 Major divisions in the brain. F, forebrain; H, hindbrain; M, midbrain. (From *Pre-Veterinary Nursing Textbook* by Masters and Bowden (2001). Reprinted by permission of Elsevier Science.)

of the nervous system – a lesion cranial to the division between brainstem and spinal cord, the C1–5 section, the C6–T2 section, the T3–L3 section, the L4–S2 section or caudal to S2. Differences between lesions of UMNs and LMNs are summarised in Table 4.1. and a summary of their use in localisation is shown in Table 4.2.

THE NEUROLOGICAL/ OPHTHALMOLOGICAL EXAMINATION

General observations

Mental status

We divide mental status into two components:

1. Level of consciousness: this can be fully conscious, depressed (easily roused), stuporous (only rousable by noxious stimuli) or comatose (unrousable).

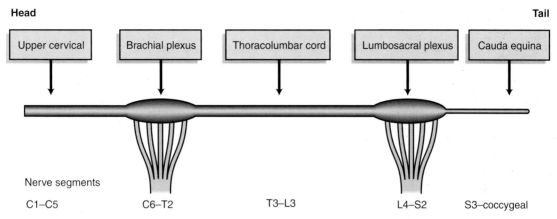

Figure 4.5   Major divisions of the spinal cord.

Table 4.1   Discriminating between upper and lower motor neurone signs

	Lower motor neurone signs	Upper motor neurone signs
Motor function	Paresis to paralysis, usually flaccid with loss of strength	Paresis to paralysis, maybe increased stiffness, loss of voluntary control
Muscle tone	Usually decreased	Usually increased
Local reflexes	Decreased to absent	Normal to exaggerated
Sensory signs	May have anaesthesia of a local segment with hyperaesthesia of surrounding tissue	Proprioceptive deficits, loss of superficial and deep pain

Table 4.2   Lesion localisation from upper (UMN)/lower motor neurone (LMN) signs

Forelimb examination	Hindlimb examination	Likely lesion localisation
Normal	Normal	Normal motor function
UMN signs	UMN signs	Brain or cervical cord C1–C5
LMN signs	UMN signs	Lower cervical cord C6–T2
Normal	UMN signs	Thoracic/upper lumbar cord T3–L3, occasionally lesions affecting sciatic nerve bilaterally may be confused
Normal	LMN signs	Lower lumbar/sacral cord, cauda equina, bilateral pelvic limb neuropathy
LMN signs	LMN signs	Peripheral neuropathy/ disorder of neuromuscular unit

may be described as appropriate or inappropriate.

Conciousness in any animal is maintained by the **ascending reticular activating system (ARAS),** a collection of neurones within the rostral brainstem which accept sensory information from cranial nerves and other sensory neurones. This system regulates consciousness by modulating cerebral activity. Thus alterations in level of consciousness usually indicate a brainstem problem or possibly a severe cerebral problem (most commonly seen with toxic or metabolic encephalopathies).

The content of an animal's consciousness tells us something about the animal's state of cerebral health rather than specifying any particular lesion.

Posture

Examination should include examination of head, trunk and limb posture.

2. Content of that consciousness (i.e. how the animal interacts with its environment): this

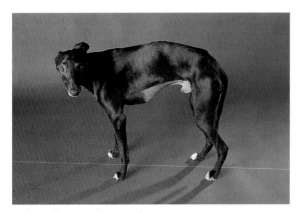

Figure 4.6 Kyphosis in a dog with suspected steroid-responsive meningitis.

Head posture should be evaluated for abnormalities such as head tilt, rotation or aversion and abnormally low or high head carriage.

Trunk posture will mainly display obvious abnormalities in the carriage of the axial skeleton which may in turn reflect specific areas of discomfort or instability. Such deviations may be referred to as kyphosis (upward arching of the thoracolumbar spine; Fig. 4.6), lordosis (ventral deviation of the thoracolumbar spine), or scoliosis (lateral deviation of the spine).

Evaluation of limb posture should include observation for increased or decreased muscle tone leading to hyper- or hypo-extension of one or more limbs, that the distal portion of each limb remains directly ventral to the primary joint of that limb (i.e. the stance is not wide-based or narrow-based) and for any feet that remain 'knuckled over' in a standing position. Wide- and narrow-based stances are commonly seen in ataxic animals and may be due to vestibular, cerebellar or proprioceptive causes of ataxia (though a narrow-based stance is infrequently seen with the first two). Knuckling usually represents proprioceptive loss to that limb and may represent either an LMN or UMN lesion.

Movement

Both voluntary movement (i.e. the animal's gait) and the presence of any involuntary movements

such as tremors or muscular spasms should be noted.

It is useful to examine the animal's gait both at walk and trotting and also to provide varying 'challenges' to its coordination by the use of different surface types, inclines and curbs where possible. Turning the animal in tight circles in both directions may also uncover subtle abnormalities of gait.

Paresis infers a deficit in voluntary movement in one or more limbs and is usually due to disruption of the voluntary motor pathways involving both UMNs and LMNs.

Paralysis (-plegia) is essentially a more severe form in which no voluntary movement is present. The prefixes **mono-** (one limb affected), **hemi-** (limbs on one side affected), **para-** (hind limbs affected), **tetra-** or **quadri-** (all limbs affected) may be applied to paresis or paralysis (-plegia).

Proprioception refers to the ability to detect the whereabouts in time and space of a limb with relation to the rest of the body and is mediated by both LMNs and UMNs under both voluntary and involuntary control.

Ataxia refers to incoordination not due solely to lack of motor control (though both may be seen together). Ataxia usually represents lesions of the proprioceptive, cerebellar or vestibular pathways.

Dysmetria infers abnormal force and range of movement. **Hypermetria** describes abnormally exaggerated ('goose-stepping') movements and is a hallmark of some cerebellar disease. **Hypometria** describes movements that are too short.

Involuntary movements most commonly manifest themselves as tremors or coarse jerking of muscle groups (**myoclonus**). Tremors may be made worse by voluntary activity such as eating and when this occurs are often referred to as **intention tremors**; these are predominantly seen in cerebellar disease, but disorders of involuntary movement may be caused by a large range of neurological diseases.

Muscle tone

Muscle bulk and symmetry are palpated and tone is assessed by passively flexing and extending each limb. Muscle strength is difficult to assess. Decreased muscle bulk (atrophy) may accompany disuse, LMN disease and disorders of the motor unit and is most obvious when rapid, severe and unilateral. Changes in muscle tone may reflect UMN disorders (muscle tone is usually increased) or disorders of the LMNs or motor unit (muscle tone decreased).

Ophthalmic examination

A thorough description of ophthalmic examination is beyond the scope of this chapter and only information relevant to neurological assessment is made here.

Examination technique

Typical neuro-ophthalmic examination is described in Box 4.3.

Before detailed examination, as with other aspects of the neurological examination, initial observation is invaluable. This is especially true of assessing vision, and a useful technique is to make the patient negotiate an obstacle course both in a fully lit and a darkened room.

Box 4.3 Neuro-ophthalmic examination protocol

1. Initially in light conditions the patient, eyes and adnexa (those structures surrounding the globe) are examined. Specifically pupil and eyelid symmetry and pupil position should be assessed
2. Pupillary light responses, menace reflex, corneal reflex, palpebral reflex and oculocephalic ('doll's eye') reflex should be assessed as part of cranial nerve examination (see below)
3. Measure tear production with Schirmer tear test strips before any topical agents have been applied to the eye. This is particularly important in cases with facial nerve involvement as it may help distinguish between peripheral and central causes of facial nerve paralysis
4. Make a detailed examination of the eye and all three eyelids using an appropriate light source and magnification. Topical stains may be used to highlight abnormalities of the corneal surface
5. A mydriatic is applied
6. In darkened conditions, make a detailed examination of the adnexa, anterior globe segment and posterior segment using both direct and indirect ophthalmoscopy

---

Interpretation

As part of the neurological examination, ophthalmoscopic assessment is essential in answering four principal questions:

1. Are there any abnormalities of the cranial nerves involved in the positioning and function of the eyes and adnexal structures?
2. Is there any evidence of ocular manifestations of systemic disease?
3. Is there any evidence of raised intracranial pressure?
4. Is there any intraocular explanation for any visual deficits?

Ophthalmic examination may reveal lesions that are reflective not only of localised ocular disease but also of systemic disease which may produce neurological signs. Examples of these are given in Box 4.4.

Cranial nerve examination

Olfactory nerve (Cn I)

Either a pleasurable or noxious odour (fish-flavoured food or alcohol is especially useful) is held in front of the animal's nose and a behavioural response (sniffing, nose wrinkling, aversion or interest) is the normal expected response. It is difficult to assess individual sides. Assessment of smell is often unrewarding and deficiencies are difficult to interpret. As in humans, non-specific rhinitis is the most common cause though structural lesions within the olfactory nerves, olfactory bulbs, cortex or limbic system may lead to signs of deficiency.

Optic nerve (Cn II)

Optic nerve function is assessed by observation of visual integrity (especially obstacle courses), visual placing responses (see later) and by the menace response (in addition to Cn VII, facial nerve) and pupillary light response (in addition to Cn III, oculomotor nerve).

For a menace response, the eye not being tested is covered and a threatening gesture is made in front of the eye being tested, taking care not to create air currents by 'wafting' a hand or

Box 4.4 Ocular manifestations of systemic disease which may be associated with neurological signs

Intraocular haemorrhage due to:
- trauma
- bleeding disorders
- neoplasia
- hypertension
- chorioretinitis

Anterior uveitis associated with:
- trauma
- viral – canine distemper, FeLV, FIV, FIP
- protozoal – *Toxoplasma, Neospora*
- rickettsial – *Borrelia, Ehrlichia*
- mycotic – principally *Cryptococcus* in the UK
- parasitic – e.g. *Angiostrongylus*

Inflammatory retinopathies:
- traumatic
- viral – canine distemper, FeLV, FIV, FIP
- bacterial – *Borrelia* spp.
- protozoal – *Toxoplasma, Neospora*
- rickettsial – *Ehrlichia* spp.
- mycotic – principally *Cryptococcus* in the UK
- parasitic – e.g. *Angiostrongylus*

Nutritional retinopathies:
- thiamin deficiency

Papilloedema due to:
- raised intracranial pressure
- lead poisoning, fern poisoning, vitamin A deficiency

Optic neuritis/papillitis due to:
- trauma
- neoplasia
- meningeal inflammation
- compression by retrobulbar space occupying lesion

Conjunctivitis due to:
- canine distemper
- *Rickettsia*

Tear film abnormalities due to:
- facial nerve palsy

FeLV, feline leukaemia virus; FIV, feline immunodeficiency virus; FIP, feline infectious peritonitis

by touching periadnexal hairs (both will stimulate the ophthalmic branch of Cn V, trigeminal). A blink is the normal expected response.

For the pupillary light response (PLR), a strong penlight is directed into each eye (in a darkened room) and the response of the pupil noted. Constriction of both the pupil into which the penlight is shone (direct response) and the contralateral pupil (consensual response) is the expected normal response.

The pathways for vision and the pupillary light response are shown in Figure 4.7. An abnormal menace or PLR response may indicate a lesion in any of these areas and only by evaluating the full neuro-ophthalmic examination can further localisation be made.

Oculomotor nerve (Cn III)

The oculomotor nerve as described above supplies a parasympathetic branch which controls pupillary constriction and therefore the PLR helps assess its integrity. Motor innervation is, however, also supplied by this nerve to several extraocular muscles (dorsal, medial, ventral rectus, ventral oblique) which maintain eye position and the levator palpebrae superioris muscle of the upper eyelid. Assessment of eye position is made by direct observation and by assessing the animal's ability to follow objects with its eyes (for instance by moving a cotton wool ball on a piece of thread in front of it with its head kept still) or by inducing normal side-to-side and up-and-down head–eye movements (and physiological nystagmus) by manipulation of the head.

With oculomotor nerve lesions, a fixed dilated pupil with normal vision, slight upper eyelid drooping (ptosis) and ventrolateral deviation of the globe (strabismus) are expected. Pharmacologic testing using pilocarpine or physostigmine may help further localise the lesion.

Trochlear nerve (Cn IV)

The trochlear nerve supplies motor innervation to the dorsal oblique muscle of the globe with the result that lesions result in a medial rotation when viewed from the front. This is most easily observed in cats with their vertically orientated pupils. In dogs, only medial rotation of a dorsal retinal vein may give a clue to a trochlear nerve deficit due to the circular pupil.

Trigeminal nerve (Cn V)

The trigeminal nerve has three branches and two functions. The maxillary, mandibular and ophthalmic branches receive sensory information from the skin of the face (see Fig. 4.8), whilst the mandibular branch also contains the motor branch innervating the muscles of mastication

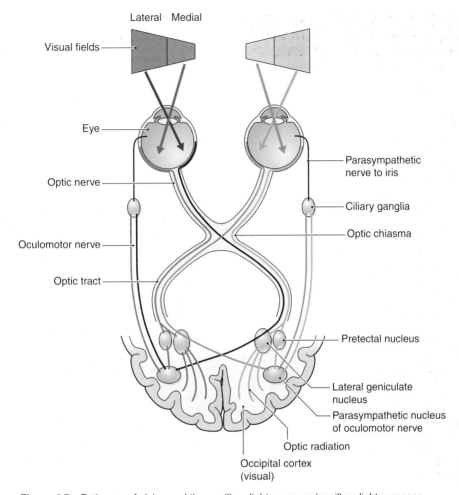

Figure 4.7 Pathways of vision and the papillary light response/pupillary light response.

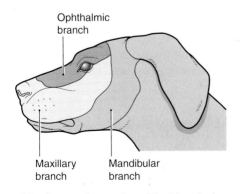

Figure 4.8 Sensory innervation of the trigeminal nerve.

(masseter, temporalis, pterygoid, rostral digastricus, mylohyoid). Sensation is tested by touch or by gentle pinching with mosquito forceps to elicit a skin-twitch response or behavioural aversion. The sites for testing are also shown in Figure 4.8. Sensation should be tested at all sites bilaterally.

The motor branch of the trigeminal nerve is assessed by palpation of the temporalis and masseter muscles. Bilateral lesions will result in an inability to close the jaw and oral dysphagia will result. Unilateral lesions may result in some dysphagia. Severe muscle atrophy of the temporalis and masseter muscles resulting in prominence of the zygomatic arch usually occurs within 1 week of a lesion occurring. This is much easier to appreciate in unilateral dysfunction.

Abducens nerve (Cn VI)

The abducens nerve innervates the lateral rectus muscle and the retractor bulbi muscles which retract the globe in response to touch. It is assessed by assessing ocular movements in the same way as the oculomotor nerve (Cn III) and by touching the surface of the cornea with a moistened swab to elicit globe retraction in the corneal reflex. The corneal reflex will also assess the sensory ophthalmic branch of the trigeminal nerve. With abducens nerve lesions, inability to follow objects as they pass laterally and medial strabismus occur as does failure of retraction with corneal contact.

Facial nerve (Cn VII)

The facial nerve supplies motor innervation to the muscles of facial expression, parasympathetic innervation to the lacrimal gland and sensations of taste from the rostral two thirds of the tongue and the palate and touch on the inner surface of the pinnae. Observation of the face for signs of asymmetry should be performed and a Schirmer tear test performed before the addition of any topical ocular medications. Taste may be assessed by touching the rostral portion of the tongue on the suspect side with a cotton wool bud which has been impregnated with atropine; the taste is extremely bitter and normal animals will react strongly to the taste, often salivating profusely. Facial nerve function is also assessed by observation of a blink during the palpebral, corneal, and menace responses.

Facial nerve dysfunction is usually unilateral and often results in striking facial asymmetry with drooping of the eyelids (ptosis), slack maxillary skin, deviation of the nasal planum, drooling, pouching and dropping of food and failure of the nostril to flare on the affected side. Corneal ulceration may result from a combination of exposure keratitis from lack of blink and decreased tear production.

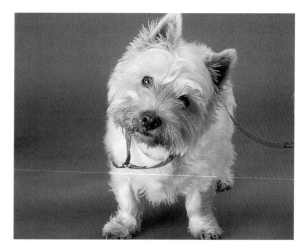

Figure 4.9   Head tilt in a West Highland white terrier.

Vestibulocochlear nerve (Cn VIII)

The cochlear portion of the nerve which is involved with hearing may be crudely assessed by observing behavioural responses to a handclap or dropping an object to the floor to make a sound.

The vestibular portion is assessed by observation for head tilt and spontaneous nystagmus (jerking of the globe from side-to-side, up-and-down, or round-and-round repeatedly) (Fig. 4.9). The direction of nystagmus should be noted as should whether it has a fast and a slow phase (and if so in which direction) or is pendulous. Spontaneous pendulous nystagmus is a normal finding in Siamese and Himalayan cats.

Hearing deficits, unless complete, are difficult to assess accurately without the use of electrophysiologic testing (brainstem auditory evoked responses, BAERs). Lesions involving the vestibular pathways may result from peripheral or central lesions. Their differentiation depends upon observations of nystagmus coupled with other cranial nerve assessment and proprioceptive responses.

Glossopharyngeal nerve (Cn IX)

The glossopharyngeal nerve innervates the muscles of the pharynx and palatine structures and also supplies sensory information from the caudal one third of the tongue and pharyngeal mucosa. Its motor functions overlap somewhat with the vagus nerve (Cn X) and assessment of both is usually undertaken together. Dysfunction of motor function is suspected by a history of pharyngeal dysphagia and is assessed by eliciting a 'gag' reflex by inserting a finger or tongue depressor towards the pharynx. Swallowing or gagging should result. Caution is strongly advised in fractious animals or when an animal's travel history makes rabies a possibility. Taste can be assessed in the same way as for Cn VII, though accurate assessment is very difficult.

Vagus nerve (Cn X)

As for the glossopharyngeal nerve the vagus innervates the muscles of the pharynx, but in addition controls laryngeal abduction and vocalisation. The vagus is also vital in providing parasympathetic innervation to the thoracic and abdominal viscera. Assessment of the gag reflex is as described for Cn IX. Failure of laryngeal abduction may result in alteration in bark (dysphonia). Assessment of parasympathetic function is difficult to perform accurately.

Accessory nerve (Cn XI)

The spinal accessory nerve provides motor innervation to the trapezius muscle and part of the sternocephalicus and brachiocephalicus muscles. Dysfunction leads to paralysis and atrophy of these muscles but even with severe atrophy it is difficult to assess and lesions of the accessory nerve appear to be rare (or rarely recognised).

Hypoglossal nerve (Cn XII)

The hypoglossal nerve provides motor innervation to the intrinsic and extrinsic muscles of the tongue. Dysfunction results in atrophy of tongue musculature and inability to retract the tongue after it is gently stretched. Assessment is made by observation of the tongue for symmetry and of range of tongue movement by provoking licking movements to either side. This may be accomplished by moistening the lips or nose with water, or by smearing food around the lips.

Postural reactions

Postural reactions are tests of an animal's ability to retain an upright posture and to maintain even load-supporting function in each limb when imbalancing forces are applied. Most postural reactions are altered by both paresis and altered proprioception. Postural reactions are sensitive tests as even minor alterations in the integrity of the nervous components of posture will result in abnormal reactions; these are often not visible by evaluation of gait alone. They are not, however, often useful in providing an anatomical localisation for lesions.

Proprioceptive positioning reaction

To test proprioception, with its weight adequately supported, the animal's foot is flexed so that the dorsal surface is in contact with the floor. A normal reaction is for the foot to be immediately replaced in a normal position. A further test is performed by placing the animal's foot on a card or piece of paper and drawing the paper laterally so that the limb is abducted. A normal reaction is for immediate in-stepping of the limb to retain a square weight-bearing posture. The first test is most useful for testing proprioception in the distal extremity whilst the proximal limb proprioception is more appropriately tested by the latter. Abnormal proprioceptive responses may result in any lesion affecting the sensory pathway from the foot being tested to the sensory cortex of the cerebrum.

Other postural reactions

Wheelbarrowing reaction

The animal is supported under its abdomen so that all its weight is carried on the thoracic limbs; care is taken not to lift the abdomen abnormally high. The animal is then walked forwards and backwards.

Extensor postural thrust

The animal is supported in an upright position caudal to the thoracic limbs and gently lowered, hindlimbs first, towards the ground. A normal reaction is a slight extension of the hindlimbs in anticipation of ground contact followed by a reflex step back until balance is restored.

Hopping, hemistanding, hemiwalking

In each of these tests both strength and coordination of limb movement are assessed. Initially the animal is supported so that only one limb is weight-bearing; this will accentuate any subtle paresis in an individual limb. The animal is then 'hopped' by gently pushing it away from the examiner, a normal reaction being a coordinated shift in position of the limb so that it is continually under the animal and bearing weight. Abnormal responses include collapsing or dragging of the limb. The reaction is tested in each limb in turn and then both limbs on each side (hemistanding/hemiwalking).

Abnormalities of voluntary motor activity (paresis/paralysis), muscle tone and proprioception may all be demonstrated by these responses.

Placing reactions

Placing reactions are usually only possible in small patients. The animal is lifted by the examiner and moved towards a surface such as a table top until the dorsal surfaces of the feet contact the table edge. A normal response to the sensory input from this contact should be a lifting and 'reaching' with both limbs being tested until the foot comes to rest on the surface. The test should be repeated with the animal's eyes covered to force more reliance on purely tactile sensory information.

Placing reactions can demonstrate subtle abnormalities in tactile sensory input and proprioception from the affected limb.

Spinal reflexes

Spinal reflexes investigate the integrity of the components of a reflex arc (i.e. an afferent sensory neurone and an efferent LMN) and also the influence of descending motor pathways. The descending UMN pathways usually have an inhibitory effect on the reflex and abnormalities of the motor pathways above the spinal cord segment of the reflex being assessed may result in an exaggerated reflex. Coventionally, spinal cord reflexes are recorded as being 0 (absent), 1 (reduced), 2 (normal), 3 (exaggerated) or 4 (myoclonus or muscle spasticity).

Myotactic (stretch) reflexes

These rely on a muscle being briefly stretched (usually by sharp contact with a tendon hammer on the tendon or muscle belly) which causes stretch within muscle spindles. This causes sensory afferent discharge to the local spinal cord segment with the descending LMN component of the arc causing a reflex contraction within the muscle. At the same time the opposing muscle group is inhibited from contracting and the result is a reflex jerk of the limb.

In the hindlimb, the most useful myotactic reflex is the patellar or quadriceps reflex, though gastrocnemius and cranial tibial reflexes may also be useful. Forelimb reflexes are very difficult to interpret as in normal animals they are often difficult to elicit. The most reproducible appears to be the extensor carpi radialis reflex, though biceps and triceps reflexes may also be attempted. Many examiners do not believe forelimb reflexes are useful to assess. It is important that when reflexes are assessed the animal is held comfortably in lateral recumbency and that only the upper limbs are tested before rolling the animal over and repeating the tests on the other side.

A summary of interpretation of myotactic reflexes is shown in Table 4.3.

Flexor (withdrawal, pedal) reflexes

With the animal in lateral recumbency the skin between the digits of the limb to be tested is gently pinched; a normal response is reflexive withdrawal of the limb. The contralateral limb should be observed for a 'crossed extensor reflex' whilst this is occurring and should not be held. The crossed extensor reflex is an abnormal forceful extension of the contralateral limb during flexion of the limb being tested. The flexor reflex

Table 4.3   Nerve segments assessed by myotactic stretch reflexes

Reflex	Sensory component (afferent arm)	Motor component (efferent arm)
Forelimb reflexes		
Flexor (withdrawal) reflex	Depends on where stimulated: Cranial surface of foot – radial nerve (C7–T1) Medial palmar surface – median/ulnar (C8–T1) Lateral palmar surface – ulnar nerve (C8–T1)	Flexor muscles stimulated by several nerves simultaneously from spinal cord segments (C6–T1)
Biceps reflex	Musculocutaneous nerve (C6–8)	Musculocutaneous nerve (C6–8)
Triceps reflex	Radial nerve (C7–T1)	Radial nerve (C7–T1)
Extensor carpi radialis reflex	Radial nerve (C7–T1)	Radial nerve (C7–T1)
Hindlimb reflexes		
Flexor (withdrawal) reflex	Depends on where stimulated: Medial digit – saphenous branch of femoral nerve (L4–6) Rest of foot – sciatic nerve (L6–S1)	Sciatic nerve (L6–S1)
Patellar (quadriceps) reflex	Femoral nerve (L4–6)	Femoral nerve (L4–6)
Cranial tibial reflex	Peroneal branch (L6–7) of the sciatic nerve	Peroneal branch (L6–7) of the sciatic nerve
Gastrocnemius reflex	Tibial branch (L7–S1) of the sciatic nerve	Tibial branch (L7–S1) of the sciatic nerve

assesses the integrity of the local reflex arc; it does not infer that an animal can feel the stimulus (unless it shows a behavioural reaction such as growling, biting or turning its head) and has an intact spinal cord. In the hindlimb the sensory and motor components of the reflex are principally maintained by the sciatic nerve (L6–S1) with the exception of the sensory component of the medial digit which is a branch of the femoral nerve (L4–6). Absence or depression of withdrawal reflexes usually indicates a lesion within the sciatic nerve. In the forelimb, the motor innervation of the reflexes is a combination of the axillary, musculocutaneous, median and ulnar nerves and tests spinal cord segments C6–T1.

The crossed extensor reflex is abnormal and is seen with UMN lesions cranial to the segment being tested on the opposite side of the spinal cord. Usually reflex extension of the contralateral limb (which occurs when the animal is standing) is inhibited in recumbency by UMNs, but when these are damaged a crossed extensor may be seen.

Panniculus reflex

Skin sensation is detected by lightly pinching the skin of the flanks with a pair of mosquito forceps from the lumbar to the thoracic region both 5–7 cm and 10–15 cm lateral to the spine. A normal expected response is a reflex twitch of the panniculus muscle under the skin. The panniculus reflex depends on the sensory integrity of the specific skin segment being tested, areas of individual sensory nerve fields being referred to as **dermatomes.** The motor component to the panniculus muscle exits the spinal cord at the C8–T1 level. The reflex should occur bilaterally if intact. Loss of the panniculus reflex below a certain level ('panniculus cutoff') can be a useful aid to further localising thoracolumbar spinal cord lesions, as can unilateral panniculus loss. If unilateral panniculus loss is accompanied by a normal bilateral response when the opposite side is tested, it is suggestive of a C8/T1 lesion on the affected side.

Anal reflex

With the tail gently elevated the anus is lightly stroked with a firm object such as the tip of a haemostat. A reflex 'wink' of the anus is expected. Both sensory and motor components of this reflex are mediated through the pudendal nerve (S1–3) and absent or reduced reflexes and a flaccid anus usually represent a lack of integrity of the sacral cord segments.

Nociception

Nociception or pain perception is a neurologically complex response resulting from stimulation of superficial or deep pain sensory pathways. Superficial pain is assessed by examining responses to gently pinching with haemostats over an area of skin to be tested. Many areas are contained within the sensory fields of many nerves and in order for testing to be meaningful an area innervated by only one sensory nerve (an 'autonomous zone') should be tested. Maps of these zones can be found in most neurological texts. Deep pain is assessed by applying stronger compressive forces to deeper tissues such as between the toes or across the digits. Deep pain sensation should only be assessed in animals with paralysis as the nerve pathways are deep within the spinal cord and will be unaffected in normally ambulatory animals. Similarly there is no merit in assessing deep pain responses in an animal with obviously normal superficial pain sensation. A normal response to pain is behavioural, i.e. anxiety, vocalising, turning, biting, snapping. Reflexive withdrawal is not an indication of pain sensation. Absence of superficial sensation may indicate a sensory field deficit. Absence of deep pain sensation in an affected limb of a paralysed animal is an ominous finding associated with severe spinal cord damage and should prompt immediate consideration of referral to a neurologist.

ENDOCRINE AND GASTROINTESTINAL TESTS

ENDOCRINE TESTS

Assessment of canine hypothyroidism

A summary of thyroid hormone stimulation and release is shown in Figure 4.10.

Total thyroxine (T_4) assay

Serum total T_4 is cheap and widely available and is traditionally used to test thyroid function. In theory T_4 levels below the laboratory reference

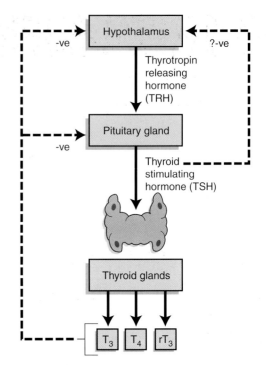

Figure 4.10 Summary of thyroid hormone stimulation and release.

range should indicate subnormal thyroid function. Its principal disadvantages as a test of thyroid function are a low specificity due to the effects of many non-thyroidal factors on total T_4 levels and normal daily fluctuation in T_4 levels. Factors which can falsely affect T_4 levels are listed in Box 4.5.

Non-thyroidal illness may contribute in many cases to the so-called 'sick-euthyroid syndrome' in which total T_4 levels are decreased by a number of mechanisms and results should be interpreted cautiously or delayed until resolution of the illness.

Free T_4 assay

Free T_4 assay is also performed on serum samples. Whilst most T_4 circulates bound to plasma proteins, a small proportion circulates unbound and is available for immediate uptake by target cells. This proportion, known as 'free T_4' or fT_4, is less markedly decreased by non-thyroidal factors, such as drug therapy or illness, and there are

Box 4.5 Non-thyroidal factors affecting *thyroxine T₄* levels

Age
- dogs <6 months old often have high T₄ levels compared with adults
- T₄ levels generally decline with age after this

Breed
- small dogs generally have higher resting T₄ levels than larger dogs
- sight hounds and other very athletic breeds often have exteremly low resting T₄ levels

Gender
- no real difference between sexes
- intraindividual variation in cycling females – highest levels during dioestrus/pregnancy

Drug therapy
- T₄ decreased by: androgens, glucocorticoids, non-steroidal anti-inflammatory drugs, anticonvulsants, salicylates, sulfonamides, mitotane, sedatives, iodinated compounds, penicillin, diazepam
- T₄ increased by: oestrogens, halothane, insulin, narcotic analgesics

Non-thyroidal illness
- will generally decrease T₄

distinct advantages to its measurement where these extrinsic factors exist. Only assay by the equilibrium dialysis method is advantageous.

Total triiodothyronine (T₃) assay

Total T₃ levels may remain within the normal range even with declining function and this assay is not recommended as an assessment of thyroid function.

Canine endogenous thyroid-stimulating hormone (cTSH)

Serum endogenous TSH is used in combination with total or free T₄ for assessment of thyroid function and monitoring thyroid replacement therapy. Loss of functional thyroid tissue results in a lack of negative feedback on the hypothalamic–pituitary axis from circulating T₄ and T₃ resulting in increased production of TSH from pituitary thyrotropes. Thus the finding of raised endogenous TSH levels, particularly in combination with a decreased total or free T₄, offers substantial evidence of thyroid dysfunction.

TSH stimulation test

The TSH stimulation test has long been held as the 'gold standard' test for the diagnosis of canine hypothyroidism. Total T₄ levels are measured before and 6 hours after the intravenous administration of 0.1 IU/kg (to a maximum of 5 IU) of bovine TSH. The normal minimum physiological response is a post-stimulation total T₄ in excess of 30 nmol/l. Equivocal results are sometimes produced. This test is not widely available in general practice.

Thyrotropin-releasing hormone (TRH) stimulation test

The TRH stimulation test has been heralded as a more practical and widely available alternative to the TSH stimulation test. Total T₄ levels are assayed before and 4 hours after the intravenous administration of 0.2–0.5 mg/dog of TRH. Higher dosages of TRH may result in clinically adverse effects such as salivation, urination, defecation, tachycardia, tachypnoea and weakness, and offer no advantage in terms of increased T₄ release. A normal response of a 1.5 times increase in the basal T₄ is generally quoted or a rise above 6 mmol/l. Increases in fT₄ may be more consistent. Interpretation of TRH stimulation tests often yields equivocal results and other than wider availability, they offer few advantages over TSH stimulation testing.

Other tests used in canine hypothyroidism

Anti-T₄ or anti-T₃ antibodies may be identified in some dogs with clinical signs of hypothyroidism and are thought to be an indication of lymphocytic thyroiditis. The finding of these antibodies in dogs with apparently normal thyroid gland function is of presently undetermined significance. Tests for anti-thyroid hormone antibodies may be useful in cases where other diagnostic tests demonstrate highly unexpected results as these antibodies can falsely elevate or depress total T₄ levels depending on the assay methodology used (this should be checked with the individual laboratory). Antibodies to the thyroglobulin protein within thyroid follicles can be detected in the serum of up to 59% of hypothyroid dogs. However, the finding of anti-thyroglobulin antibodies in a large number of dogs with non-thyroidal illness and in normal euthyroid dogs suggests that this assay is of limited value until further work has been undertaken.

Total T_4 assays may also be used to monitor therapeutic response to thyroid hormone supplementation. A serum sample taken 3–8 hours after dosage should yield a result within the target range of 30–70 mmol/l if T_4 supplementation is adequate. TSH levels, if elevated prior to T_4 supplementation, should also return to normal with successful supplementation.

Assessment of feline hyperthyroidism

Total T_4/T_3 levels

Levels are assayed in serum as a screening test for feline hyperthyroidism. In hyperthyroid feline patients total serum T_4 levels and to a certain extent T_3 levels are usually elevated. Similar to the situation in canine hypothyroidism, however, many hyperthyroid cats have T_3 levels which fall within the normal range, therefore T_4 assays are preferred. Measurement of free T_4 appears to offer little advantage over total T_4 assessment except where depression of T_4 by non-thyroidal factors is suspected. A small percentage of cats with clinical hyperthyroidism may have T_4 levels which fall within the upper limit of the normal feline range due to early disease, daily fluctuation or concurrent non-thyroidal disease.

T_3 suppression test

This is used to assess thyroid function in cats with equivocal T_4 levels. A serum sample is taken to evaluate basal T_4 and T_3 levels. The owner or veterinary staff then administer one 25 µg tablet of T_3 p.o., TID for 48 hours and then on the third day a final 25 µg tablet is given followed by blood sampling 2–4 hours later. This is again assayed for T_4 and T_3, the former to assess the degree of suppression and the latter to assess whether the T_3 has been satisfactorily administered and absorbed.

In normal cats the administration of exogenous T_3 inhibits TSH release from pituitary thyrotropes by negative feedback and so serum T_4 levels decrease. In hyperthyroidism, the thyroid tissue autonomously secretes T_4 without the stimulatory influence of TSH and it is this difference which is the basis of the T_3 suppression test. In normal cats, dramatic suppression of T_4 levels should result whereas in the presence of hyperthyroidism, little response is seen.

TSH/TRH stimulation tests

Due to the independence of T_4 secretion by adenomatous thyroid tissue from pituitary stimulation, the administration of TSH or TRH in hyperthyroid cats should result in minimal or no increase compared with normal individuals. However, both tests frequently result in equivocal results and neither can be recommended as particularly useful in the diagnosis of feline hyperthyroidism.

Other tests for feline hyperthyroidism

Where it is available nuclear scintigraphy may be invaluable for the diagnosis of hyperthyroidism in cases where test results are equivocal but clinical signs are highly suggestive of disease.

Tests of canine adrenal function

Canine adrenal function tests are utilised for the diagnosis of hyperadrenocorticism (Cushing's disease), both naturally occurring and iatrogenic, and of hypoadrenocorticism (Addison's disease). A summary of the pituitary–hypothalamic–adrenocortical axis is shown in Figure 4.11. It should be noted that, whereas the diagnosis of hypoadrenocorticism on the basis of adrenal function testing is usually unequivocal, the highly variable specificity and sensitivity of tests utilised in diagnosing hyperadrenocorticism may lead to a high incidence of false positive and false negative results and often multiple tests need to be performed.

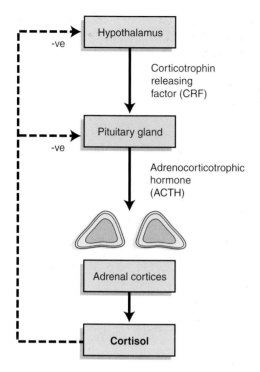

Figure 4.11 Summary of cortisol stimulation and release.

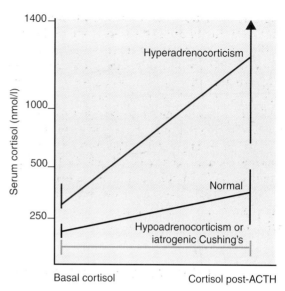

Figure 4.12 Typical adrenocorticotrophic hormone (ACTH) stimulation test findings.

ACTH stimulation test

This test is used as a screening test of hyperadrenocorticism, for diagnosis of iatrogenic hyperadrenocorticism, for diagnosis of hypoadrenocorticism, and for monitoring therapy. Serum cortisol levels are assayed before, and 60–90 minutes after, the intravenous administration of synthetic ACTH. A dose of 0.25 mg synthetic ACTH is given to dogs >5 kg body weight and 0.125 mg to dogs <5 kg body weight. A basal level of 20–250 nmol/l and a post-stimulation cortisol value of <660 nmol/l is expected in normal dogs. Hyperadrenocorticism is indicated by post-stimulation values of >660 nmol/l and hypoadrenocorticism is indicated by failure of stimulation of cortisol release by ACTH administration and a pre- and post-stimulation level of <20 nmol/l (Fig. 4.12). Iatrogenic hyperadrenocorticism due to exogenous glucocorticoid administration also results in failure to stimulate cortisol production after administration of synthetic ACTH. Approximately 85% of dogs with pituitary-dependent hyperadrenocorticism and 50% of dogs with adrenal-dependent hyperadrenocorticism will be correctly identified by a normal test result. False-positive results may also sometimes be seen in dogs with severe nonadrenocortical illnesses.

ACTH stimulation tests may also be used to monitor dogs undergoing mitotane or other chemotherapy for the treatment of hyperadrenocorticism. A target pre- and post-stimulation cortisol level of <120 nmol/l signifies effective suppression.

Urine cortisol:creatinine ratio

This test is performed on a urine sample collected at home (to minimise elevation of cortisol release through stress of hospitalisation) and is a useful screening test for hyperadrenocorticism. Long-term increases in cortisol release may be detected by this test. Urine cortisol is stable in postal samples and a ratio of $>10 \times 10^{-6}$ is supportive evidence of hyperadrenocorticism. However, though the test is very sensitive, many dogs with non-adrenal illness will also have an elevated value. It should, therefore, not be used as a sole diagnostic test for hyperadrenocorticism, but is a useful and cost-effective screening test.

Low-dose dexamethasone suppression test (LDDST)

This test is also a useful screening test for hyper-adrenocorticism. Serum samples are collected for cortisol assay before, and 3 and 8 hours after, the intravenous administration of 0.01 mg/kg of dexamethasone sodium phosphate (which does not cross-react with cortisol assays). Only very small volumes of dexamethasone are needed and care must be taken to dose accurately. In normal dogs, the exogenous administration of cortico-steroids results in negative feedback of pituitary ACTH secretion and thus suppression of adrenal cortisol release; in these animals 3 and 8 hour samples should both be severely depressed, e.g. <20 mmol/l. In dogs with functional pituitary tumours, ACTH release by the functional mass is generally only temporarily suppressed by exogenous corticosteroid administration, and dogs with adrenocortical tumours (which are persistently cortisol secreting) experience no such suppression. In dogs with hyperadrenocorticism, cortisol levels either fail entirely to suppress at 3 and 8 hours (which is the situation in virtually all adrenal-dependent cases, and approximately 20% of pituitary-dependent cases) or the 3-hourly sample is suppressed but cortisol levels have increased by 8 hours (the usual situation in pituitary-dependent hyperadrenocorticism) (Fig. 4.13).

LDDST does not reliably differentiate between pituitary and adrenal-dependent hyperadreno-corticism. False-positive results can be found in dogs with severe non-adrenal illnesses and this should be borne in mind when performing the test if a concurrent disease has already been identified (e.g. uncontrolled diabetes mellitus)

Tests to discriminate between pituitary-dependent and adrenal-dependent hyperadrenocorticism

Traditionally the high-dose dexamethasone suppression test (HDDST) has been used to distinguish between pituitary-dependent hyper-adrenocorticism (PDH) and adrenal-dependent hyperadrenocorticism (ADH) but this should only be performed once a diagnosis of hyperadreno-corticism has been confirmed. Theoretically the

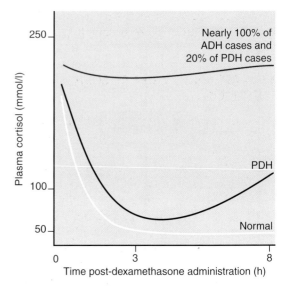

Figure 4.13 Low dose dexamethasone suppression test findings to discriminate between adrenal-dependent hyperadrenocorticism (ADH) and pituitary–dependent hyperadrenocorticism (PDH).

administration of a higher dose of dexamethasone (0.1 mg/kg dexamethasone sodium phosphate intravenously) with cortisol samples measured at 0, 3 and 8 hours should result in no suppression with ADH but suppression with PDH. However, approximately 25% of dogs with PDH do not suppress, and whilst if suppression is seen a diagnosis of PDH is likely, if no suppression is seen ADH *or* PDH is still possible.

The measurement of endogenous ACTH levels can be a useful discriminatory test, cases of PDH theoretically producing very high levels, well above the reference range of 20–80 mg/ml, and dogs with ADH should have levels well below this range due to feedback suppression of pituitary ACTH release due to high endogenous cortisol levels. Equivocal results falling within the normal range are unfortunately often found and the hor-mone is extremely labile and must be transported and interpreted rapidly after immediate freezing acording to the laboratory's requirements.

Ultrasound of both adrenal glands by a skilled ultrasonographer is useful for the detection of adrenal tumours, though in some cases both glands cannot be satisfactorily imaged. Advanced imaging techniques such as computed tomography (CT) or magnetic resonance imaging (MRI) can be invaluable, though expensive, in the unequivocal diagnosis of pituitary-dependent hyperadreno-corticism.

Tests for feline adrenal gland dysfunction

Adrenal function testing in cats is inherently more problematic than in dogs as responses to ACTH administration and dexamethasone suppression seem to be affected by more inter-individual variation. Responses to ACTH administration are usually measured with two samples taken at 1–3 hours post-ACTH administration and ACTH stimulation, as in dogs it is inherently less sensitive than dexamethasone suppression. Dexamethasone suppression is usually performed with both 0.01 and 0.1 mg/kg dexamethasone intravenously as a percentage of normal cats will fail to suppress cortisol release with the lower dosage.

A rare entity seen occasionally in cats and extremely rarely in dogs is hyperaldosteronism (or Conn's syndrome) in which hypokalaemia +/− hypernatraemia results from an aldosterone-secreting adrenocortical tumour. Aldosterone levels are assayed before and after ACTH administration and grossly elevated levels are indicative.

Diagnostic tests of endocrine pancreatic disease

Fructosamine and glycosylated haemoglobin

Serum fructosamine and glycosylated haemoglobin levels can be assayed to provide a longer-term assessment of glycaemic control than is afforded by single blood-glucose measurements. These analytes represent the irreversible binding of glucose to albumin or haemoglobin. Only fructosamine is widely available commercially. It allows an objective measurement of glycaemic control over the preceding 2–3 weeks to be made and is especially useful in patients in which stress-induced hyperglycaemia may make a single blood-glucose sample difficult to interpret (particularly cats). It is also a valuable tool in the long-term monitoring of glycaemic control in cats and dogs who are receiving daily insulin therapy (Table 4.4).

Table 4.4 Guidelines for serum fructosamine interpretation

Glycaemic control	Canine	Feline
Excellent	<350 µmol/l	<300 µmol/l
Good	<500 µmol/l	<400 µmol/l
Fair	<600 µmol/l	<500 µmol/l
Poor	>600 µmol/l	>500 µmol/l

Insulin

Diagnosis of insulinoma is dependent on documenting fasting hypoglycaemia with a concurrently high or inappropriately normal serum insulin level. The pancreatic islet cells are exquisitely sensitive to subnormal serum glucose levels and insulin secretion should rapidly reduce in the face of such hypoglycaemia. Thus a normal insulin level in the face of hypoglycaemia reflects an inappropriate insulin response and may be supportive evidence of insulinoma. Normal canine serum insulin levels are commonly reported as 5–20 µIU/ml, and while levels in excess of this range in the face of hypoglycaemia support a diagnosis of insulinoma, levels in the 10–20 µIU/ml range may also be consistent with insulinoma.

Diagnostic tests for parathyroid gland disease

Parathyroid hormone (PTH)

The diagnosis of primary hyperparathyroidism is dependent on the documentation of a concurrently raised serum calcium level and PTH level. Similarly to glycaemic homeostasis, calcium homeostasis is an exquisitely sensitive system, and PTH release by the parathyroid glands, which ultimately results in raised serum calcium levels, should sharply decline with increased levels of calcium. Thus PTH levels raised above the normal reference range of 10–60 mg/ml in the dog or 3–25 mg/ml in the cat, in the face of concurrent hypercalcaemia, is supportive of primary hyperparathyroidism. Care must be taken if concurrent azotaemia is documented since PTH is renally excreted and impaired renal clearance may lead to a false elevation. PTH is assayed in serum or plasma but, like endogenous adrenocorticotrophic hormone (ACTH), is very labile and must be stored and transported under exacting conditions.

Similarly a diagnosis of primary hypoparathyroidism is supported by a finding of concurrently reduced serum calcium and subnormal PTH in an animal showing appropriate clinical signs. Obviously, due to the lability of PTH, one must be confident of proper sample handling to interpret a low PTH assay result properly. Low serum calcium levels due to hypoalbuminaemia are a frequent cause of misinterpretation and a low corrected calcium level or ionised calcium should be documented if PTH assay is to be performed.

PTH assays may also be used in the supportive diagnosis of hypercalcaemia of malignancy (in which PTH is usually appropriately suppressed by circulating hypercalcaemia) and in renal secondary hyperparathyroidism (in which hyperphosphataemia, raised PTH levels, but normocalcaemia are generally seen).

Diagnostic tests of growth hormone deficiency or excess

Documentation of pituitary growth hormone (somatotropin) deficiency or excess is important in the diagnosis of pituitary dwarfism or acromegaly, respectively. Growth hormone assays are not readily available in the UK and often require the use of laboratories abroad. Where available, pituitary dwarfism may be diagnosed by the documentation of failure of growth hormone increase after stimulation with exogenously administered growth hormone releasing hormone (GHRH), clonodine or xylazine. The individual laboratory concerned should be contacted for test protocols as these vary between institutions.

More widely available is the insulin-like growth factor-1 (IGF-1) assay. IGF-1 is produced intra-hepatically after stimulation of growth hormone and may be used to assess growth hormone levels indirectly. The normal range is described as 200–1000 mg/ml for dogs and cats with levels <50 mg/ml consistent with growth hormone deficiency and >1000 mg/ml consistent with growth hormone excess.

Tests of release and responsiveness of anti-diuretic hormone (ADH)

Water deprivation test

The water deprivation test is used in establishing a diagnosis of failure of release (central diabetes insipidus) or renal responsiveness (nephrogenic diabetes insipidus) to ADH in the investigation of polyuria/polydipsia and diagnosis of primary polydipsia.

NB The water deprivation test is potentially extremely dangerous in animals with obligatory water loss. It must *only* be performed in animals in which all other causes of polyuria/polydipsia have been definitively excluded and which show no evidence of azotaemia or dehydration. Close monitoring is mandatory and animals must never be left unattended overnight during this test.

A 12-hour fast is recommended. If excessive polyuria/polydipsia has been occurring, gradual reduction in water availability over the preceding 3 days (100 ml/kg day 1, 80 ml/kg day 2, 60 ml/kg day 3) will help reduce the effects of renal medullary washout. The animal's urinary bladder is catheterised and emptied, urine specific gravity and preferably osmolality are measured, as are plasma osmolality, packed cell volume (PCV), total protein and blood urea nitrogen (BUN); the animal is weighed. All water is withheld and weight and urine specific gravity (SG) are measured by catheterising and emptying the bladder every 1–2 hours.

The test is ended when 5% bodyweight has been lost and urine SG exceeds 1.030 in the dog or 1.025 in the cat. The test should be abandoned should *any* signs of illness be seen. Failure to concentrate the urine above an SG of 1.010 is strongly suggestive of diabetes insipidus.

ADH response test

In order to differentiate central and nephrogenic diabetes insipidus once a water deprivation test has been failed, DDAVP (synthetic ADH) is administered i.v., s.c., or i.m. at a dose of 2 µg for dogs <15 kg and cats, and 4 µg for dogs >15 kg. The bladder continues to be catheterised every hour for 2–4 hours and urine and plasma osmolality and urine SG measured. An increase in urine SG of >1.025 or osmolality of >10% is an indication of central or partial nephrogenic diabetes insipidus.

After both these tests small quantities of water should be introduced gradually to avoid water toxicity.

GASTROINTESTINAL TESTS: ASSESSMENT OF ROUTINE LABORATORY FINDINGS IN THE PRESENCE OF GI DISEASE

Haematology

Although often normal in gastrointestinal (GI) disease, a complete blood count may offer specific diagnostic clues in some cases; examples are shown in Table 4.5.

Total protein, albumin and globulin

Mild hypoalbuminaemia and compensatory hyperglobulinaemia are frequently seen in many debilitated animals. Severe hypoproteinaemia from starvation alone is rarely seen and should prompt a search for sources of decreased protein production (namely hepatic disease) or increased loss (protein-losing enteropathies and protein-losing nephropathies). Urinary protein loss can be quantified by urine-protein:creatinine ratios and in cases of protein-losing nephropathy a hypoalbuminaemia/normoglobulinaemia is usually seen. Protein-losing enteropathies are characterised by loss of albumin and globulin (panhypoproteinaemia), whilst the magnitude of globulin in hepatic disorders may be normal, increased or decreased. Liver function testing is ultimately required in most cases.

Urea and creatinine

Urea may be elevated due to recent feeding, GI bleeding or dehydration and renal azotaemia should be distinguished by assessment of urea and creatinine with simultaneous urine SG determination in a fasted sample. Low urea may reflect hepatic insufficiency.

Table 4.5 Haematological changes that may be seen with gastrointestinal (GI) disease

Red blood cell indices

Normocytic, normochromic, non-regenerative anaemia	May be seen due to anaemia of chronic disease in patients with many illnesses or in the first 48–72 hours after acute GI haemorrhage
Macrocytic, hypochromic, regenerative anaemia	May be seen with GI haemorrhage
Microcytic, hypochromic anaemia	May be seen with iron deficiency due to chronic GI blood loss (e.g. due to parasitism) in some hepatic disease especially portosystemic shunting. May be regenerative or non-regenerative
Relative polycythaemia	May be seen due to haemoconcentration in cases of dramatic or prolonged GI fluid loss. Most dramatic examples seen with canine haemorrhagic gastroenteritis

White cell indices

Neutrophilia	An increased white cell count, usually composed principally of neutrophils, may indicate ongoing GI tract inflammation, though more usually this is within normal limits. A band shift represents severe ongoing inflammation and is most typically seen in infectious GI disease such as parvovirus. In severe cases the band shift may exceed the mature neutrophil count (degenerative left shift) and is a poor prognostic sign. Toxic neutrophils may be seen with gram-negative sepsis accompanying bacterial translocation in severe GI disease
Neutropenia	Neutropenia in association with GI disease most typically represents excessive neutrophil sequestration as a result of severe inflammation
Lymphocytosis	Usually reflects inflammation
Lymphopenia	May reflect stress response, loss due to lympangiectasia or viraemia, particularly in cats
Monocytosis	Typically represents ongoing inflammation
Eosinophilia	May reflect GI parasitism

OTHER BIOCHEMICAL ANALYTES

While alanine aminotransferase (ALT) and alkaline phosphatase (ALKP) are often considered markers of hepatocellular damage and cholestasis respectively, both may become non-specifically raised with a number of extra-hepatic GI disorders with no evidence of hepatic pathology.

Calcium may be decreased in pancreatitis but the most usual reason for hypocalcaemia is concurrent hypoalbuminaemia. Cholesterol may be found to be decreased in hepatic insufficiency or increased in cases of severe cholestatic disease.

Electrolytes and blood gas analysis

These tests, if available, are extremely useful in the assessment of the acid–base balance and electrolyte levels of anorexic, vomiting and diarrhoeic animals as well as in monitoring for iatrogenic electrolyte depletion through inappropriate fluid therapy.

Faecal analysis

Gross examination

Gross examination gives information as to the consistency, colour and shape which may aid further diagnostic endeavours (see Box 4.6 and Fig. 4.14).

Microscopic faecal analysis is performed to assess the presence of micro-organisms and intestinal parasites, in cytological evaluation of inflammatory cells and potentially may aid the diagnosis of malabsorption.

Faecal parasitology

Ova, oocysts, trophozoites and larvae of many nematodes and protozoa can be identified by direct smear examination. However, many nematode ova and protozoal cysts and oocysts are best identified by faecal flotation using a faecal flotation test as described in Box 4.7. For many intestinal parasites, immediate examination of faeces is preferred and due to the intermittent nature of the shedding of some of these (in particular *Giardia* spp.) a minimum of 2–3 faecal examinations is recommended.

> **Box 4.6** Significance of gross findings on faecal analysis
>
> Abnormalities of consistency
> - Diarrhoea of small intestinal origin, frequently very watery and large volumes. Large intestinal diarrhoea frequently has an increased mucus content and may appear to be encased 'in a sausage skin'
>
> Abnormalities of colour
> - Very pale faeces may be due to increased faecal fat content in cases of malabsorption (steatorrhoea) or due to lack of bile-derived pigment in complete biliary obstruction (acholic faeces). Some medications such as antacids and antibiotics may cause lighter faeces
> - The presence of fresh blood is indicative of large intestinal haemorrhage and is seen diffusely in the stool in inflammatory lesions, but may cause a linear 'stripe' in bleeding mass lesions
> - Dark, black and tarry stools may indicate melaena due to haemorrhage within the upper GI tract and digestion of haem pigments. Medications such as charcoal, bismuth and salicylates as well as meat-rich diets may also darken the faeces
>
> Abnormalities of shape
> - Thin and flattened faeces may indicate intestinal narrowing due to intra- or extraluminal mass lesions

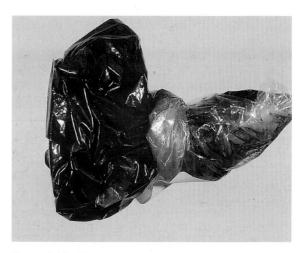

Figure 4.14 Melaenic stool sample in a dog with thrombocytopenia.

Faecal microbiology/virology

Historical findings of onset of GI signs after kennelling, mixing with other affected dogs, ingestion of spoiled foods or bloody diarrhoea accompanied by signs of systemic illness should prompt consideration of infectious causes. Many potential pathogens can be isolated from the intestines of normal asymptomatic dogs and cats and interpretation of positive findings must always be very cautious. The findings of large numbers of neutrophils, bacterial spores (especially *Clostridium* spp.) or intercellular bacteria on microscopic examination of fresh faeces or cytology of rectal scrapes may suggest pathogenic bacterial involvement. *Salmonella, Clostridium perfringens, Campylobacter jejuni* and enteropathogenic *E. coli* are the most commonly isolated bacterial enteric pathogens in the UK. Diagnosis is often hampered by the need for exacting microbiological technique and the need for very fresh samples.

The most common viral intestinal pathogens isolated in the UK are canine and feline parvovirus and enteric coronaviruses. An in-house canine faecal enzyme-linked immunosorbent assay (ELISA) kit is available for the detection of canine parvovirus in the UK.

Faecal occult blood

Testing for occult blood may be performed where occult GI bleeding is suspected. Animals must be fed on a diet free of red meat for at least 3 days prior to testing and certain drugs, iron supplements and vegetable haem-proteins will cause false positives.

Faeces as an indicator of malabsorption

The finding of large amounts of undigested starch, fat and muscle fibres in faeces may be supportive, but is not diagnostic of malabsorption. Faecal

proteolytic activity, measured by the ability of faecal trypsin to digest gelatin on X-ray film, is an extremely unreliable test for exocrine pancreatic insufficiency and is not recommended.

DIAGNOSTIC TESTS FOR EXOCRINE PANCREATIC DISEASE

Tests for pancreatitis

Amylase and lipase

Amylase and lipase are enzymes which, whilst produced by the pancreas, are not pancreas-specific, being also found within the gastric and small intestinal mucosa. Thus elevations may be seen with any GI tract inflammation and levels also increase with decreased glomerular filtration as both are renally excreted. Lipase is reportedly more pancreas-specific in dogs, though levels can be elevated by corticosteroid administration. Both enzymes are relatively insensitive markers of pancreatic disease, often remaining within the reference range during episodes of pancreatitis.

Trypsin-like immunoreactivity (TLI)

TLI is an assay for both trypsin and trypsinogen and offers significant advantages over amylase and lipase assessment in terms of specificity as these analytes are produced solely in the pancreas. During pancreatic inflammation TLI levels have been found to rise and decline relatively quickly, thought to be due to a short half-life, though levels may remain raised for longer during cases of chronic 'smouldering' pancreatitis. In the UK canine TLI assays are readily available but assays for feline TLI are only currently available in the US.

Other tests for pancreatitis

Supportive evidence for pancreatitis may include clinical signs, radiographic and ultrasonographic evidence of pancreatic inflammation and heterogenicity, variable leucocytosis, mild hypocalcaemia, azotaemia and hyperlipidaemia. Ultimately histopathology is the only truly definitive diagnostic test.

Tests for exocrine pancreatic insufficiency (EPI)

Trypsin-like immunoreactivity

The TLI test has become the accepted test of choice for the diagnosis of EPI, a subnormal result indicating the presence of EPI. It should be noted that there is no cross-reactivity between canine and feline TLI tests and the normal feline TLI range is significantly higher than that for dogs.

Faecal proteolytic activity

As mentioned previously this test is not as reliable as the TLI test as faecal proteolytic enzyme concentrations fluctuate with time such that many normal cats and dogs will sometimes have very low levels of faecal proteolytic enzymes. This assay is no longer recommended.

Diagnostic tests for intestinal function and bacterial overgrowth

Serum folate and cobalamin (B$_{12}$)

These two water soluble vitamins may be assayed to gain indirect information about small intestinal absorptive function and the possible presence of small intestinal bacterial overgrowth (SIBO). Their use in the cat is not well described and they are most useful in canine patients.

Folate absorption occurs in the proximal small intestine and since it is plentiful in most canine diets (making nutritional deficiency unlikely), lowered serum levels may reflect proximal small intestinal disease. Folate levels may become increased in SIBO as a result of folate synthesis by intraluminal bacteria, though again this must be occurring within the proximal small intestine for serum levels to reflect this production as this is the principal site of the folate receptors.

In contrast, cobalamin is principally absorbed in the distal small intestine after first undergoing a series of steps in which carrier proteins are first bound, then broken down by proteases then rebound to allow receptor-mediated absorption. Low levels of cobalamin may be seen in distal small intestinal disease (SIBO) as a result of bacterial competition for cobalamin substrate if present in high enough numbers, or in EPI as a result of failure of pancreatic proteases releasing protein-bound cobalamin. Since they can be affected by the presence of EPI a trypsin-like immunoreactivity test should be performed simultaneously.

Other tests for SIBO

The 'gold standard' test for SIBO is quantitative culture of duodenal juice aspirated endoscopically. This is a technically demanding and time-consuming test that is only available at certain research institutions. A diagnosis of SIBO *cannot* be made by faecal culture.

Other tests for malabsorption

Other tests for intestinal malabsorption are usually confined to research institutions but may become accessible in general practice.

Most rely on tests of carbohydrate malabsorption by detecting levels of hydrogen in expired air after the feeding of a carbohydrate meal. Normal mammalian cells do not metabolise carbohydrate to release hydrogen, though bacteria within the gut do. Thus increases in the amount of hydrogen absorbed and expired may reflect either an overgrowth of bacteria, or a lack of intestinal carbohydrate absorption allowing an increased amount of carbohydrate substrate to be utilised by the intestinal bacteria. This may be helpful in the diagnosis of intestinal malabsorption or of SIBO.

Another test which is becoming commercially available is the α-1 protease inhibitor (α-1-PI) test as an assay for protein-losing enteropathy. α-1-PI has a molecular weight comparable with albumin and thus is lost into the intestinal lumen in amounts paralleling those of albumin in protein-losing enteropathies but unlike albumin, it is not further degraded by luminal bacteria.

DIAGNOSTIC TESTS FOR HEPATOBILIARY DISEASE

Enzymatic tests

Alanine aminotransferase

ALT is an enzyme found within the intracellular cytosol of hepatocytes and is considered liver-specific in dogs and cats. Rises usually reflect the degree of damage to hepatocytes and cytosolic enzyme leakage but offer little information regarding specific diagnosis and prognosis. The latter can be inferred by serially monitoring ALT levels which should gradually return to normal after an acute, self-limiting hepatocellular insult. Levels of ALT may be raised by corticosteroids and also mild rises (2–3 times the upper normal range) may be seen with non-hepatic disease causing 'secondary reactive hepatopathy' such as intestinal inflammation or sepsis.

Aspartate aminotransferase (AST)

AST is not liver-specific in the dog or cat, being found in a variety of tissues. In hepatocellular injury rises do, however, often parallel those seen in ALT. Much intracellular AST within the hepatocytes is bound to mitochondria, prompting speculation that rises in AST may reflect more severe hepatocellular injury. The test, however, appears to offer few advantages over ALT assays.

Alkaline phosphatase (ALKP, SAP)

ALKP is a membrane-bound enzyme which is found in hepatocytes and also in biliary epithelial cells. ALKP is found in a number of tissues but, with the exception of bone, the half-life of ALKP found in extrahepatic sites is too short to be clinically significant. Rises in ALKP usually reflect intra- or extrahepatic cholestasis. The importance of two additional forms of ALKP (isoenzymes), the steroid- and bone-isoenzymes, should always be borne in mind when interpreting abnormal results. The bone-isoenzyme may cause mild to moderate elevation in ALKP in animals which are growing or which have destructive bone disease. Steroid-induced rises in ALKP are usually seen with any exogenous corticosteroid administration and may be dramatic but increases can also be caused by endogenous cortisol release. The half-life of ALKP in cats is significantly shorter than in dogs and even mild elevations are more significant in feline patients.

Gamma glutamyltransferase (GGT)

GGT usually parallels changes seen in ALKP in the dog and does not appear to offer any signifi-

cant advantages. In the cat, however, it may be more sensitive though less specific, and may also be useful in the diagnosis of feline hepatic lipidosis in which, in contrast to most feline cholestatic disease, GGT does not usually become raised in parallel with ALKP. The mechanism for this is unknown.

Bilirubin

Total bilirubin levels reflect a balance between the release of haem-pigment from effete red blood cells, hepatocellular uptake, conjugation within the liver, and biliary excretion. Essentially, rises in total bilirubin may reflect increased production overwhelming hepatocellular uptake (for example in massive haemolysis), reduced hepatocellular uptake due to hepatocellular dysfunction, or extrahepatic obstruction to biliary secretion. It is important to attempt to discern whether hyperbilirubinaemia (jaundice) is due to pre-, intra-, or extrahepatic causes and this is usually achieved by a combination of haematological and biochemical testing and imaging of the liver and extrahepatic structures by ultrasound. Total bilirubin rarely, if ever, offers specific diagnostic information but is more an indication for further investigation. There is no diagnostic merit in determining the proportion of conjugated and unconjugated bilirubin ('Van den Bergh fractionation').

Assessment of liver function

Enzymatic tests may offer information about hepatocellular damage or cholestasis but offer no direct information about liver function. Function tests may be divided into direct and indirect tests.

Direct function tests – bile acid stimulation test

The bile acid stimulation test (BAST) relies on assessing the integrity of the enterohepatic circulation of bile acids. These are synthesised from cholesterol within the liver and are secreted via the biliary system into the intestine where they are later reabsorbed within the ileum and recycled to the liver via the portal circulation. Thus abnormal liver function resulting in a failure of adequate re-uptake, or mixing of the hepatic portal circulation with the systemic circulation (as is seen with portosystemic shunting) will result in rises in serum bile acids. Serum levels are assessed after a 12-hour fast and again 2 hours after feeding (which should stimulate gall bladder contraction and thus bile acid release). The greatest magnitudes of rise are usually seen in portosystemic shunts though abnormal results do not usually offer specific diagnostic information other than the presence of abnormal hepato-cellular function or of abnormal portal circulation. Abnormal BAST results are most productively followed up by liver biopsy.

Indirect evidence of hepatocellular dysfunction

Decreases in albumin, cholesterol and urea may all be seen in hepatic dysfunction due to failures in synthesis. Glucose levels may also be sub-normal. All of these are somewhat ominous findings if accompanied by direct evidence of hepatocellular dysfunction as their production is usually well preserved until hepatic dysfunction is advanced and hepatic failure is imminent.

Serum ammonia levels

Ammonia levels may be assayed in cases of suspected hepatic encephalopathy (HE) due to portosystemic shunting or severe hepatocellular dysfunction since it is the one toxin associated with HE that can be biochemically evaluated routinely. However, samples should be assayed within 1 hour of collection and should be kept on ice. Red blood cells and muscle contain large amounts of ammonia and any haemolysis or recent muscular activity may falsely raise levels. Any abnormal results should be interpreted cautiously.

FURTHER DIAGNOSTIC TESTS FOR THE ASSESSMENT OF GASTROINTESTINAL AND HEPATOCELLULAR DISEASE

Imaging studies using radiography with or without the use of radiographic contrast agents such as barium or barium-impregnated polyspheres may offer further information, as may ultra-sonographic determination of normal intestinal

'layering' and thickness. Properly constructed and adhered-to dietary exclusion trials and re-challenges are time-consuming and expensive but remain the only suitable diagnostic test for the evaluation of dietary intolerances; blood 'allergy-tests' currently marketed are not specific enough to be diagnostically useful.

Ultimately, however, all of these diagnostic endeavours seldom lead to a specific diagnosis and evaluation of pathological material by a veterinary pathologist is often required for a definitive diagnosis to be made.

BODY FLUID COLLECTION

CEREBROSPINAL FLUID COLLECTION

Indications

Cerebrospinal fluid (CSF) is a clear, acellular, supportive and nutritive fluid surrounding the brain and spinal cord. It is usually collected by needle centesis from one of two dilatations in the subarachnoid space: the cerebellomedullary cistern (cisternal puncture) or the caudal lumbar subarachnoid space (lumbar puncture). CSF collection and analysis are most useful for the diagnosis of infectious and inflammatory disorders of the CNS and when multifocal disease is suspected. Other conditions such as CNS neoplasia, degenerative diseases and vascular disorders may also produce alterations in CSF characteristics but these are by no means consistent. An example of diseases in which CSF analysis may be useful is given in Box 4.8. CSF collection and analysis are often performed in combination with contrast spinal radiography as placement of a spinal needle in the subarachnoid space facilitates the injection of contrast material around the spinal cord (the myelogram).

Contraindications

Contraindications to CSF collection are:

- an animal with an unstabilised disease which renders it unlikely to survive general anaesthesia

---

Box 4.8 Examples of disorders in which cerebrospinal fluid (CSF) analysis may be useful

Infectious central nervous system (CNS) disease
- bacterial meningitis
- protozoal meningitis
  - *Toxoplasma gondii*
  - *Neospora caninum*
- fungal meningitis
  - *Cryptococcus neoformans*
  - various opportunistic fungi
- rickettsial meningitis
  - especially *Ehrlichia* spp. *Borrelia*
- viral meningitis
  - canine distemper virus
  - feline infectious peritonitis
  - rabies virus
- parasitic meningitis

Inflammatory CNS disease
- steroid-responsive meningitis–arteritis
- granulomatous meningoencephalomyelitis
- eosinophilic meningitis
- non-suppurative encephalomyelitis
- feline polioencephalomyelitis
- pug dog encephalitis
- necrotising meningitis
- traumatic inflammation

Neoplastic CNS disease
- it should be noted that with the exception of CNS lymphoma, neoplastic cells rarely exfoliate into the CSF

Degenerative CNS disease
- usually mild and non-specific changes

Vascular CNS disease
- usually mild and non-specific changes

Traumatic CNS disease
- usually mild and non-specific changes

- the presence of an unstable cervical spine fracture
- the presence of raised intracranial pressure (ICP).

A thorough physical, neurological and ophthalmological examination should always be performed prior to CSF collection and cervical radiographs taken where regional trauma has occurred. In the presence of raised ICP, collection of CSF, either from the cervical or lumbosacral subarachnoid space, may result in shifts in the brain parenchyma caudally with catastrophic compression of the brainstem ('herniation'). Signs at or soon after collection include respiratory depression or arrest, failure to regain consciousness and uni- or bilaterally unresponsive mydriasis.

In this situation aggressive attempts to reduce ICP such as the administration of mannitol and the reinduction of anaesthesia and hyperventilation should be performed.

Equipment needed

- Yale spinal needle with stylet (size dependent on size of patient but 20–22 G and 1.5–3.5 inch (3–8 cm) needle usually sufficient)
- sterile gloves
- collection tubes.

Technique

Technique for CSF collection is shown in Box 4.9 (Fig. 4.15). The reader is referred to several excellent reviews of anaesthesia management during neurological procedures listed in the Further Reading section. Due to the caudal flow of CSF, lumbosacral collection is usually indicated when a lesion caudal to the cerebellomedullary cistern is suspected or when a lumbosacral myelogram is to be performed. It is technically more difficult than the cerebellomedullary site sampling and generally yields a lower volume of fluid and a higher risk of haemorrhagic contamination.

CSF is collected into an ethylenediaminetetraacetic acid (EDTA) sample tube for cytology and plain tubes for bacteriological and biochemical examination.

Handling and storage

CSF is hypotonic when compared with serum and cells within it rapidly swell and burst due to osmotic lysis soon after collection. For best results analysis should ideally be performed within 30 minutes of collection after cytocentrifugation (to concentrate the generally low cellular content) by a veterinary cytologist or haematologist. In the practice setting such cases are often referred to a centre with this expertise on hand or arrangements can sometimes be made with a local hospital haematology laboratory for handling CSF samples. A less ideal but alternative solution is to centrifuge a sample at $1500\,g$ for 7–10 min, pipette off most of the fluid and to resuspend the sample in a drop of the patient's own serum.

Box 4.9 Cerebrospinal fluid collection technique

1. *Patient assessed* prior to procedure
2. *Corrective measures to reduce intracranial pressure undertaken if necessary*
3. *General anaesthesia induced* with close attention to agents used and ventilation
4. *Patient preparation* by wide clipping and surgical skin preparation overlying the cerebellomedullary or lumbosacral sites. If patient temperament allows, clipping prior to induction should be considered
5. *Collection*

CEREBELLOMEDULLARY CISTERN COLLECTION
1. Animal in lateral recumbency
2. With the endotracheal cuff deflated and an assistant monitoring respiration, another assistant should flex the neck 90° keeping the bridge of the nose parallel to the surface that the animal is lying on (Fig. 4.15B)
3. Wearing sterile gloves the operator inserts the spinal needle (with stylet in place) in a direction parallel with the bridge of the nose and the table top at a point half way along an imaginary line which joins the occipital protuberance and a point midway between the wings of the atlas (Fig. 4.15C)
4. The needle is slowly advanced through the skin, subcutis and overlying muscle until a depth is reached whereby the cistern is approached. The

stylet is then removed and the needle very slowly advanced, checking for cerebrospinal fluid (CSF) flow at the hub, until it is felt entering the cistern. A sudden loss of resistance is often felt at this point by the operator. If bone is encountered the needle is redirected or withdrawn completely.
5. CSF is collected by allowing it to drip passively from the hub into collecting vessels (Fig. 4.15D)

LUMBOSACRAL COLLECTION
1. The animal is positioned in lateral recumbency with the hindlimbs firmly flexed cranially
2. The recommended point of collection is the L5–6 intervertebral space
3. The needle is inserted as described for cerebellomedullary collection alongside the dorsal spinous process of L6 and directed cranially and ventrally to penetrate the ligamentum flavum between L5 and L6. It is then advanced until it touches the floor of the vertebral canal, thus fluid is generally collected from the ventral subarachnoid space in this area, the needle passing through the cauda equina. A slight twitch of the hindlimbs may occur as the cauda equina is penetrated but this is usually of no neurological consequence
4. Fluid is collected as before

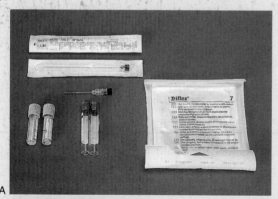
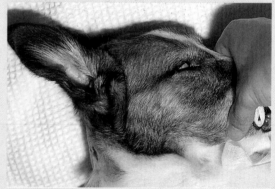
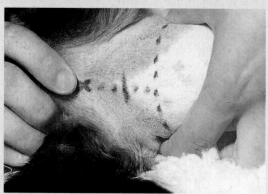
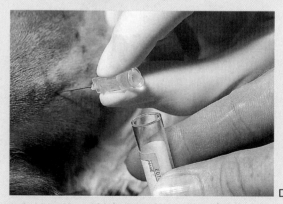

A B C D

Figure 4.15 Cerebrospinal fluid collection technique. (A) Equipment needed for CSF collection. (B) Neck positioning during CSF collection. (C) Bony reference points for CSF collection. (D) CSF being collected from the needle hub.

Another alternative, and one which often quite adequately concentrates cells, is to manufacture a home-made sedimentation chamber by affixing a tube (such as a sawn-off 5 ml syringe base with the plunger removed) to a clean microscope slide and smearing Vaseline or another occlusive lubricant around the base to form an air-tight seal. CSF is allowed to settle within the chamber for 30 minutes before discarding the supernatant. The slide with adherent cells is then air-dried and stained (e.g. with 'Diff-Quick' or Wrights-Giemsa) and examined.

Analysis

Normal and abnormal CSF characteristics are shown in Table 4.6. Other diagnostic tests that may be performed include:

- CSF culture
- CSF immunoelectrophoresis

- CSF canine distemper virus or coronavirus titres, usually in combination with serological tests.

PERICARDIOCENTESIS

Indications

Pericardiocentesis is the removal of fluid from the pericardial sac via a pre-placed catheter and drainage set. It is primarily a therapeutic procedure to relieve cardiac tamponade but may occasionally be diagnostically useful. Fluid accumulates most commonly due to idiopathic pericardial effusion or due to haemorrhage from a neoplasm especially at the heart base. Other less common causes include right-sided heart failure, pericardial infections, left atrial rupture, coagulopathy and trauma.

Table 4.6 Normal and abnormal cerebrospinal fluid findings

	Normal	Neoplastic	Infectious inflammatory	Non-infectious inflammatory
Colour and turbidity	Clear and colourless	Usually clear and colourless	Clear to cloudy depending on cell count	Clear to cloudy depending on cell count
Nucleated cell count/μl	<2–3	Usually normal to increased	Depends on aetiology – increased, usually >100 in bacterial and fungal, usually less marked in viral, protozoal, parasitic	Usually very increased in GME and steroid-responsive meningitis, less so in traumatic, vascular and degenerative lesions
Differential cell count	Mononuclear cells	Cells rarely exfoliate except where lymphoblasts predominate. A neutrophilic predominance may be seen with necrotic CNS tumours	Depends on aetiology: • bacterial meningitis – neutrophilic predominance with signs of degeneration • viral and protozoal – usually mixed with mononuclear predominance except FIP in which neutrophils predominate. Protozoa may be seen • fungal – usually mixed. Organisms may be seen • parasitic – usually eosinophilic predominance	Usually neutrophilic predominance in steroid-responsive meningitis GME usually demonstrates mononuclear predominance with large 'foamy cells' – however occasionally neutrophils predominate Eosinophilic meningitis may be seen without parasitic/infectious cause Red cells and erythrophagocytosis may be seen with recent haemorrhage
Protein (mg/dl)	<25	Increased but usually <100	Increased and usually >100 except with viral infections	Variably increased

GME, granulomatous meningoencephalomyelitis; CNS, central nervous system; FIP, feline infectious peritonitis.

Contraindications

Pericardiocentesis is contraindicated in cases where pericardial effusion does not exist and this obviously relies on good-quality imaging and interpretation for the diagnosis of effusion. Differentiation from other causes of cardiomegaly (e.g. dilated cardiomyopathy) and from globular cardiac silhouette due to breed is essential. Ultrasound evaluation is usually required for definitive diagnosis.

Equipment needed

- a long (minimum 7 cm) 14–16 G over-the-needle catheter (an 18–20 G may be used in small dogs and cats)
- 3-way tap, syringe and extension tubing
- scalpel
- local anaesthetic
- gloves.

If large amounts of fluid are being drained the catheter will sometimes collapse under pressure. This can be prevented by introducing a sterile dog urinary catheter of suitable diameter through the over-the-needle catheter once placed within the pericardial sac. Several manufacturers also market especially designed pericardiocentesis catheters.

Technique

The technique of pericardiocentesis is described in Box 4.10.

Monitoring

It is useful for the patient to be connected to an ECG during the procedure to monitor for ventricular extrasystoles (Fig. 4.16). The occurrence of these is usually an indication that the epicardium has been contacted by the catheter stylet and should prompt slight withdrawal and repositioning of it. During successful removal of pericardial fluid (which may be several hundred millilitres), ECG R-wave height should increase and an improvement in peripheral pulse quality should be felt.

Box 4.10   Pericardiocentesis technique

1. The patient is gently but firmly restrained, either in sternal recumbency or slightly tilted so that the right hand side of the thorax is uppermost. Light sedation may be required.
2. An area of the 5th to 6th intercostal space on the right-hand side at the level of the costochondral junction is widely clipped and surgically scrubbed. The point of insertion (just cranial to the adjacent rib) is infiltrated with local anaesthetic right down to the pleura.
3. A small stab incision with a scalpel is made and the over-the-needle catheter is slowly advanced medially and slightly dorsally until some resistance at the pericardial sac is met. The needle is then advanced through the sac (at which point a slight 'popping' sensation is often felt), and fluid should begin to accumulate at the hub of the needle.
4. This is then withdrawn and the needle, three-way tap and extension tubing are connected.
5. Fluid is then withdrawn and samples collected for cytology and culture.

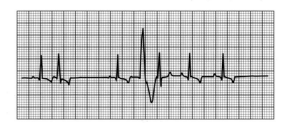

Figure 4.16   Ventricular extrasystole seen due to hepicardial contact during pericardiocentesis.

Initially a small amount of the fluid is withdrawn and allowed to stand in a container containing no anticoagulant. Fluid from the pericardial space (unless caused by a very recent atrial tear or active bleed) should not clot and any clots that form should make one suspicious that drainage of ventricular blood is occurring. The catheter should be replaced or the procedure abandoned and the diagnosis reviewed.

Analysis

Samples should be collected for cytology, bacteriology, protein estimation, SG and pH. Most pericardial effusions have a PCV well below that of peripheral blood, and if the PCV is similar, penetration of the ventricle during pericardiocentesis or very recent and active haemorrhage should be suspected. Cytological evaluation is unfortunately disappointing as an aid to diagnosing neoplastic effusions, even when performed by an excellent cytologist, and every effort should be made for thorough ultrasonographic examination of the heart base and associated structures. This is best performed before drainage as the pericardial fluid offers excellent contrast. Strongly inflammatory cytological pictures may be seen with infectious pericardial effusions and in effusion due to feline infectious peritonitis. Effusion pH measurement has been cited as being useful in differentiating neoplastic from non-neoplastic effusions but has recently been brought into question.

URINE COLLECTION
Cystocentesis

Indications

Cystocentesis is the removal of urine by direct puncture of the urinary bladder through the body wall with a needle or over-the-needle catheter for the collection of urine. It is, with practice, easily and rapidly performed and is well tolerated in most conscious animals. The principal advantages of cystocentesis are the ability to extract urine at the time of the operator's choosing (and not having to wait for spontaneous voiding) and the lack of contamination of urine samples either with bacteria from the external genitalia or from the local environment, both of which are common in free-catch urine samples (especially when owner-delivered). Cystocentesis is, for this reason, the urine collection method of choice for most urinalysis but especially for urine culture.

Cystocentesis may also be performed as a short-term therapeutic endeavour in cases of lower urinary tract obstruction during the initial stabilisation phase of treatment. This is not without its risks but can be a useful measure to prevent bladder overdistension and post-renal obstruction whilst fluid therapy is given; it must, needless to say, be swiftly followed by definitive relief of the obstruction by passage of a urinary catheter.

Contraindications/risks

Cystocentesis should not be performed where a coagulopathy or other bleeding disorder exists, and is relatively contraindicated where the urinary bladder cannot adequately be palpated. An overtly distended urinary bladder is at risk of rupture from forceful palpation and urine may additionally leak intra-abdominally through areas of bladder wall devitalised due to pressure necrosis. Care should be taken, especially in cats, that ventrally positioned and mobile kidneys are not mistaken for the urinary bladder.

Technique

Few patients require sedation for cystocentesis and in some cases (such as unrelieved lower urinary tract obstruction) sedative or anaesthetic procedures may be risky. The site of needle puncture may be clipped and prepared with surgical spirit, though some operators are unconvinced of the need for this. Good restraint by an experienced assistant is essential. Cystocentesis may be performed by blind palpation or with ultrasound guidance. A 5–10 ml syringe attached to a 1 inch, (2.5 cm) 23-G needle is usually the only equipment required. In cats and male dogs the patient is gently but firmly restrained in a comfortable position in which the caudal abdomen is easily accessible to the operator. With one hand the caudo-ventral abdomen is palpated until the fluid-filled urinary bladder is felt and this is gently held in position against the abdominal wall. The needle is slowly inserted into the bladder through the ventral or ventrolateral body wall in cats and the ventrolateral body wall in male dogs (taking care to avoid the penis and the caudal superficial epigastric vessels which are often prominent in this area). The bevel of the needle should ideally be orientated facing caudally to prevent trauma to the bladder wall as the structure reduces in size. Sufficient fluid should be removed for urinalysis; it is seldom necessary or desirable to empty the whole bladder as this will increase the risk of iatrogenic trauma and urine leakage. In female dogs, a useful technique is to perform cystocentesis 'blind' with the bitch lying in dorsal recumbency and comfortably supported there. An imaginary cross is visualised connecting the most caudal four nipples and the needle inserted perpendicular to the skin in the midline exactly at the point of intersection of this cross and the urinary bladder will invariably be entered.

Handling and analysis of samples

Urine samples should ideally be analysed in-house and immediately as storage, cooling and transport often result in artefactual information, particularly the precipitation of crystalline material which often occurs during cooling. Samples should be collected into sterile universal containers for immediate analysis and samples for culture may be collected into boric-acid containers unless they are to be received by the laboratory within 12 hours. Complete urinalysis should include gross examination, SG, protein quantification, dipstick testing and examination of a centrifuged sediment sample.

Catheter collection

Urinary bladder catheterisation involves the passage of a man-made (usually polypropylene) urinary catheter via the urethra. Advantages of the procedure include giving diagnostic information about sites of urinary tact obstruction, allowing urine collection without the need to await spontaneous voiding and in those animals where cystocentesis is not possible (e.g. very obese animals) or undesirable, allowing monitoring of urine output, facilitating diagnostic imaging procedures such as contrast radiography and finally to facilitate relief of lower urinary tract obstruction. Disadvantages of the procedure include the need for heavy sedation or general anaesthesia in many animals (essential in cats), equipment and time costs, the risk of contamination of samples and the urinary bladder with bacteria inoculated from the external genitalia and distal urethra and finally the risk of iatrogenic trauma caused by passage of the catheter.

Male dogs are generally simple to catheterise once the penis has been extruded from the prepuce. With the penis grasped in one hand the lubricated tip of a sterile catheter is slowly fed up the urethra until urine is seen to emerge from the tip of the catheter. A little resistance may be felt as the tip passes through the os penis; it is vital, as with all urinary catheter procedures, that the catheter is never forced but gently advanced and manipulated to avoid catastrophic urethral trauma.

Female dogs and cats generally require sedation or general anaesthesia. In female cats it can be useful to have the cat in sternal recumbency and to use a catheter with a wire guide slightly curved ventrally at the tip to allow passage into the urethra on the ventral wall of the vagina. In bitches this can also be a useful technique as can the use of a speculum to visualise the urethral orifice. The author prefers to insert a lubricated, gloved finger to palpate the orifice and positions it immediately cranial to the orifice before passing the catheter so that it is deflected downwards into the lumen.

Male cats always require some form of general anaesthesia for safe passage of a urinary catheter and the potential for life-threatening iatrogenic damage if this procedure is improperly performed cannot be overemphasised. The cat's penis undergoes an s-shaped flexure caudal to the pelvis and this must be straightened in order to allow safe passage of a catheter. The penis is extruded from the prepuce and the tip of the lubricated catheter is inserted. The prepuce is then grasped and drawn caudally which will straighten the flexed penis to allow gentle advancement of the catheter.

Analysis is performed as for cystocentesis.

Free-catch samples

Free-catch samples are usually collected by the owner at home or by clinic staff if an animal spontaneously voids. Advantages of free-catch samples are the ease of collection and minimal requirement for time, equipment, restraint or sedation. Disadvantages are the requirement for the animal to urinate spontaneously and the contamination of many samples which occurs, particularly with bacteria from the external genitalia and distal urethra, but also from inappropriate non-sterile containers. Samples collected should be mid-stream and have had no contact with any other surfaces. The timing of collection may alter the urinalysis. For example early-stream samples are most likely to contain material from the lower urinary tract such as urethral plugs, crystals, bacteria and haemorrhage; these samples are also most likely to be contaminated with debris from the external genitalia. Mid-stream samples are probably appropriate for most examinations whilst end-stream samples contain prostatic fluid.

PROSTATIC WASH AND CATHETER BIOPSY

This technique can be useful in obtaining material for culture and cytological examination from dogs with suspected bacterial prostatitis or with prostatic neoplasia. The techniques are often combined and are described in Box 4.11.

Box 4.11   Prostatic wash and catheter biopsy

Prostatic wash technique
1. A sterile urinary catheter is first placed within the bladder which is completely emptied and flushed 2–3 times with sterile saline to ensure complete emptying. Some authors recommend that the last portion to be removed is retained as a 'pre-wash' sample to compare with subsequent prostatic wash fluid.
2. The catheter is then withdrawn distal to the prostate as determined by digital palpation and the prostate is then digitally massaged per rectum for 1–2 minutes in order to facilitate fluid secretion.
3. 5–10 ml of sterile saline is then injected through the urinary catheter with digital occlusion of the urethra around the catheter and is then advanced into the bladder for aspiration of post-prostatic massage fluid. This can then be analysed cytologically and submitted for culture.

Prostatic urethra catheter biopsy technique
1. A urinary catheter with side holes is essential for this. The catheter is advanced within the urethra until it lies within the area bound by the prostate as determined either by rectal digital palpation or radiographically.
2. A syringe with a small amount of sterile saline is attached to the catheter and with suction applied the catheter is rapidly passed back and forth within the prostatic urethra in order to remove suctioned portions of epithelial tissue.
3. Cytological preparations are then made from the material gained.

TRANSTRACHEAL WASH AND BRONCHOALVEOLAR LAVAGE

Lavage samples from the trachea and the bronchial tree allow cytological assessment and bacterial culture in cases where coughing and pulmonary parenchymal disease are present. They are most useful in cases where bacterial bronchopneumonia is present and in the diagnosis of inflammatory airway diseases such as pulmonary infiltration with eosinophils (PIE). Interpretation of lavage samples must be undertaken cautiously as there is much normal variation in airway cytology and the technique is only semiquantitative. In particular, interpretation of bacteria derived from the trachea should be based on a knowledge that there is a normal commensal population within the upper respiratory tract.

Transtracheal lavage

Transtracheal lavage involves the installation of sterile saline into the trachea before aspiration to obtain material for cytology and bacteriology. Tracheal samples may be gained by placing a sterile catheter through the lumen of an endotracheal tube in anaesthetised patients, though this will usually result in contamination from the distal ET tube and pharynx. Transtracheal lavage requires the placement of a catheter directly into the trachea, so bypassing the pharyngeal area and associated contaminant organisms, and is surprisingly well tolerated in most conscious cats and dogs. It is therefore a useful technique in patients where general anaesthesia is contraindicated or undesirable. The technique is described in Box 4.12 (Fig. 4.17).

Bronchoalveolar lavage

Similar to transtracheal lavage, bronchoalveolar lavage (BAL) describes the introduction and then aspiration of sterile saline within the respiratory tract to gain material for cytological and bacteriological examination. BAL samples can either be gained 'blind' by the introduction of a sterile catheter via the endotracheal tube or via the biopsy port of an endoscope during bronchoscopy. The latter has several advantages including

Box 4.12 Transtracheal lavage technique

1. An area overlying the cricoid cartilage is clipped and scrubbed and the cricothyroid ligament (palpated as a depression cranial to the cricoid cartilage and in the midline) is infiltrated with local anaesthetic.
2. With the animal gently restrained by an assistant standing behind it and raising its head vertically, a small stab incision is made in the overlying skin with the tip of a scalpel blade and a 14–16 G short over-the-needle catheter is placed into the tracheal lumen. Usually minimal objection to this occurs.
3. Once the catheter is in place, the stylet is removed and an appropriately sized sterile suction catheter or sterile urinary catheter is advanced through the hub of the catheter to a depth approximating the bronchial bifurcation.
4. 0.5 ml/kg of sterile saline (with no bacteriostatic agent) is then injected through the catheter and then rapidly aspirated. The volume yielded from aspiration is usually much less than that introduced.
5. Material gained should be collected in an ethylenediaminetetraacetic acid container for cytology and in a sterile universal container for culture.

Over-the-needle catheter placed through cricothyroid ligament into the tracheal lumen

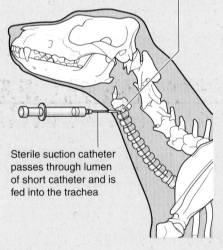

Sterile suction catheter passes through lumen of short catheter and is fed into the trachea

Figure 4.17 Transtracheal lavage technique.

the ability to 'marry' cytological findings with the gross inspection of the lower respiratory tract seen at bronchoscopy and also the ability to direct the lung-lobe from which washings are obtained according to the most radiographically affected region. Well maintained equipment and thorough knowledge of bronchoscopic anatomy are essential to this. Disadvantages of per-endoscopic BAL include the expense and expertise needed to perform thorough bronchoscopic evaluations and the need for scrupulous sterilising techniques for endoscopic channels if contamination of samples is not to take place. With the blind technique a sterile catheter is placed through the endotracheal tube and continually fed through until resistance is met; this usually occurs when the flushing tube has encountered an airway of smaller diameter than the tube. With the animal in lateral recumbency, the most dependent lung lobe should be intubated by the tube if the catheter is advanced slowly.

With either technique, once the flushing catheter has been pre-placed in the desired airway and cannot be advanced further, 1 ml/kg of warm, sterile, additive-free saline is flushed down the tube and rapidly re-aspirated. Coupage of the appropriate side of the chest by an assistant can greatly enhance diagnostic yield. Samples are again submitted for cytology and bacterial culture.

It is essential that antibiotics are withdrawn for at least 5 days before such procedures or that they are performed prior to commencement of antibiotics.

THORACOCENTESIS

Indications

Thoracocentesis (removal of fluid from the pleural space via a needle, catheter or chest drain) may be both a diagnostic and a therapeutic procedure. It is indicated whenever pleural fluid is demonstrated on thoracic radiographs or when fluid is suspected on the basis of physical examination in the severely dyspnoeic animal and for the relief of pneumothorax. It should always be remembered that animals with pleural space disease (especially cats) are in a fragile state of respiratory compromise and any diagnostic or therapeutic endeavours should be undertaken in a calm and expedient way at a time when the animal is most able to withstand them. Supplemental oxygen therapy and patience are the two most helpful resources to have at one's disposal when dealing with these patients.

Technique

The procedure is usually performed in conscious animals; occasionally light sedation is needed in distressed animals though in severely compromised patients general anaesthesia may be safer, quicker and more easily controlled. The technique is described in Box 4.13.

Fluid analysis is invaluable in the diagnosis of the underlying cause for the effusion and classification of pleural effusions is shown in Table 4.7.

ABDOMINAL PARACENTESIS

Indications/contraindications

Abdominal paracentesis (collection of fluid from the abdomen) should always be performed when there is evidence of abdominal fluid accumulation (i.e. ascites) but should also be considered in cases of acute abdominal pain, where peritonitis is suspected, and in cases of shock due to trauma (especially abdominal) which is

Box 4.13 Thoracocentesis technique

1. An area over the 7th–8th intercostal space on the desired side of the thorax is widely clipped and surgically scrubbed. The preferred point of entry for drainage of fluid is at approximately the costochondral junction, whilst a more dorsal location is preferred for the removal of air.
2. The area is infiltrated with local anaesthetic down to the pleural tissue as this can be very sensitive. A small stab incision with a scalpel blade is made to ease transcutaneous passage of the drainage catheter.
3. In cats and small dogs a butterfly catheter may be used but in most larger animals an over-the-needle catheter of as wide a bore as possible should be used to facilitate drainage of fluid and to minimise the risk of collapsing of the catheter lumen as suction is applied. In large dogs a 14–16 G catheter can often be used and the creation of additional side holes in the catheter with a sterile scalpel blade can be helpful.
4. The needle/catheter is placed through the intercostal tissues just cranial to the adjacent rib to avoid the neurovascular bundle coursing down the caudal edge of each rib, until it is felt to 'pop' through the pleural space. Some discomfort is often felt by the animal at this point and firm but gentle restraint should be given by an assistant.
5. A drainage system such as a three-way tap, syringe and extension set should then be connected and the fluid slowly aspirated.
6. Fluid should be collected for cytology, biochemistry and bacteriology in appropriate sterile containers.

Table 4.7 Diagnosis of thoracic and abdominal fluid accumulations

	Pure transudate	Modified transudate	Exudate	Chyle
Colour	Clear, watery	Serous/serosanguineous, may be cloudy	Serosanguineous, sometimes creamy, cloudy or flocculent	Milky white or 'strawberry milkshake', opalescent
Total protein	<25 g/l	25–50 g/l	>30 g/l	>25 g/l
Specific gravity	<1.017	1.017–1.025	>1.025	>1.018
Nucleated cell count/μl	<1000	500–10 000	>5000	Variable
Differential cell count	Predominantly mononuclear cells (mesothelial cells, lymphocytes, macrophages)	Mesothelial cells, macrophages, neutrophils, lymphocytes, red blood cells	Neutrophils (may be degenerative with intracellular bacteria in cases of sepsis), macrophages, lymphocytes, mesothelial cells	Lymphocytes (predominant cell type in early disease), neutrophils (usually appear in chronic disease), mesothelial cells
Lipid content	None	None	None	Fluid triglycerides > serum, cholesterol < serum
Bacteria	No	No	Yes, if septic	Rarely

unresponsive to fluid therapy. Contraindications and risks are relatively few. The major risk is of abdominal organ laceration such as of the spleen or bladder, but if performed carefully this risk should be low and is more of a cause of concern in giving false results than in causing harm to the patient.

Technique

There are three principal ways of performing abdominal paracentesis – needle centesis, catheter centesis and diagnostic peritoneal lavage (DPL). With all of these techniques, the principal drawback is that of gaining a false-negative result (i.e. finding no fluid when some is present). This can be due to several reasons but is most often due to small quantities of fluid being present and 'pocketing' in limited areas, or occlusion of the drainage needle or catheter by falciform or omental fat. If the former is suspected, ultrasound-guided aspiration of pocketed fluid may be useful. DPL is most useful in cases where a limited amount of peritoneal fluid is suspected, such as in cases where pancreatitis or early septic peritonitis is suspected.

Regardless of the exact technique used the patient (usually fully conscious) is best restrained in left lateral recumbency to allow the spleen to fall away from the centesis site and avoid its puncture. The bladder should preferably be emptied prior to abdominal paracentesis. A site two fingers' width caudal to the umbilicus (to avoid the falciform fat in this area) and in the midline is aseptically prepared and, if a catheter is to be placed, infiltrated with a local anaesthetic. An 18–20 G 1 inch (2.5 cm) needle or 14–16 G 2.5 inch (6 cm) catheter with additional side-holes cut with a sterile scalpel blade is then placed through the midline linea alba and any fluid emerging is collected as it drips from the hub. If no fluid is obtained then gentle suction may be applied with a syringe but this often results in the tip of the needle or catheter becoming plugged with fat. Should no fluid be obtained then another side may be sampled or the animal gently rolled so that the needle or catheter is in a more dependent position.

If DPL is to be performed, 20 ml/kg of warmed sterile, preservative-free saline is infused via the pre-placed catheter and the animal gently rolled from side to side. As much of the fluid as possible is then withdrawn and collected in appropriate sterile containers for analysis.

Handling and analysis of samples

Samples should be collected for cytology (in an EDTA pot), and in sterile containers for biochemistry and culture. Cytological examination should be performed immediately before cellular degeneration starts to occur, particularly in DPL samples. Cytology should include measurement of PCV in grossly haemorrhagic samples and a differential white blood cell count. The finding of large numbers of degenerative neutrophils and intra- or extracellular bacteria should prompt suspicion of a ruptured GI tract and rapid surgical intervention may be necessary. The differentiation of abdominal fluid as pure transudate, modified transudate or exudate may be made on the basis of cytology and fluid-specific gravity and protein quantification (see Table 4.7). This is often invaluable in diagnosing a cause for the fluid accumulation. Protein quantification may be especially helpful in aiding diagnosis of feline infectious peritonitis. Measurement of fluid bilirubin and creatinine may be useful in the diagnosis of bile and urine peritonitis respectively, levels far in excess of those in peripheral blood being diagnostic.

ARTHROCENTESIS FOR SYNOVIAL FLUID ANALYSIS

Indications/contraindications

Arthrocentesis is principally indicated in patients with palpable joint effusions (be they single or multiple) and is invaluable as a diagnostic aid in ruling out polyarthropathies in cases of pyrexia of unknown origin. Provided it is performed in a strictly aseptic manner there are few contraindications to arthrocentesis though in patients with coagulation disorders haemarthrosis may develop.

Table 4.8 Normal and abnormal synovial fluid analysis

	Normal	Degenerative joint disease	Infectious inflammation (septic arthritis)	Non-infectious inflammation (usually immune-mediated)
Colour/turbidity	Clear, straw-coloured	Light yellow, clear or slightly turbid	Turbid to purulent, may be yellow or blood-tinged	Variable appearance, may be slightly turbid and blood-tinged
Viscosity	Viscous	Viscous	Reduced	Reduced
Nucleated cell count/µl	0–3000	0–3000	30 000–250 000	Variable but usually >5000
Differential cell count	Predominantly mononuclear cells (usually lymphocytes, synoviocytes, macrophages)	Lymphocytes macrophages, synoviocytes, <12% neutrophils	Usually neutrophils predominate (>90%). Many degenerative changes are often seen, though rarely intracellular organisms	Variable but usually neutrophils (non-degenerate) predominate

Technique

Most patients require some form of sedation or even short-acting general anaesthesia for arthrocentesis, as the procedure is a painful one. Strict asepsis must be maintained and the skin over any joint to be sampled must be clipped and surgically prepared.

A sterile 22–25 G $\frac{5}{8}$–1 inch (1.5–2.5 cm) needle and 2–5 ml syringe are the only equipment needed. The extensor surface of any joint to be sampled is preferred due to the paucity of blood vessels and nervous structures. The joint is held by an assistant in a flexed position to 'open' the joint space and the needle is inserted with guidance by digital palpation of the joint space. Fluid is removed by gentle suction. Overtly bloody samples may represent haemarthrosis but more usually represent iatrogenic haemorrhage and may be unsuitable for analysis.

Sample handling and analysis

If only small volumes are produced, a smear should be made for cytological evaluation. Larger volumes are collected in EDTA sample tubes for cytological evaluation and in sterile plain tubes for culture. Samples are analysed for volume, appearance (colour, turbidity, viscosity), cell cytology and differential nucleated cell count, mucin clot test and aerobic/anaerobic culture.

Normal and pathological criteria are shown in Table 4.8.

TISSUE BIOPSY TECHNIQUES

INTRODUCTION

The practice of collection of cellular material for diagnostic evaluation has become well established in veterinary medicine and there are numerous disease conditions in which a definitive diagnosis can only be made after appropriate evaluation of pathological material. Tissue biopsy is usually undertaken as dictated by the clinical setting of the patient and, whilst an invaluable diagnostic aid, should not be undertaken hurriedly without first considering the animal's history and clinical examination findings. Tissue specimens may be obtained post-mortem (necropsy specimens) or in the live patient (biopsy).

In the live patient, biopsy material is used to provide information concerning the nature of abnormal tissue identified by physical examination or other diagnostic evaluation and may ultimately lead to a definitive diagnosis being made. It also has the potential to offer information concerning the extent, behaviour and prognosis for a particular disease entity and this information is especially important in the evaluation of patients with cancer as it may allow their owners to make a more informed decision regarding treatment options.

It is important however, to realise that there are several limitations to tissue biopsy techniques and steps that can be taken to minimise these. Whilst in an ideal world all biopsy material would lead to a definitive diagnosis, frequently non-diagnostic or (even worse) misleadingly diagnostic results may be obtained. Currently there are many excellent diagnostic laboratories in the UK that offer a fast and cost-effective pathology service with a high level of expertise and the establishment of a good rapport between the clinic and laboratory is important if the most is to be made from this resource. However, even the most experienced of pathologists are only as good as the material that they receive and it is in the selection of technique, the collection and handling of material, and in transport and communication, that most problems arise.

Types of biopsy available

There are many collection methods for biological material but in general sampled tissue may comprise solid pieces of biological material or aspirated cells which are spread on a slide for examination. Solid tissue is usually submitted for histopathological evaluation which allows assessment not only of the cell type and morphology, but also the local architecture. This is extremely important in the assessment of some diseases as sometimes determination of cell type alone does not allow sufficient information for a diagnosis to be made. Cellular aspirates are evaluated cytologically; that is, cell type and morphology may be determined but because the aspirated cells are discontinuous with the surrounding tissue, important architectural information may be missed. In many cases cytological and histopathological evaluation may, however, be complementary and the combination of the two may yield excellent diagnostic results.

Patient assessment

Any tissue biopsy technique should only be undertaken after thorough evaluation of the animal and an assessment of what one expects to gain from the procedure and whether it is of any risk to the animal. Principal risks come in the form of haemorrhage from local blood vessel laceration or undetected bleeding disorders, damage to adjacent structures through inappropriate positioning of instruments and seeding of neoplastic material by disruption of a tumour bed. Other considerations may be the need for patient analgesia or general anaesthesia and whether only a partial surgical biopsy (incisional) is to be taken or whether complete excision of abnormal tissue as both a diagnostic and therapeutic endeavour is appropriate.

DESCRIPTION OF CYTOPATHOLOGY TECHNIQUES

Techniques for fluid collection for cytology are described in Chapter 3.

Impression smears

Impression smears may give excellent cytological information and are usually collected from superficial lesions such as ulcerated skin lesions or from excised surgical material. The harvest of cells gained tends to rely on the degree to which they are likely to exfoliate from the tissue (which tends to be less in firm masses) and also relies on adequate preparation of the surface to be sampled. The surface should be gently blotted dry of exudate with sterile gauze swabs and a clean, dry microscope slide is gently 'rocked' over the exposed surface rather than 'dabbed'. Very cellular samples may be too thick to examine adequately and gentle spreading of cells using a 'draw-back and push' or 'pull-apart' method may be required (see Fig. 4.18).

Fine needle aspiration

Fine needle aspiration is a rapid, simple, inexpensive and easily learned technique which is well tolerated in most normal animals without the need for sedation or anaesthesia unless deep intracavity structures are sampled. Superficial lesions may be sampled by palpation alone whilst intracavity structures generally require the guidance

'Draw-back and push' method

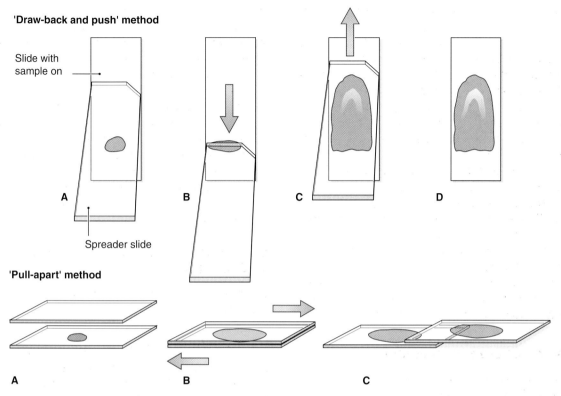

Slide with sample on

Spreader slide

A   B   C   D

'Pull-apart' method

A   B   C

Figure 4.18   Preparation of cytological smears.

of imaging such as radiography or ultrasono-graphy. Whichever technique is used, the principles are the same. The technique is described in Box 4.14.

With firm lesions such as lymph nodes, an alternative is to collect many small 'core' specimens in the cylinder of a needle without a syringe attached by repeatedly stabbing it into the tissue to be sampled and then expelling the contents using a syringe as before.

With either method, the most common causes of non-diagnostic samples are blood contamination and clotting, failure to sample the tissue intended/representative tissue and unreadable slides due to very cellular and thick preparations or damage due to excessive force used in smear making. The presence of blood within the hub of the needle should alert the operator to the likelihood of blood contamination and the procedure should be repeated in a different site using fresh equipment.

Slides with smears on them should be properly air-dried and labelled and either stained in-house or sent to the laboratory unstained dependent on the laboratory's preference. Air-tight slide containers are invaluable for safe transportation.

Bone marrow aspiration

Cytological examination of bone marrow is generally indicated in cases of non-regenerative anaemia, single or multiple cell-line cytopenias, where abnormal cells are found circulating on peripheral blood smears, staging of some tumours (e.g. lymphoma) and in cases of hyper-proteinaemia, hypercalcaemia and fever of unknown origin. Bone marrow aspirates result in the collection of the non-adherent elements of the bone marrow. Larger core samples comprising haematopoietic cells, fat and trabecular bone may also be obtained concurrently (see later) and will give more architectural information when

Box 4.14   Technique for fine needle aspiration

1. The site to be aspirated is clipped and cleaned and if a body cavity is to be entered should be aseptically prepared.
2. A 5–10 ml syringe with a 21–25 G needle and several clean dry microscope slides are all that is required. After fixation of the tissue to be aspirated with one hand (mobile structures should be tensed against the skin surface to avoid risk of contamination of interposed tissues and damage to other structures) the needle attached to the syringe is briskly inserted into the centre of the structure.
3. The syringe plunger is withdrawn to a suction of 3–5 ml rapidly several times or held out so that vacuum is maintained. The needle may be repositioned within the tissue with the vacuum still applied in several directions so that more than one site is sampled; it is however essential that the vacuum should be released prior to exiting the tissue as failure to do this will result in cells being aspirated into the barrel of the syringe where they will be irretrievable.
4. Once several aspirations have been performed, suction is released and the needle and syringe are removed.
5. The needle is then detached *prior* to aspirating 3–5 ml of air into the syringe and then reattached. Holding the bevel of the needle downwards over a clean slide, the air is then forcefully expelled from the syringe creating a 'spray' of cellular material on to the slide.
6. Spreading is then performed using either the 'pull-back and push' method or the 'pull-apart' method (Fig. 4.18).

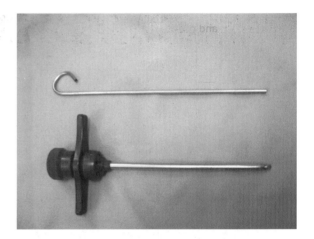

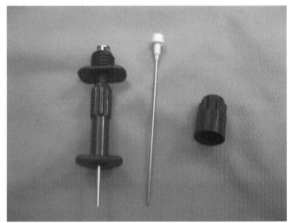

Figure 4.19   Types of bone marrow needle.

examined by a histopathologist. In some cases of cytopenias, inadequate cellular samples may be obtained by aspiration alone and core samples are required for further diagnosis; in most cases, however, the two samples are complementary and it is the author's preference always to obtain both concurrently.

For bone marrow aspiration an aspiration needle, anticoagulant, clean dry microscope slides, sterile gloves and a scalpel blade are required. Several types of bone marrow needle, both for aspirates and core samples, are available; examples are shown in Figure 4.19. Both comprise an outer needle and an inner stylet to prevent cores of cortical bone and fat blocking the needle upon entry. Biopsy needles may be cleaned and resterilised but become increasingly difficult to use as they blunt with repeated use. In some patients, bone marrow aspiration may be accomplished with sedation and local anaesthe-

sia, but in many (and in the author's preference), short-acting general anaesthesia greatly facilitates the procedure and is preferable for patient comfort (especially if core biopsies are taken).

The technique of aspiration is shown in Box 4.15 (Fig. 4.20).

Contraindications are relatively few and even in profoundly thrombocytopenic animals, haemorrhage appears to be of minimal risk.

DESCRIPTION OF TISSUE BIOPSY TECHNIQUES

Tru-Cut biopsies

Tru-Cut biopsies are cores of tissue obtained by the use of a wide-bore needle device comprising an inner cutting rod (obturator) containing a trough in which tissue is collected, and an outer

Box 4.15 Bone marrow aspirate technique

1. For aspiration and core collection a site over the proximal humerus or femur or the wing of the ilium is selected (the wing of the ilium may allow more productive sampling in older animals in which the long bone medullary cavity may become less active and more fat filled, but this site can be more challenging in obese animals).
2. The bone and the periosteum are liberally infiltrated with local anaesthesia and the site is surgically prepared (the operator should treat the procedure as a sterile one, especially since leucopenia is frequently present).
3. The needle with the stylet is removed and a sterile 20 ml syringe is first primed by repeated 'washing' of the syringe barrel with a suitable anticoagulant such as acid citrate dextrose (ACD) then the stylet replaced in the needle.
4. The needle is then advanced through a small nick made in the overlying skin parallel to the direction of the bone being sampled and advanced with firm pressure and a back and forth rotatory movement into the medullary cavity. An assistant should brace the bone being entered as quite considerable force is often needed and care should be taken that no bending of the needle occurs.
5. When fully lodged within the proximal medullary cavity (at which point rocking of the needle should move the entire animal!) the stylet is removed and the anticoagulated syringe attached.
6. Brief, firm aspiration is then performed until marrow enters the hub of the syringe. Non-adherent marrow elements appear similar to peripheral blood.
7. The syringe is then disconnected and drops of marrow are placed on to slides which are then tilted to allow the liquid component to run off. Small gritty bone marrow spicules should be left adherent to the slide and should be appreciated as refractile grains if it is held up to the light. The remaining marrow can be gently smeared across the remaining slide using previously described methods.

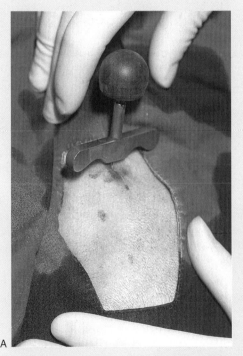
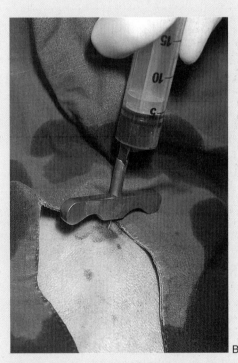

A   B

Figure 4.20 Bone marrow aspirate technique. (A) Here, an Islam aspiration needle inserted in the proximal humerus. Note the stylet is still in place during the insertion process. (B) The stylet has now been removed and aspiration into a pre-coagulated syringe is occurring with a short application of moderate suction.

cutting sheath (cannula) which, when advanced over the needle, cuts the tissue specimen loose and protects it during withdrawal (Fig. 4.21). The Tru-Cut device may be manually operated, self-firing or be fired using a spring-loaded device

(Fig. 4.22). The principle of operation is the same for each method.

After immobilisation of the structure to be sampled the obturator is advanced into the tissue so that the tissue fills the specimen trough. The

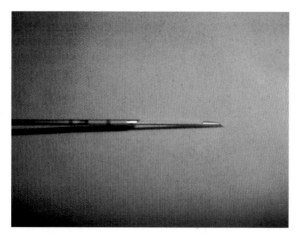

Figure 4.21 Cannula and obturator of the 'Tru-Cut' biopsy device.

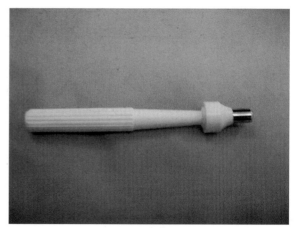

Figure 4.23 A punch biopsy device.

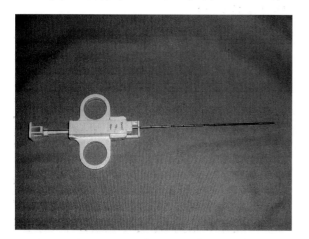

Figure 4.22 'Tru-Cut' device mounted in a spring-loaded biopsy gun.

cannula is then rapidly advanced over the obturator, so sectioning off a core of tissue within it. The whole structure is then removed and the cannula retracted to allow the tissue sample to be removed. With automated and spring-loaded biopsy 'guns', these steps occur rapidly once a trigger is depressed after the device has been 'cocked'.

Tru-Cut devices are extremely useful in obtaining tissue from solid abdominal and thoracic structures such as masses and parenchymal organs, such as the liver and renal cortex. Ultrasound guidance, general anaesthesia and an experienced operator are mandatory and the coagulation status of any patient should be confirmed before this is undertaken.

Punch biopsies

Punch biopsies are cylindrical specimens obtained from superficial lesions by the use of a disposable biopsy punch which comprises a cylindrical cutting blade on a handle (Fig. 4.23). Punch biopsies are particularly indicated for the diagnostic evaluation of skin lesions and the margin between normal and abnormal tissue is the most useful site to biopsy as are fresh lesions rather than old, traumatised or resolving ones. Punch biopsies are *not* suitable for obtaining gastrointestinal biopsies. The technique for punch biopsy is given in Box 4.16.

Surgical biopsies

Surgical biopsies have the advantages of needing very little specialised equipment, the ability to obtain large specimens of tissue, hopefully containing representative material upon which an accurate diagnosis can be made, and in the case of excisional biopsies are both diagnostic and therapeutic if the whole lesion is removed. The decision as to whether to remove part of a lesion in order adequately to plan a definitive surgical procedure to remove it, or whether to attempt excision in toto as a first endeavour is one that is

Box 4.16 Technique for punch biopsy

1. Punch biopsies of skin lesions may be performed under general anaesthesia or sedation and local anaesthesia with adrenaline-free lidocaine (lignocaine) administered through a fine needle to avoid traumatic artefact. The surface should *not* be scrubbed, merely clipped and if deemed necessary wiped with alcohol.
2. The biopsy punch is orientated perpendicular to the skin and gently rotated back and forth or with a continuous rotatory movement until the subcutis is reached.
3. The plug of tissue is then very carefully elevated with a fine needle if it is still attached and released from the subcutis with fine scissors.
4. Biopsy sites are then closed with a single interrupted non-absorbable suture.

based on clinical judgement and by assessment of the extent of abnormal tissue by palpation and by imaging (radiography, ultrasound, MRI, CT) including the proximity of other vital structures. Evaluation of cytological material may also provide useful information.

Whichever type of surgical biopsy is undertaken, thorough pre-operative patient evaluation (including evaluation of coagulation status as necessary), planning of the procedure with respect to possible future surgical procedures, proper sample handling, labelling and communication are all vital in establishing a diagnosis. Where incisional biopsies are taken, particularly if a malignancy is possible, seeding of local normal tissues with neoplastic cells should be anticipated and adequate labelling of samples to aid the pathologist is essential.

Bone marrow core biopsies

Bone marrow core samples are taken with a larger-bore needle than is used for an aspirate sample such as a Jamshidi needle. The needle with stylet in place is advanced into the medullary cavity of the bone as described for aspiration. The stylet is then removed and the needle advanced a further 2–3 cm. It is then rotated rapidly to break off the distal portion of trabecular bone within the cavity of the needle. The needle is then withdrawn and the stylet is passed *retrograde* down the lumen

of the needle to push the core specimen out of the handle end to avoid distorting it. Adequate samples are red in colour and 1–2 cm in length. The technique is shown in Figure 4.24. Jamshidi needles may also be used to obtain cortical bone samples from radiographically diagnosed destructive bone lesions.

Other types of tissue biopsy

Suction catheter biopsy technique is described under prostatic sampling in the section 'Body Fluid Collection'. Endoscopic biopsy is described later in the appropriate section.

TISSUE BIOPSY HANDLING AND TRANSPORT

A source of great frustration to pathologists and clinicians alike is failure of a diagnostic sample being obtained, not by poor selection of technique or sampling error, but because of injudicious handling or misinformative samples.

In general, cytological preparations on slides (smears) require little preparation other than rapid air drying. Alcohol fixation is seldom needed unless Trichrome stains are to be used. If in doubt the cytologist who is performing the cytologic assessment should be consulted *prior* to making smears. Samples should be clearly labelled, preferably on the slide (small adhesive labels are invaluable for this) and the slide container. Most laboratories are happy to supply plastic air-tight slide transporters which allow safe transport of multiple slides with little risk of breakage.

Larger tissue specimens should be fixed in a suitable preservative agent to prevent cellular autolysis and degeneration. For most samples 10% formalin is the fixative of choice, though for certain examinations (e.g. ultrastructural examination of nerve samples) other agents such as glutaraldehyde may be required. Again, if in doubt, the laboratory should be contacted prior to tissue biopsy collection. An adequate volume of fixative per unit volume of tissue is required for adequate penetration by the fixative and very large or thick specimens should be carefully sectioned prior to fixation. If this is performed it

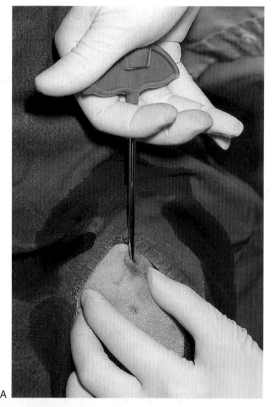

A

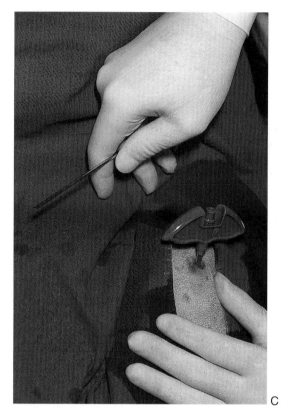

C

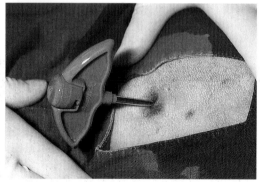

B

Figure 4.24 (A) A Jamshidi needle with the stylet in place is being inserted in the proximal humerus. (B) The needle is firmly inserted into the proximal humeral medulla with the stylet in place but not the full depth of the instrument. (C) With the stylet removed, the needle is inserted 3–4 cm deeper with firm rotatory movements and then a core of marrow is broken off before removal.

is *essential* that the pathologist is given as much information as possible regarding the site of excision, the gross appearance, the planes of sectioning and the portions of tissue submitted to give adequate orientation. Multiple specimens should be individually labelled and submitted in separate containers. Containers should be of adequate size so that tissue is not compressed or distorted in any way and should be undamaged, plastic, watertight and sealed in an impervious

bag with adequate absorptive material to contain any leaked fluid. All packages should be clearly labelled as containing pathological material and postal regulations strictly adhered to.

Finally, each cytological or histopathological specimen submitted should be accompanied by legible, unambiguous and expansive documentation (usually on the laboratory's own forms) to provide the pathologist with as much clinical information as possible. This will not only allow him or her to give as accurate an assessment as possible but also demonstrates a strong commitment to maintaining a good working relationship between clinic and laboratory and encourages a good quality of practice.

BASICS OF CYTOLOGICAL INTERPRETATION

Cytological evaluation requires a systematic approach and a degree of operator experience that is usually best performed by a dedicated cytopathologist. However, the rapid interpretation of cytological preparations in the practice setting can be invaluable when treatment decisions need to be made expediently (e.g. in the dog with a septic abdomen) or out of normal working hours, and can also be of great personal interest. A suggested approach is outlined below:

1. Collect samples for cytological evaluation as carefully as possible, namely by:
   a. making sure that the region of interest, and not adjacent structures, is sampled
   b. making sure cytological smears are prepared carefully and rapidly air-dried or fixed
   c. making sure staining is performed completely and evenly and that stains are kept in good working order/replenished regularly
   d. keeping microscopic equipment clean and in working order.
2. Establish that a suitable number of intact cells are present on the smear.
3. Evaluate the smear initially under low power to determine whether all areas are similarly representative or whether there is unevenness in distribution of cell type which may be misleading if examined in isolation.
4. Evaluate cells in areas of good cellular quantity and quality.
5. Initially determine whether the predominant cell type is inflammatory or non-inflammatory (tissue cells).
6. In the case of inflammatory cell predominance an inciting aetiology should be sought.
7. In the case of tissue cells predominating evaluate for cell type to determine the originating tissue type (e.g. epithelial, mesenchymal cell, round cell) and whether any characteristics of malignancy exist.

Table 4.9 Classification of inflammatory tissue

Type of inflammation	Predominating cell type	Features
Neutrophilic inflammation/ suppurative inflammation	Neutrophils	May be sterile (e.g. immune-mediated polyarthritis) or induced by micro-organisms/foreign material Intracellular organisms may be seen Presence of degenerate neutrophils (wider, irregular, light-staining nuclei, cytoplasmic vacuolation) should prompt an extensive hunt for an inciting organism. Care should be taken not to mistake old, or damaged, neutrophils for degenerate neutrophils
Granulomatous and pyogranulomatous inflammation	Mixture of macrophages and neutrophils	Larger inciting agents such as fungi or foreign bodies should be considered Neutrophils are found more frequently than macrophages on aspirates and impression smears than on tissue samples as they exfoliate more easily
Chronic inflammation	Mixture of cell types, e.g. neutrophils, plasma cells, macrophages, fibroblasts	Usually seen in long-standing inflammatory states
Eosinophilic inflammation	Eosinophils are usually rare and only marginally increased numbers may be significant	May be seen with parasitic, or immune-mediated tissue reactions

Inflammatory cytology

In inflammatory states tissue cytology mostly comprises one or more of the following cell types: neutrophils, macrophages, eosinophils, lymphocytes, plasma cells, and the type of inflammation often describes the predominating cell type (see Table 4.9).

When an inflammatory cell predominance is found, a search for an inciting agent such as bacteria, fungi, yeasts, foreign bodies, parasites and protozoa should be made. Failure to identify causative material or organisms suggests either that the inflammation is sterile or that the examination has been inadequate to identify a causative agent either through unrepresentative tissue, poor staining or examination technique or agents which are extremely difficult to identify. Certain characteristics such as the finding of degenerate or toxic neutrophils (which often will have granular cytoplasm, intracytoplasmic inclusions or hypersegmented nuclei) may suggest a higher likelihood of a causative organism. Cartoons of basic inflammatory cells are shown in Figure 4.25.

Tissue cell cytology

The cytological characteristics of different cell types are shown in Table 4.11 (Fig. 4.26). In most cases the cell type of origin is not clear-cut but must be made on the basis of the predominating cell-characteristics in cases of mixed type. Once an assessment of cell-type has been made the next diagnostic step is to try to determine whether the cells represent a normal or hyperplastic population or whether they are showing any criteria which may make malignancy a consideration. Characteristics of malignancy are shown in Box 4.7.

Bone marrow cytology and histopathology

Evaluation of bone marrow samples should always be performed by a haematopathologist, though a basic understanding of the interpretation of such results is essential. It is vital that a peripheral blood sample is also examined

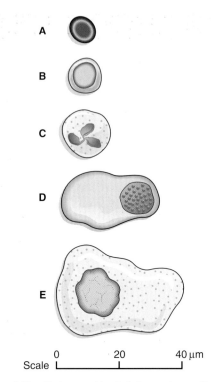

Figure 4.25 Cartoons of basic inflammatory cells. (A) Erythrocyte. (B) Small lymphocyte. (C) Neutrophil. (D) Plasma cell. (E) Macrophage.

on the same day that an aspirate or core marrow sample is taken and that pertinent clinical examination and historical findings are also submitted to the examining haematopathologist.

Initially aspirates are examined under low power to assess cellularity, adequacy of spicule numbers for interpretation and that the sample is heterogeneous (i.e. contains representative numbers of maturing cells from all red, white and platelet lineages and is not overly contaminated with blood). The proportion of fat spaces to cells is examined (this proportion increases dramatically in elderly animals and also in some disease states such as aplastic anaemia) and the number and morphology of megakaryocytes (platelet precursors) evaluated. Megakaryocytes usually cluster around the bone marrow spicules and 5–10 are usually found associated with each particle. More than one half of the megakaryocytes should be mature and granular, higher proportions of immature cells usually being seen

Table 4.11 Cytological characteristics of different tissue cell types

Category	Examples	Features
Epithelial	Adenoma Adenocarcinoma Transitional cell carcinoma	Many cells exfoliated (usually in clusters), round or polygonal cells with round nucleus and moderate to abundant cytoplasm. May form ducts or pallisades
Mesenchymal	Haemangiosarcoma Fibrosarcoma Osteosarcoma	Spindle-shaped cells with elongated bodies and tails of cytoplasm. Not many cells exfoliate. Nuclei are oval to elongated. Often only single cells seen or very dense clumps with indistinct borders
Round cell	Lymphoma Plasmacytoma Mast cell tumour Histiocytoma	Cells are small, round, and are usually discrete cells. Where cells are close together the margins between them are usually well defined

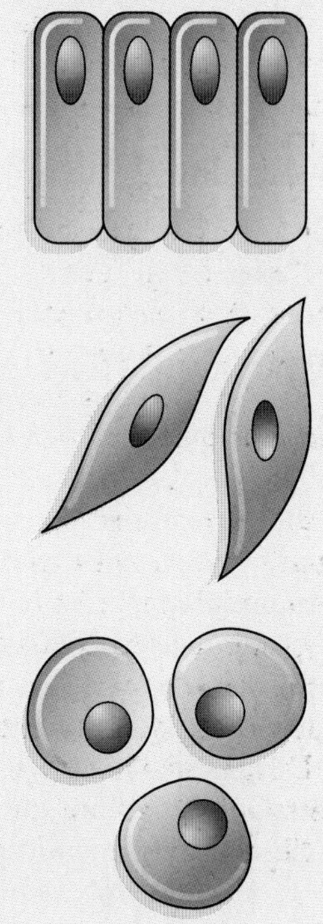

Figure 4.26 Cytological characteristics of different tissue cell types.

Box 4.7 Characteristics of malignancy

Cellular criteria
- Hypercellularity of sample
- Variability in cell size and shape

Nuclear criteria
- High or variable nuclear:cytoplasmic ratio
- Variation in nuclear size
- Multinucleated cells particularly if accompanied by nuclear size variation
- Large nucleoli
- Coarse nuclear chromatin
- Variation in size and shape of nucleoli
- Increased numbers or abnormally shaped mitotic figures

Cytoplasmic criteria (not highly specific)
- Vacuolation
- Increased basophilic staining (blue) of cytoplasm

with increasing demand such as in immune-mediated thrombocytopenia.

Next, iron stores are evaluated by the degree of brown–black staining seen with Wright's stain; chronically iron-deficient states usually produce an appreciable decrease in the amount of stained tissue.

Finally, under high power, the proportions and morphology of the maturing series of red cells (rubriblasts, prorubricytes, rubricytes, metarubricytes), and white cells (lymphoid and myeloid cells originating from common precursors and maturing through several stages, e.g. myeloblast, promyelocyte, myelocyte, metamyelocyte, band and segmented). Most of the white cell precursors are difficult to differentiate until they have reached a relatively mature stage in which they are well committed to their ultimate lineage. The myeloid:erythroid ratio is calculated and a distribution percentage of the precursor cells calculated (the myelogram). Usually a greater proportion of the cells are found in more mature stages as progenitor cells lead to a mutiplication in cell numbers as they mature.

PART
2

Endoscopy

Edward J. Hall

INTRODUCTION

Endoscopy (the word is derived from the Greek *endo-* = within and *skopein* = look) refers to the technique used to look within body cavities. Now, with increasingly sophisticated equipment, it is possible, not only to look but also to record images, collect fluid and tissue samples, and undertake surgical treatments.

There are two main types of endoscope – flexible and rigid – which are self-explanatory descriptions of their ability to bend within body cavities. Both work by transmitting light from a light source to illuminate the body cavity and transmitting the resulting image to the operator.

To accomplish this, an endoscope system has four main components:

- a light source
- a light-transmitting rod or cable (may be incorporated within the endoscope)
- an insertion tube (part inserted in patient)
- a facility for viewing the image (may be incorporated within endoscope).

The illuminating light and image are carried either by rigid glass rods and lenses or by flexible optical glass fibres (fibre-optics). In flexible endoscopes the illumination is always carried by fibre-optics, but the image is either carried by fibre-optics (fibre-optic endoscope) or captured by a video chip (video-endoscope).

PRINCIPLES OF ENDOSCOPY
Rigid endoscopy

With rigid endoscopes, their rigidity aids insertion into a body cavity but limits their use to sites where the scope can be inserted in a straight line.

They can be as simple as a hollow tube through which the unmagnified image is viewed directly (Fig. 4.27A). A removable blunt obturator may be used to prevent trauma during insertion. If a magnifying lens is attached over the viewing end, inflation with a simple rubber bulb pump is possible (e.g. proctoscope, Fig. 4.27B), but the lens must be removed to allow insertion of instruments through the tube.

Solid, rigid endoscopes have a rod/lens telescope system to improve image quality, with better light transmission, greater magnification and a wider field of view. However, instruments must be inserted alongside it or through a parallel port (e.g. laparoscopy).

The most frequently used rigid endoscope in veterinary practice is the 2.7 mm diameter telescope with a 10–30 degree viewing angle or 'arthroscope' (Fig 4.27C). As well as arthroscopy it can be used for urethrocystoscopy, rhinoscopy, otoscopy and avian coelioscopy.

Flexible endoscopy

A flexible endoscope can be inserted around bends (e.g. into the intestine), although the ability to steer the tip is required. Flexibility depends on the illumination being carried by fibre-optics and the image is carried either by fibre-optics or electronically by wires in video-endoscopes.

The image bundle of a standard fibre-optic endoscope is 0.5–3.0 mm in diameter and contains 20 000–40 000 fine glass fibres, each 6–10 μm in diameter. Each individual glass fibre is coated with glass of lower optical density ('cladding') to prevent leakage of light. Light focused on to the face of each fibre is transmitted by repeated total

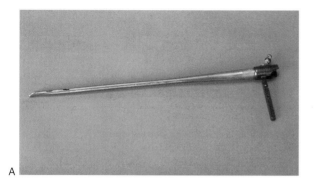

A

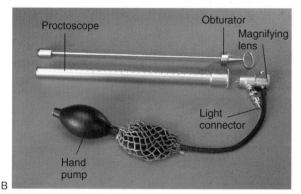

B

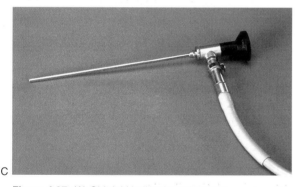

C

Figure 4.27 (A) Old rigid hollow bronchoscope. (B) Hollow rigid proctoscope, with obturator for atraumatic insertion, and magnifying window with light connector, and hand pump for insufflation. (C) Rigid arthoscope with 10 degree viewing angle suitable for rhinoscopy.

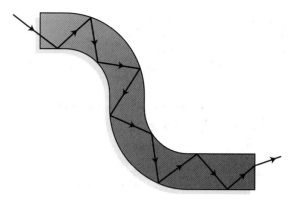

Figure 4.28A Transmission of light through optical glass fibre by total internal reflection.

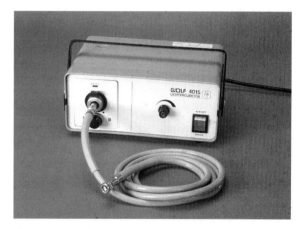

Figure 4.28B Simple portable light source and detachable flexible light guide.

internal reflection (Fig. 4.28A), and transmits a single spot of uniform colour and brightness.

Illumination cables

In flexible endoscopes the fibre-optic illumination cable (also known as the 'light guide') is usually included in the umbilical cord and insertion tube. For some older models, and for rigid endoscopes, light guides are available as separate detachable cables (Fig. 4.28B). Cables may be used interchangeably with a variety of endoscopes if adapters are available to ensure a correct fit.

Image bundles

Faithful transmission of an image depends on the spatial orientation of the individual glass fibres being the same at both ends of the bundle, i.e. 'coherent'. To be coherent, the bundles have individual fibre faces fixed in an identical pattern at either end (Fig. 4.28C). If a small group of fibres in the image bundle is broken a black dot is seen in the image. The illuminating cable only contains non-coherent fibres as transmission of the illumination is all that is required.

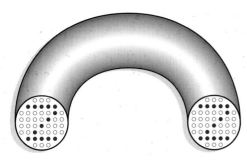

Figure 4.28C Faithful transmission of image by coherent fibre-optic bundle.

The cladding and the space between the fibres of the image bundle cause a dark 'packing fraction' which is responsible for the fine mesh apparent in the image. Furthermore, the lower size limit of fibres has now been reached; with fibres any narrower there is massive loss of light. Thus the number of image fibres (and hence image quality) is now limited by the diameter of the endoscope; narrower scopes inevitably have fewer fibres and poorer image.

Optical system

In fibre-optic endoscopes, a fixed distal lens gives a depth of focus from 10–15 cm down to 3 mm, and focuses the image on to the image bundle. The image is then reconstructed at the top of the bundle and transmitted to the eye via a focusing lens in the eyepiece.

Video-imaging

Video-endoscopes are mechanically similar to fibre-optic endoscopes, but with a charged couple device (CCD) or 'chip' and supporting electronics mounted at the tip. To-and-fro wiring replaces the image bundle, and further electronics and switches occupy the site of the eyepiece on the hand piece.

The subtleties of different CCD systems in design and performance are beyond the scope of this book. However, in essence a CCD chip is an array of up to 100 000 individual photo-cells (pixels) receiving photons reflected back from the patient surface and producing electrons in proportion to the amount of light received. The resultant 'electronic image' is processed and displayed on a monitor.

The functional characteristics of the two types of flexible scope are described below.

Fibre-optic endoscope

- Satisfactory image quality
- portable
- wide range of sizes available
- moderate cost

but

- faceted image as many fibres make up the composite image
- decreasing the diameter of the insertion tube reduces the resolution
- fragile
- requires attachable CCD camera for video capability.

Video-endoscope

- Excellent image quality (photographic quality)
- integral video capability
- no need to hold instrument close to endoscopist's eye
  — hygienic advantages
  — easier to rotate
- image visible to assistant and observers
- even smaller pixels and better resolution feasible in the future

but

- not readily portable
- very small diameters not yet available due to size of CCD
- high cost.

USES OF ENDOSCOPY

Endoscopes can be used for diagnostic and therapeutic purposes.

Diagnosis

- Direct viewing
- sampling
- collection of body fluid for cytology and culture
- lavage for cytology and culture
- brush cytology
- punch biopsy.

Therapy

The types of procedures most commonly performed in veterinary medicine are:

- foreign body removal
- stricture dilatation
- feeding tube placement
- polypectomy.

Rigid endoscopes can be used for:

- nasopharynx – anterograde rhinoscopy
- oropharynx – pharyngoscopy
- larynx – laryngoscopy
- ears – otoscopy
- vagina and cervix – vaginoscopy
- urinary tract – urethrocystoscopy (direct in female only; percutaneous prepubic insertion in males)
- joints – arthroscopy
- peritoneal cavity – laparoscopy
- pleural cavity – thoracoscopy.

Flexible endoscopes can be used to examine a number of organ systems:

- airways
  — nasopharynx – anterograde and retrograde rhinoscopy
  — larynx – laryngoscopy
  — trachea/bronchi – tracheoscopy and bronchoscopy
- upper GI tract
  — oesophagus – oesophagoscopy
  — stomach – gastroscopy
  — duodenum – duodenoscopy
  — jejunum – enteroscopy
- lower GI tract
  — rectum – proctoscopy
  — colon and caecum – colonoscopy

  — ileum – ileoscopy
- urethra/bladder – urethrocystoscopy.

Bronchoscopy, oesophagoscopy, cystoscopy and proctoscopy are preferably performed with flexible endoscopes as the image is better. However, for foreign body removal, a rigid hollow tube may be preferred. For example, sharp bone fragments can be pulled from the oesophagus into the endoscope before removal.

CONTRAINDICATIONS FOR ENDOSCOPY

Endoscopy requires general anaesthesia, and in some instances may be too dangerous to perform. It may also be an inappropriate way to reach a diagnosis, e.g. gastroduodenoscopy cannot diagnose pancreatitis as a cause of vomiting and diarrhoea. Specific contraindications include:

1. poor anaesthetic risk
   a. relative
      i. poor cardiopulmonary reserve
      ii. resting expiratory effort
      iii. pleural disease
      iv. severe pulmonary parenchymal disease
      v. pulmonary hypertension
      vi. uraemia
   b. absolute
      i. uncorrected bleeding disorder
      ii. non-reversible hypoxaemia
      iii. unstable cardiac arrhythmias
      iv. cardiac failure
2. poorly prepared patient
   a. not starved/cleaned out
   b. inadequate investigations prior to endoscopy.

COMPLICATIONS OF ENDOSCOPY

Although endoscopy is minimally invasive there is the potential to do harm to the patient, although this is fortunately rare, or to damage the equipment.

Patient harm

- Hypoxaemia

- cardiac arrhythmias
- bacteraemia/fever
- haemorrhage
- perforation
  — (tension) pneumothorax
  — mediastinitis
  — peritonitis
- induced airway irritation
- failure to get adequate biopsies.

Damage to the equipment

- Damaged insertion tube cover
  — wear and tear
  — bitten
  — snagged on tooth
- perforated biopsy channel by inserting biopsy forceps with the endoscope retroflexed
- broken fibres.

DESIGN AND STRUCTURE OF FLEXIBLE ENDOSCOPY SYSTEM

The main parts of an endoscopy system (Fig 4.29) are:

- light source
- air/water pump
- suction
- endoscope
- endoscopic accessories.

Light source (Figs 4.28B, 4.29)

Historically small, heat-emitting, incandescent light bulbs were used in the tip of rigid endoscopes, and are still used in some otoscopes, for example. However, by using fibre-optics, 'cold light' can now be transmitted through the endoscope to illuminate the patient.

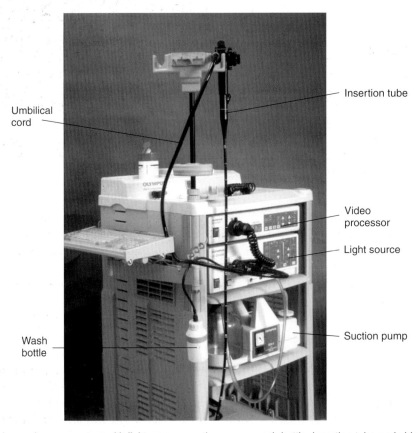

Figure 4.29   Video-endoscopy system with light source, suction pump, wash bottle, insertion tube and video processor.

The main types of bulbs now in use vary in their power, their resemblance to white light, and their cost:

- tungsten–halogen
  - relatively cheap
  - last ~250 hours
  - not very bright (150 watts)
  - red/yellow colour
- xenon arc
  - expensive
  - last 400–1000 hours
  - brighter than halogen (150–300 watts)
  - colour reproduction resembles sunlight as whole spectrum reproduced.

Light is focused on to the face of the light bundle, and filters and/or a mechanical diaphragm control the intensity of the transmitted light. For CCD video-endoscopes rotating filters in front of the xenon light source produce alternating coloured light that a video processor eventually turns into a composite coloured image.

Insufflation/suction

The light source for flexible endoscopes usually also houses an air pump for insufflation (i.e. distension of the body cavity by introduction of gas through the endoscope) and a water reservoir for feeding water to the endoscope tip for washing during use. A separate suction pump is attached to flexible endoscopes.

Endoscope

A flexible endoscope has a protective plastic covering, and in modern scopes is completely watertight so that it can be fully immersed for cleaning (Fig. 4.30). It comprises:

- umbilical cord
- hand piece
- insertion tube.

Umbilical cord

This attaches the insertion tube to the light source via a light-guide plug-in connector (Fig. 4.31) and carries:

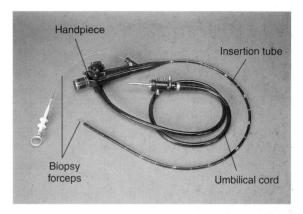

Figure 4.30 Fibre-optic gastroscope showing umbilical cord, hand piece and insertion tube, with biopsy forceps inserted through accessory channel.

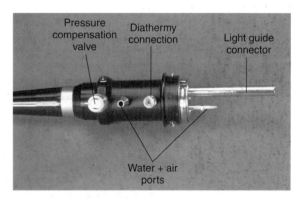

Figure 4.31 Umbilical cord showing light guide connector, air/water and suction ports, diathermy connection and pressure compensation valve.

- light-guide from light source
- air–water channel from air inflation pump and water reservoir (housed with light source)
- S-connector if diathermy accessories are being used
- the image to video processor (video-endoscope only)
- pressure compensation valve.

This permits equalisation of pressure between the inside and outside of the protective sleeve of the endoscope during ethylene oxide sterilisation or transport by aeroplane, and allows attachment of a leakage tester.

Hand piece

It is designed to be held in the left hand (Fig. 4.32) and bears all the controls for the endoscope:

*   Air/water control valve (blue). Insufflation is activated by placing a finger over a hole in the top of the valve, diverting the flow of air from the inflation pump to the endoscope tip. Irrigation, and hence cleaning of the lens, is activated by depressing the valve fully.
*   Suction control valve (red). Activated by depressing the valve, it allows suction from the tip of the endoscope into the suction pump attached to the umbilical cord.
*   Opening of accessory (biopsy) channel. Allows insertion of biopsy forceps down the insertion tube. It is covered by a disposable rubber seal that allows insertion of accessories without allowing leakage of air from the body cavity.
*   Eyepiece (fibre-optic endoscope only, Fig. 4.32A). Lens system to permit direct visualisation, with dioptre ring allowing focusing for individual users. Locking pins allow attachment of CCD camera for display on monitor.
*   Iris, illumination and video controls (video-endoscope only, Fig. 4.32B).
*   Tip deflection control wheels or levers. The inner wheel is moved by the right hand (or left thumb) and controls left–right tip deflection by anti-clockwise/clockwise motion respectively. The outer wheel is moved by the left thumb/fingers and controls up–down tip deflection by anti-clockwise/clockwise motion respectively. The wheels may be locked by friction brakes so that tip deflection is maintained; each control wheel can still be turned safely but is stiffer (Figs. 4.32A,B). Bronchoscopes have two-way tip deflection controlled by a lever (Fig. 4.32C).

Insertion tube

This is the part of the instrument that is inserted in the patient. The umbilical cord and hand controls are usually integral to the insertion tube. The insertion tube (Fig. 4.33A) carries:

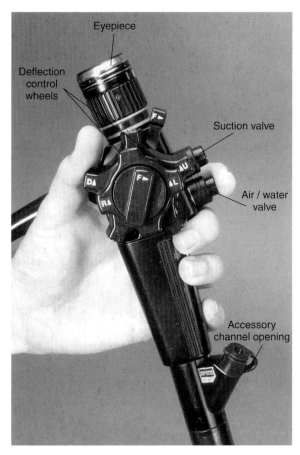

Figure 4.32A Hand piece of gastroscope.

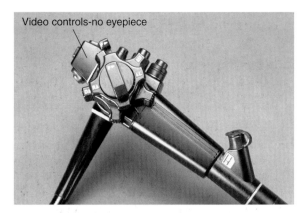

Figure 4.32B Hand piece of video-gastroscope.

*   air/water channel
*   accessory/biopsy channel
*   light and image guides

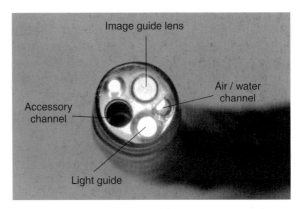

Figure 4.33A Tip of endoscope showing light guide, lens, accessory channel and air/water channel.

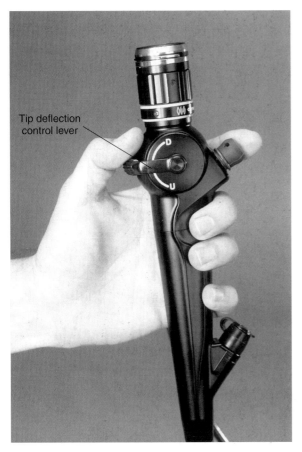

Figure 4.32C Hand piece of bronchoscope showing lever controlling two-way tip deflection.

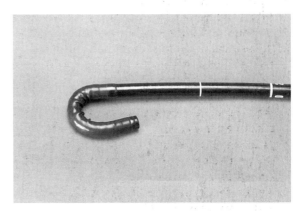

Figure 4.33B Tip of endoscope showing retroflexion in the bending section.

- deflection cables
- objective lens at tip.

The last few centimetres have tip deflection capability and are known as the 'bending section' (Fig. 4.33B).

The utility of any flexible endoscope depends on its length and diameter with respect to the size and position of the body cavity being intubated, and the size of the biopsy channel. Ideally the scope should be as narrow as possible but contain the widest diameter instrument channel possible, yet these two features tend to be mutually exclusive. Since the size of veterinary patient also varies widely, an endoscope that is a compromise of these features is usually used.

The tip diameter of flexible endoscopes varies from 1 mm to 15 mm. Scopes smaller than 3 mm

diameter usually don't have an accessory (biopsy) channel or any means of deflecting the tip; they are used in a manner similar to rigid endoscopes, although their flexibility allows them to be pushed around bends, e.g. rhinoscopy, otoscopy.

The length of flexible endoscopes varies from 15 cm for a simple instrument with no controls or accessory channel to enteroscopes several metres long. In general, bronchoscopes are 50–100 cm, and gastroscopes 100–150 cm long. The most common size of gastroscope used in small animal medicine has a tip diameter between 7 and 9 mm and is 1 metre long.

In larger endoscopes, control knobs on the hand piece facilitate tip deflection. Gastroscopes have four-way tip deflection (up, down, left, right); it is important that there is at least 180 degree deflection (often up to 210 degrees) in at least one plane to give the ability to look back (retroflexion). Tip deflection is usually at least 90 degrees in all other directions.

Gastroscopes are usually too large a diameter (because of the incorporation of four cables for steering) for very small patients or procedures such as bronchoscopy, rhinoscopy, urethrocystoscopy, etc. Dedicated bronchoscopes only have two-way tip deflection controlled by a lever (Fig. 4.32C), and a smaller or absent accessory channel.

Image display, capture and storage

For a single user, a fibre-optic endoscope with direct observation at the eyepiece may be adequate, but shared viewing on a monitor allows an assistant to help the procedure more readily and is ideal for teaching. Everyone can see the image transmitted either directly from a video-endoscope or from a CCD camera attached to the eyepiece.

Capture and storage of the image are important for medical records, and permit it to be shown to colleagues and clients. Devices available (Fig. 4.34) include:

- video tape recorder and printer
- digital stills recorder
- slide camera.

Endoscopic accessories

Hollow, rigid endoscopes allow insertion of simple instruments, e.g. crocodile-type biopsy

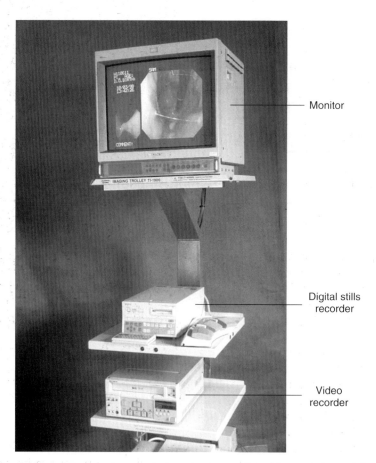

Figure 4.34 Recording equipment for an endoscopy system showing monitor, video recorder and digital stills recorder on a movable trolley.

forceps through the tube. Solid, rigid endoscopes can only be used with instruments that are inserted alongside them or through adjacent access/parallel ports, e.g. laparoscopic and arthroscopic instruments.

There are numerous instruments/accessories that can be inserted via the accessory (biopsy) channel of flexible endoscopes. The accessories obviously must be small enough in diameter to pass down the channel, and of sufficient length to pass out at the tip of the insertion tube. Some endoscopes have a colour coding on the accessory channel port and the accessory handle to aid matching.

Accessories are used for diagnostic and therapeutic purposes.

Diagnostic accessories (Fig. 4.35)

- Biopsy forceps (Fig. 4.35A,B)
- cytology brushes (Fig. 4.35C)
- wash and collection tubes (+ suction trap)
- injection/aspiration needles (Fig. 4.35C).

The diagnostic yield is improved if bigger biopsies can be taken. Thus, using an endoscope with the largest available biopsy channel, which will take the biggest biopsy forceps, is ideal. The biopsy channel can vary from 1.8 to 3.7 mm, and biopsy forceps are available in a variety of sizes to fit.

There are a number of designs for the jaws of biopsy forceps:

- Round or oval/ellipsoid cups (Fig. 4.35A). Oval cups have a larger surface area and theoretically achieve a bigger biopsy.
- Smooth-edge or alligator or rat tooth. Serrated edges theoretically permit better grasping of tissue.
- Non-fenestrated or fenestrated. Fenestrations in the cups allow the biopsy to bulge out when the jaws are closed and reduce the amount of tissue that is crushed.
- With or without spike (Fig. 4.35B). A spike between the cups allows the forceps to be lodged in the tissue, so that they don't slip away from the area of interest as the jaws are closed, but may increase tissue crush artefact.

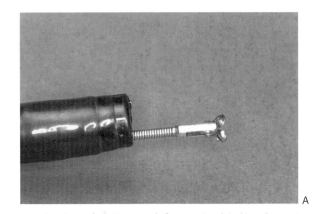

A

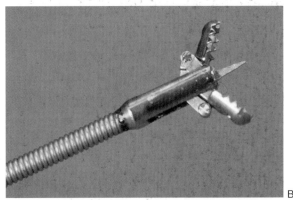

B

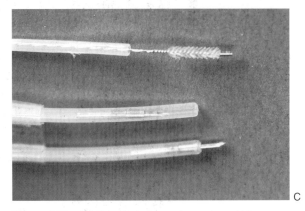

C

Figure 4.35 (A) Fenestrated, round cup-shaped biopsy forceps extending from distal tip of endoscope. (B) Fenestrated, ovoid biopsy forceps with spike and serrated cups. (C) Cytology brush and injection needle before and after extrusion from the tip of catheter.

- Rotatable. Their construction allows rotation of biopsy cups by rotation of the handle, enabling better-directed biopsy of masses.

- Swing-jaw. Swing-jaws allow the cups to turn to face the tissue and achieve a deeper bite.
- Disposable or re-usable. With care re-usable forceps can be used for many procedures, justifying their significantly greater expense.

The benefits of all these modifications are unclear. Generally, the size and quality of the biopsy depend on the size of the forceps cups, the pressure exerted on the tissue, and the skill of the endoscopist. Excess pressure exerted by the assistant on the handle to close the jaws does not improve the biopsy quality, but can damage the forceps.

Therapeutic accessories

The types of instrument available are:

- grasping forceps (Fig. 4.36A)
  — alligator jaws
  — rat tooth
  — rubber-tipped for sharp pins
  — pronged forceps (2-, 3-, 4- and 5-prong, W-shaped)
- wire retrieval baskets (Fig. 4.36B,C,D)
- magnetic probe for metallic objects
- balloon catheters/dilators
- coagulating electrodes, forceps, scissors
- polypectomy snares ± diathermy
- injection/aspiration needle
- operative lasers.

ROLE OF THE ENDOSCOPY NURSE

Endoscopy *cannot* be done safely single-handed; the operator is reliant on an assistant. The endoscopy nurse is crucial in setting up the procedure, assisting during endoscopy, and in clearing up and maintaining the equipment.

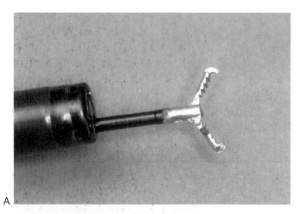

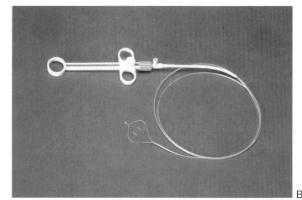

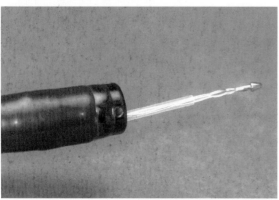

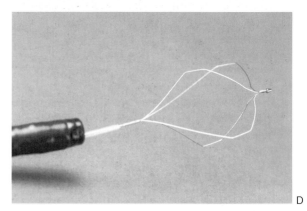

Figure 4.36 (A) Rat tooth grasping forceps extending from distal tip of endoscope. (B) Basket forceps with handle. (C) Basket forceps being inserted through endoscope. (D) Basket forceps being expanded.

Pre-procedure

Check equipment set-up

- Anaesthesia machine and anaesthetics
- light source
- suction
- endoscope
- ancillary instruments (e.g. biopsy forceps)
- preparation of disinfecting and rinsing solutions.

Arrange specimen supplies

- Biopsy pots
- slides
- laboratory forms.

Patient preparation

- Oral cleanser and enemas for colonoscopy
- check bodyweight
- assist with placing i.v. catheter
- assist with premedication and induction of general anaesthesia.

Procedure

Monitoring

- Depth of anaesthesia
- cardiovascular status
- respiratory function
- degree of gastric distension.

The endoscopy nurse also assists with sample procurement.

Post procedure

- Patient monitoring during recovery
- completion of lab forms
- equipment clean-up and storage
  — leakage testing
  — washing
  — disinfection
  — rinsing
  — drying
  — storage
- preparation of patient for discharge.

THE ENDOSCOPIC PROCEDURE
Patient preparation

For airway endoscopy no special patient preparation is required other than the standard withholding of food before anaesthesia.

For upper GI endoscopy again no special preparation is needed, but for the lower GI tract extensive preparation (oral cleansers, enemas) is needed. Oral cleansing with polyethylene glycol/electrolyte solutions (e.g. Kleanprep™, Colyte™) given by gavage at 30 ml/kg on three occasions is very effective at cleansing the GI tract. Warm water enemas rarely clean the whole colon effectively, and addition of surfactants or irritants to aid evacuation may cause artefactual histological changes in the mucosa.

Sedation and anaesthesia

General anaesthesia is required for nearly all endoscopy, except perhaps for proctoscopy. A cuffed endotracheal tube is always used, as there is a danger of inhalation of material draining from the nasopharynx or refluxed from the stomach. The patient's cardiovascular and respiratory function should be assessed and supported as necessary.

The safest anaesthetic regime is the one the operator and nurse are most familiar with. Premedication should aid smooth induction and recovery, and pethidine and acetylpromazine, or ketamine or buprenorphine is often used depending on the species. After induction with an intravenous agent, anaesthesia is maintained by inhalation agents. Thiopental or propofol can be used for induction; halothane and isoflurane are suitable inhalation agents.

Anaesthesia for bronchoscopy

The presence of the insertion tube within the major airways can seriously compromise the oxygenation of the patient. Thus the most important principle is to prevent hypoxia, and the endoscope may have to be repeatedly withdrawn temporarily to reinstitute adequate ventilation.

The dangers are most significant in cats and toy-breed dogs. It must also be remembered that anaesthetics inhibit the normal mucociliary escalator, aggravating any airway disease.

Acetylpromazine is a suitable premedicant for dogs and cats. In cats, low doses of ketamine can augment it and in dogs added butorphanol is also helpful as an anti-tussive.

ECG monitoring and pulse oximetry are recommended and an i.v. catheter should be placed. Furthermore the procedure is carried out as quickly as possible; all equipment is made ready before the procedure.

Endoscopy often elicits coughing and gagging, which predispose to trauma both to the patient and to the endoscope, and predispose to hypoxia. Reflex coughing can be abolished by deeper anaesthesia, which ideally is produced by short-acting agents (e.g. propofol, Saffan, halothane, isoflurane). This allows rapid recovery and restoration of the cough reflex. As extubation may be needed to enable insertion of the endoscope, an intravenous agent that can be topped up is preferred.

After induction, intubation and oxygenation (± inhalation agent) should be performed before beginning bronchoscopy. Nitrous oxide is avoided if continuous oxygenation is not possible, as diffusion hypoxia may develop undetected.

When the bronchoscope is in situ for a significant time, hypoxia will develop and positive pressure ventilation is required. Ventilation can be achieved down hollow rigid bronchoscopes by the Venturi effect (injecting oxygen down the tube entrains air flow through the scope). However, this is not possible with flexible bronchoscopes. Pulse oximetry can be helpful to determine when the bronchoscope must be withdrawn and ventilation recommenced.

To increase the time available for bronchoscopic intubation, endotracheal tube intubation and ventilation with 100% oxygen for 5 minutes before and after bronchoscopy have been recommended (known as **apnoeic diffusion oxygenation**) but carries a major risk of hypoxia. Instead, in smaller patients, the endotracheal tube is withdrawn to allow insertion of the bronchoscope, but oxygen continues to be supplied

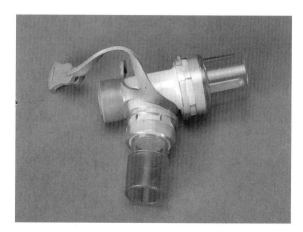

Figure 4.37 Elbow connector to permit passage of oxygen during bronchoscopy.

through a small catheter inserted alongside the bronchoscope; this is adequate for patients <15 kg for maintenance of oxygenation for up to 10 minutes, although CO_2 will rise in this time. Nevertheless, the oxygenation of the patient must be closely monitored, and bronchoscopy interrupted for ventilation with oxygen if there is suspicion of hypoxia. In larger dogs the bronchoscope can be inserted down the endotracheal tube through an air-tight gasket with ventilation maintained by bag compression through an elbow connector (Fig. 4.37).

Anaesthesia for gastroscopy and colonoscopy

Sedation and general anaesthesia are simpler and tailored to the health status of the patient. Nitrous oxide is not used as an anaesthetic gas because a hollow viscus is being inflated with air, and nitrous oxide would diffuse into the viscus ('third-space effect') and cause over-distension. Diazepam may be given during gastroscopy when pyloric intubation or distension of inflamed tissue causes a pain response (tachycardia, etc.) even though the level of unconsciousness is adequate, when a greater depth of anaesthesia might be dangerous.

Patient positioning

* Anterograde rhinoscopy – sternal recumbency is easiest

- retrograde pharyngoscopy – sternal or lateral recumbency
- tracheo-bronchoscopy – sternal recumbency is best; the head is rested on a sandbag
- gastroscopy – left lateral recumbency to allow air to rise into the antrum, permitting visualisation of the pylorus
- percutaneous endoscopic gastrotomy (PEG) tube placement – right lateral recumbency for tube placement through the left flank
- colonoscopy – left or right lateral recumbency to permit drainage of fluid away from the area of colon being examined.

If the endoscope is being inserted per os, a mouth gag *must* be used.

Endoscopic biopsy and sample collection methods

The most common procedure performed by endoscopy, other than mere visualisation of a lesion, is punch biopsy. Biopsies are routinely collected even if the organ looks grossly normal, as microscopic changes may be present. It is also possible to perform brush cytology, fluid collection and lavage through a flexible endoscope, and these are safer than biopsy in bronchoscopy because of the dangers of haemorrhage within the airway.

Brush cytology

Cytology brushes within sterile sheaths can be inserted down the accessory channel and used to abrade the area being investigated by exfoliating some cells. After withdrawal the brush is smeared on a clean glass slide for fixation, staining and microscopy.

Fluid aspiration

Fluid can be aspirated through a sterile catheter inserted down the accessory channel for cytology and culture.

Lavage

During bronchoscopy, washings of the smaller airways can be obtained by broncho-alveolar lavage. The bronchoscope is advanced into a

bronchus as far as possible and a sterile catheter is inserted through the accessory channel.

Sterile saline is then instilled and rapidly aspirated back whilst an assistant performs external coupage on the chest to dislodge secretions. In medium-size dogs about 20 ml of saline may be infused very safely, but only 1–2 ml is usually recovered. The process is then repeated in the opposite lung. The samples are submitted for cytology and culture.

With narrow bronchoscopes the biopsy channel may be too narrow to permit any tube. Lavage is then performed directly down the biopsy channel, and suction applied directly to the biopsy channel with a syringe or from the suction pump, with a suction trap to collect any aspirated material. The endoscope must be cleaned and disinfected beforehand to avoid contaminants.

Needle aspiration

Masses visualised endoscopically can be aspirated with needle catheters.

Endoscopic biopsy

During rigid endoscopic bronchoscopy, rigid biopsy forceps can be inserted through hollow scopes, or adjacent to the telescope. For flexible endoscopy, flexible biopsy forceps are passed down the accessory (biopsy) channel. They are never forced or passed when the endoscope tip is retroflexed as this might cause damage to the channel and leakage. During GI endoscopy the forceps enter the accessory channel through a rubber seal (Fig. 4.38B) that helps maintain the insufflation of the viscus; this is not necessary during bronchoscopy.

Once the forceps can be seen exiting the tip of the scope by the operator the assistant is asked to open the forceps' jaws by manipulation of the handle. The forceps are then directed to the biopsy site and the assistant is told to close the jaws. This process is more readily coordinated if the endoscopist and assistant can see the image on a monitor. Opening or closing the jaws is performed by gentle manipulation of the handle; excessive pressure only serves to stretch the wire inside the forceps and damage them. The forceps must never be withdrawn with the jaws open.

Once the tissue is grasped the forceps are withdrawn sharply to avulse the biopsy. In the GI tract multiple biopsies are taken at each site (e.g. 6–10 specimens). This is because the pieces are quite small and only some will be adequate for histopathological diagnosis. However, the number taken at bronchoscopy is limited by the problems of haemorrhage.

There are several methods described for handling biopsies before fixation in formalin. Some operators remove the biopsy from the cups with a 25 gauge needle, and may even try to orient the tissue on a piece of moistened lens paper or card (or even a slice of cucumber) before fixation. However, such manipulation often causes damage to the biopsy. The simplest method, of simply immersing the forceps tip directly in formalin to release and fix the biopsy, is usually as good. Of course, the forceps cups must be rinsed in water before the next biopsy.

CARE OF ENDOSCOPES AND ACCESSORIES

The fibre-optics of endoscopes (and the CCD of video-scopes) are fragile and liable to damage even when there are no external signs of damage. Therefore extreme care must be used when using, cleaning and storing endoscopes as repairs can be very expensive.

Cleaning, disinfection/sterilisation

Cleaning and disinfection of any endoscope should be performed immediately after the procedure. The principle is to remove organic debris by thorough washing and brushing with detergent solution before disinfection/sterilisation. The disinfectant used depends on local safety rules and Control of Substances Hazardous to Health (COSHH) regulations.

Flexible endoscopes must *never* be sterilised with heat. Heat will cause serious damage to the optical system and protective sleeve.

The disinfectants available are:

- ethylene oxide gas
- immersion in:
  — gluteraldehyde (Cidex, Gigasept)
  — 70% ethyl alcohol or
  — non-aldehyde compounds such as MedDis (Trigene-related) or Dettol Endoscope Disinfectant (discontinued).

Cleaning endoscope

External cleaning

- Immediately after use, take a secure hold of the endoscope and wipe down the insertion tube with a soft cloth or gauze square.
- Flush the air/water channel for 10–15 s to eject any refluxed material.
- If available, use the appropriate air/water channel cleaning adapter to force flush with water and air for at least 10 s (Fig. 4.38A).
- Remove all valves, caps and hoods and clean separately.

Brushing

- Immerse the instrument (totally) in warm water and neutral detergent; ensure it is a fully immersible endoscope, and cap the electrical contacts on a video-endoscope.
- At this stage carry out a leakage test (see below).
- Use the port cleaning brush to clean the biopsy and suction port openings and also carefully clean the distal end of the endoscope (Fig. 4.38B).
- Suck detergent individually through the suction/biopsy channels or, if available, use an all-channel suction cleaning adapter (Fig. 4.38C).
- Pass the cleaning brush three times each through
  — the biopsy port and down the insertion tube
  — the suction port and down the insertion tube
  — the suction port and down the umbilical tube.

NB Clean the brush head *each* time it emerges from the endoscope.

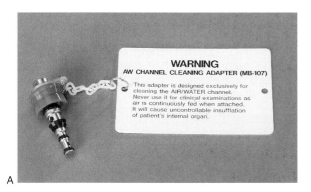

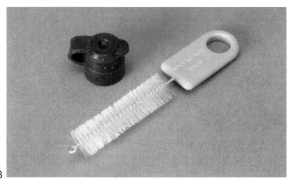

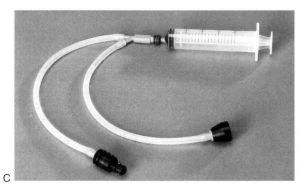

Figure 4.38 (A) Air/water channel cleaning adapter to force flush channels. (B) Port cleaning brush and disposable rubber seal for accessory channel. (C) All-channel cleaning suction adapter for flushing endoscope with detergent, water or disinfectant.

Flushing

- Re-immerse the endoscope
- irrigate all channels sequentially with:
  — detergent
  — disinfectant
  — clean water.

NB Ensure adequate irrigation/contact times.

Drying

- Dry the external surface of the endoscope. The use of an alcohol wipe is recommended to assist drying.
- Remove residual fluid from all channels: blow air through air/water channels and aspirate air through the suction/biopsy channel. The use of a little 70% ethyl or isopropyl alcohol prior to blowing/aspirating is recommended to assist the drying process.
- Hang scope vertically in a ventilated cupboard.

Leakage testing

Any leak in the outer protective sleeve of the endoscope will allow entry of water into the inside of the endoscope. This will impair the image by fogging and, more importantly, it may cause weakening and subsequent breakage of the glass fibre bundles as well as electrical damage in video-scopes. Early detection of leaks is essential to minimise the risk of damage, and leakage testing is ideally performed after every use of the endoscope.

The leakage tester is connected first to the pressure compensation valve on the umbilical cord, and then to an air pump, which is either in the light source or an external hand pump. As air is pumped into the protective sleeve, it can be seen to inflate slightly. Immersion of the whole endoscope will then detect any leak by the tell-tale rise of small air bubbles (as for checking a bicycle inner tube for punctures).

The most likely leakage sites are:

- the bending section of the insertion tube
- the seals around the control wheels
- damage to the biopsy channel caused by incorrect accessory insertion
- anywhere the outer sleeve may have been traumatised by the patient's teeth.

After completion of the leakage test, the tester is disconnected from the insufflator for a few seconds *before* its removal from the pressure compensation valve: this allows the sleeve to deflate and prevents any water being sucked into the endoscope. If the endoscope fails the leakage test, it should not be used again until repaired.

Cleaning/disinfecting flexible accessories

- Disassemble the accessory into its component parts (if applicable).
- Immerse the accessory in a bowl of warm detergent solution and thoroughly wash the sheath and all moving parts using a soft brush. If the accessory has a luer-lok connector, flush the lumen of the sheath with cleaning solution using a 10 ml syringe.
- Rinse in clean water, and flush if applicable.
- Ultrasonically clean all parts; ensure all lumens are pre-filled with cleaning solution.
- Rinse all parts carefully, including internal lumen, to remove residual debris and cleaning solution.
- Carefully dry with a gauze swab and air flush any lumens with a syringe.
- Lubricate all moving parts using a suitable silicone oil.
- Disinfect/sterilise the accessory by:
  — cold immersion followed by thorough rinsing, or autoclave, ensuring the temperature does not exceed 138 C, or ethylene oxide gas sterilisation followed by thorough aeration.
- Store in a clean, dry, well ventilated location, maintained at room temperature. Never store accessories in the endoscope carrying case or coil them tighter than a diameter of 15 cm.
- Examine accessories carefully before use and discard them if they are kinked or display faults. Damaged accessories can cause major damage to endoscopes.

Rules and techniques to help prevent damage to endoscopes (Fig. 4.39)

- Endoscopes should only be used by qualified personnel.
- They should always be transported in their protective suitcases.
- When outside the patient, both the hand

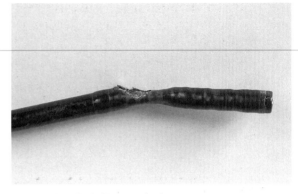

Figure 4.39 Irreparable damage to gastroscope caused by incorrect handling allowing the insertion tube tip to be crushed by a trolley.

piece and insertion tube tip must be supported.
- Never swing, knock or crush the insertion tube.
- Do not leave unattended on a work surface.
- Never force the insertion tube into the patient.
- Always use the correct-size accessories.
- Never forcibly insert an accessory when the bending section is deflected to avoid damage to the channel.
- Foreign objects should not be pulled through the accessory channel.
- Clean *properly* after use.
- *Never* use heat to clean an endoscope.
- Extreme cold makes the glass fibres more fragile.
- Hang vertically when not in use, preferably in a lockable, ventilated cupboard; if stored in the suitcase the endoscope will not dry properly so that bacteria and fungi may grow; it will also eventually adopt the coiled shape permanently.

Rules and techniques to help prevent damage to accessories

- Always inspect forceps, etc., prior to use for evidence of damage, and remove from use if detected.
- Never use excessive force to open or close the cups.

- Always hold the insertion portion close to the biopsy channel valve and insert in sections of no more than 5 cm.
- Clean properly immediately following use.
- Ultrasonic baths are essential to remove debris from the inner operating wire and cups so that movement does not become restricted.
- Silicone lubricating oil helps maintain smooth movement.

- Placing heavy objects on top of instruments can cause damage.
- Store biopsy forceps as straight as possible to prevent kinking of the coil sheath.
- Never coil to a diameter of less than 15 cm as this will damage the insertion portion; attempted opening of the cups whilst coiled will also cause damage.

PART 3

Electrocardiography

Alasdair Hotston Moore

INTRODUCTION

What is the electrocardiogram?

The ECG is a graphical recording of the electrical activity of the heart. The majority of the tissue of the heart is cardiac muscle, which is a specialised type of striated muscle. Within this are particular areas that are responsible for the initiation of the heart beat and its propagation throughout the remainder of the heart. The heart beat results in changes in the electrical charge of the muscle fibres. Although the change in the electrical charge of each fibre is too small to be detected at the body surface, since large parts of the heart are activated at once, the changes within these areas can be detected at the body surface and it is these that form the basis of the ECG. The machine that detects and records these changes is an electro-cardiograph, the technique is termed electro-cardiography and the resulting graph or trace is known as an electrocardiogram. The output may be as a trace on a strip of paper or as a line on a screen (oscilloscope or liquid crystal display). Some machines may also store the output elec-tronically for later analysis or be able to transmit to other equipment (e.g. a personal computer).

As the heart beat occurs in an area of heart muscle, the surface membrane of the muscle fibres initially depolarises and this is responsible for the largest changes noted in the trace. Subsequently these muscle fibres repolarise to return to their resting state and this repolarisation also produces a detectable change but this is typically of a smaller magnitude than the changes of depolarisation. All of these electrical changes are quite small and are easily masked by other muscular activity, particularly movement of the limbs or shivering, movement of the patient or other electrical fields in the area of the patient (such as those generated by electrical apparatus). Changes detected by the ECG due to these other sources are known as **artefacts**.

INDICATIONS FOR MAKING AN ECG

The ECG can be used to detect changes in the size of the heart (or typically its individual chambers), change in position of the heart, disturbances in the order in which the chambers depolarise (dysrhythmias), the influence of changes in the internal environment on the heart beat (most commonly due to alterations in the electrolyte status of the patient) and the effects of other systemic disease on the heart beat. In humans, changes in the ECG due to restriction of blood supply are an important diagnostic aid in patients with coronary heart disease; this type of disease is uncommon in animals and these types of change are less important in veterinary electro-cardiography.

Electrocardiography is also commonly used as a monitoring aid during anaesthesia and in the

Table 4.12 Common indications for electrocardiography

Indication	Examples
Investigation of suspected congenital heart disease/cardiac murmurs	Patent ductus arteriosus, aortic or pulmonic stenosis, atrioventricular valve dysplasia, ventricular septal defects
Investigation of suspected acquired heart disease	Degenerative valve disease (endocardiosis), hypertrophic or dilated cardiomyopathy, pericardial effusion, dysrhythmias
Investigation of syncope, seizures and collapse	Dysrhythmias, congenital or acquired heart disease
Investigation of weakness	Dysrhythmias, congenital or acquired heart disease
Investigation of suspected dysrhythmias	Ventricular tachycardia, atrial tachycardia, atrial fibrillation, ventricular fibrillation, heart block
Assessment of patients with systemic disease	Shock, septicaemia, gastric dilation/volvulus, splenic disease, hyperkalaemia, hypoadrenocorticism
Monitoring during anaesthesia	Tachycardia, bradycardia, hypoxia, dysrhythmias
Monitoring of the critically ill patient	Tachycardia, bradycardia, hypoxia, dysrhythmias, electrolyte or acid–base disturbances

intensive care unit. In these situations (compared to diagnostic electrocardiography, as described above), changes in the trace are of more interest than absolute values. Features of interest include dysrhythmias, effects of hypoxia, electrolyte imbalance and acid–base disturbance, and changes in heart rate.

The common indications for electrocardiography are summarised in Table 4.12.

PERFORMING THE ECG

Patient preparation

The animal should be calm and relaxed. Movement due to struggling or other voluntary movement, shaking or exaggerated respiratory efforts will produce artefacts. Chemical restraint of the patient may produce alterations in heart rate and rhythm and should be avoided. In some cases, it may be preferable to compromise and allow the patient to adopt a relaxed position rather than forcing the animal into the preferred posture. If sedation is used, it should be recorded on the trace. Combinations of acepromazine and opiates given at low doses have been used successfully even in patients with cardiac disease. One suggestion is acepromazine (0.05 mg/kg) and pethidine (2 mg/kg) given by subcutaneous injection. The α-2 adrenergic agonists (xylazine and medetomidine) and atropine should be avoided in sedating these patients as these all produce significant changes in the electrical activity of the heart.

Precautions for producing a diagnostic ECG (elimination of artefacts)

Positioning

Dogs are positioned in right lateral recumbency with the limbs gently extended in a neutral position. The patient should be gently restrained and reassured to avoid shivering, muscle twitching or anxiety.

For dogs that cannot be restrained in this way without distress, sternal recumbency or a standing position can be used, but this must be noted on the trace. This position may affect interpretation of the recording and so is really only suitable for investigation of heart rhythm rather than a full diagnostic evaluation.

Cats are most commonly encouraged to adopt a relaxed sternally recumbent position. This is the standard position and is preferred to enforced lateral recumbency to avoid struggling. Purring will produce significant artefacts and must be discouraged, although this may prove problematical.

When electrocardiography is used for anaesthetic monitoring, the operator does not control the patient position but in this context it is the heart rate and rhythm which are of most interest, and these can be assessed regardless of patient position.

Producing electrical contact

Since the recording depends on the detection of small electrical currents within the body, excellent contact between the electrodes of the machine and the patient's tissues is required. The cables can be connected to the patient with crocodile clips, plates, needles or adhesive pads. Whichever is used, it is critical that contact is directly with the patient and not on to hair. If clips or needles are used, the hair can simply be parted, but if plates or pads are used then the hair is clipped. The skin is cleaned with spirit to improve adhesion if self-adhesive pads are used and electrode gel and light bandages are used with plates. Pads are most useful if a long period of recording (an ambulatory ECG) is required, otherwise the alternatives are convenient. To improve contact between clips and the skin, either spirit or electrode gel is applied around the clip.

Placement of contacts

The position of the contact is important to produce a recording that can be interpreted according to established criteria. The contacts are away from underlying muscle masses. The standard ECG uses four electrodes that are applied to the skin of the limbs. The exact position of the electrodes is not critical but suggested positions are for the forelimbs the skin folds cranial or caudal to the elbow, and for the hindlimbs the precrural skin folds or adjacent to the hocks. The cables are led away from the electrodes without becoming entangled and avoiding placing them over the trunk, which may result in respiratory artefacts. The leads are labelled or coloured to allow the operator to place each lead on the correct limb (see Table 4.13). Occasionally, additional information

Table 4.13 Position of standard limb cables

Limb	Standard colour code	US colour code	Medical label
Right fore	Red	White	RA
Left fore	White	Black	LA
Left hind	Green	Red	LL
Right hind (earth)	Black	Green	RL

is obtained by placement of the 'chest leads'; these are usually only used by specialists and are not considered further. Electrocardiographs used during anaesthesia and in the intensive care unit generally only have three cables and electrodes, with no earth. The other three can be positioned in the standard way, although this is not critical and the positions can be varied, as the situation requires. As a matter of course, the three electrodes should be placed evenly around the heart, for example on the two forelimbs and one hindlimb, or on two forelimbs and the dorsum.

Avoiding electrical interference

A common cause of interference in the recording (see below) is the effect of electrical fields generated by nearby equipment. To minimise this mains interference, all non-essential electrical equipment in the room should be turned off; fluorescent lights are an important cause of problems. Artefacts can also arise if the patient cables are tangled or wrapped around the supply cord to the electrocardiograph. Positioning the patient on a nonconducting tabletop is also helpful. Good contact between the electrodes and the skin (see above) also reduces electrical artefacts. In the context of anaesthetic monitoring, common causes of electrical interference are electrical heating pads and electrosurgical (diathermy) equipment. In this case, the use of electrode gel is also recommended, since if spirit is used for contact, electrical interference will become apparent as the spirit evaporates.

Machine controls

There are three controls on most machines that can be set by the operator. These are paper or trace speed, calibration setting and the filter. In addition, there may be a marker button which produces a calibration spike. There may also be a control to set the position of the baseline of the trace to ensure it can be displayed in its entirety. The trace speed controls the rate at which the trace moves across the screen or the paper advances. Another way of considering this is that a faster speed spreads the heart beats across a longer line. This results in complexes that are wider and may be easier to interpret but fewer can be recorded on the screen or paper. The paper speed should be written on the trace if it is not automatically recorded. A common procedure is to record part of the trace at a high speed (e.g. 100 mm/s) and then a longer period at a lower speed (e.g. 25 mm/s, the 'rhythm strip').

The calibration setting or amplitude sets the height of the complexes recorded compared to the strength of the intrinsic electrical activity. Typically a setting of 1 cm/mV is chosen, but this may be reduced to 0.5 cm/mV if the complexes are very large or increased to 2 cm/mV if they are very small (typically in cats and if there is fluid within the thorax). The amplitude should be recorded on the trace: if this is not done automatically, the marker button is used to mark a 1-mV-high spike on the trace. The machine may incorporate a filter to reduce the effects of artefacts, notably 50 Hz interference from other electrical equipment. Use of the filter can reduce the size of complexes and result in the loss of some information. Initially, these artefacts should be investigated and eliminated by other means if possible; if they cannot be controlled, the filter can be used, but it should be noted on the trace.

On some machines, the position of the baseline is set manually. This is done to keep the entire complex on the paper. If the trace still falls outside the limits of the paper, the amplitude is reduced.

HOW IS THE ECG PRODUCED?

Electrical activity in the heart

The conduction system in the heart (Fig. 4.40) must be understood to allow interpretation of the trace. The normal heartbeat is generated in the sino-atrial (SA) node, a specialised area in the wall of the right atrium. This is the pacemaker of the heart, although if diseased other sites can act as the pacemaker. A wave of depolarisation spreads from here rapidly over the right and left atria. To reach the ventricles, the wave must pass through the atrioventricular (AV) node. It is delayed in the AV node and then enters the bundle of His, a specialised area of cardiac muscle

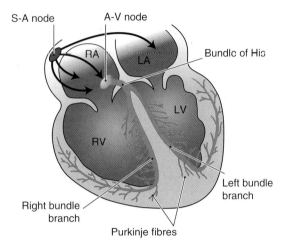

Figure 4.40 Conduction system of the heart.

that conducts it rapidly down the interventricular septum and into the left and right bundle branches. These finally branch into the Purkinje fibres that spread throughout the ventricles. As the wave leaves these specialised areas it results in rapid depolarisation of the entire left and right ventricles.

Lead systems

The machine develops a trace by monitoring the change in polarity (charge) at the body surface. Since it is the polarity that is detected, the machine needs to compare two points on the surface. The most straightforward way of doing this is to compare each pair of electrodes (excluding the earth). This gives rise to the three 'limb leads' (leads I, II and III). Comparing any single electrode to the remaining pair can derive further information. This gives rise to a further three leads, known as the augmented limb leads (aVR, aVL and aVF). The ways in which these leads are constructed is shown in Figure 4.41 and the diagram indicates the way in which this allows the machine to assess the heart in several planes.

Mean electrical axis

Using the lead system to assess the heart in several planes means that a calculation of the orientation of the bulk of the heart muscle within the thorax can be made. For example, if the left

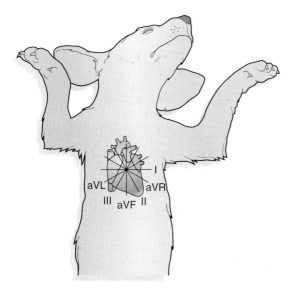

Figure 4.41   The lead system. The standard and augmented lead systems are superimposed over the heart, each represented by a line. The ECG recording for each lead is the electrical activity in the direction of the corresponding line.

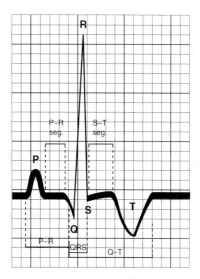

Figure 4.42   Example of a lead II ECG trace with the major deflections (waves) and intervals marked.

ventricle increases in size (dilation or hypertrophy), the sum of the electrical activity of the heart moves to the left and this is reflected in a change in the mean electrical axis (MEA).

THE P WAVE, QRS COMPLEX AND T WAVE

The ECG is usually principally assessed in lead II and the waves as they appear in this lead will be discussed (see Fig. 4.42). The P wave is the first part of the ECG complex. It results from depolarisation of the atria. The right atrium begins to depolarise before the left, but usually only a single wave, which is positive in lead II, is detectable. On some machines, and if the P wave is increased in duration, a dip in the P wave may be present, indicating the change in contribution of the bulk of activity from the right to the left atrium. Once the atria are depolarised the baseline returns to a neutral position during the PR interval as the wave of repolarisation is delayed in the AV node. The QRS complex appears as the ventricles depolarise, and depolarisation of the atria is hidden by this larger activity. Depolar-

isation of the ventricles is complicated, but the R wave, by definition, is the first positive deviation in the baseline. Any previous negative deviation is the Q wave and any subsequent negative deviation is the S wave. Once depolarisation of the ventricles is complete, the baseline returns to a neutral position during the 'ST segment' of the ECG. Changes in the ST segment can be recognised (such as slurring or depression below the baseline), and may indicate heart disease but less importance is attached to these than is in human cardiology. More significance is attached to alterations in the ST segment occurring during a period of examination or anaesthesia.

The ST segment is terminated by the T wave, which represents repolarisation of the ventricles. The T wave is rather variable in size and polarity. Finally, the baseline returns to a neutral position before the next cardiac cycle. If the heart rate is high, parts of the complexes can become superimposed.

SIMPLE INTERPRETATION

Artefacts

The presence of artefacts both reduces the quality of the trace and may also lead to erroneous interpretation. It is therefore important that the person

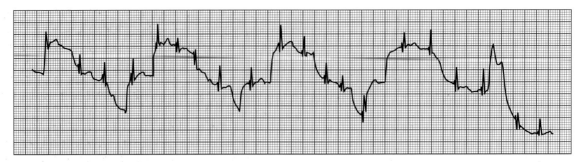

Figure 4.43 Respiratory movement artefact. Note the large variation in baseline position on the trace at a frequency of 30 cycles/s, consistent with respiratory rate. (Same dog as Fig. 4.42 but this is lead I, 2.5 cm/s, 1 cm/mV).

recording the ECG can recognise these so that they can be eliminated if possible, or ignored if recognised as unimportant.

Movement of the animal can produce several types of artefact. One of the commoner is respiratory movements (Fig. 4.43). These typically result in variation in the baseline height and can be recognised as a regular rise and fall in this, which may be large enough to result in the trace moving outside the recordable area of paper or screen. Artefacts due to other movements of the patient are less easy to recognise and may appear as bizarre complexes, for example. One way in which to distinguish them from dysrhythmias is that the underlying rhythm is unchanged, that is, the QRS complexes continue at the same rate, without the rhythm being 're-set' by the extra complex. If a true extra complex occurs, the heart rhythm is interrupted and then may restart at the same rate, but after a pause. The artefact can also be recognised as such by concurrent observation of the patient and by palpation of the peripheral pulse. Artefacts due to electrical interference (Fig. 4.44) are most commonly due to detection of the 50-cycle/s field produced by mains equipment. This results in a fine variation in the trace, most obvious in the baseline. One common feature is the inability to distinguish the P wave and an erroneous diagnosis of atrial fibrillation may be made. The artefact is worsened by poor electrical contact and can often be eliminated by improving this (e.g. application of electrode gel) or switching off nearby equipment. Activating the filter will usually eliminate the artefact but may lead to the loss of information, particularly with small complexes (cats).

Several general rules can be applied to the recognition of artefacts:

- Consider the possibility of respiratory movement, which is common and may be eliminated by adjusting lead position. It is easily recognised but can be difficult to eliminate, particularly in anxious patients.

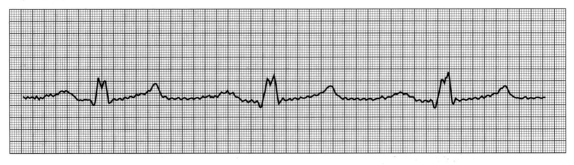

Figure 4.44 Electrical interference artefact. Note the fine variation in the baseline at 50 cycles/s. Lead II, 10 cm/s, 1 cm/mV. Also shows P waves and small QRS complexes.

- Consider the possibility of mains interference. Again, it is easily recognised and can often be eliminated with care or by use of the filter if necessary.
- If bizarre changes are seen in the ECG, first check for patient movement and then check the peripheral pulse. If a steady pulse or apex beat is detected, then the changes must be artefactual. If isolated bizarre complexes are seen, check whether these affect the underlying rhythm; true extra complexes usually do, but artefacts do not.

Changes in wave size and duration

Changes in wave size and duration provide essential information from the ECG. Knowledge of how the waves are produced (above) gives an introduction to understanding how these changes can be interpreted. Size of the waves can be reduced by either a reduction in the bulk of cardiac muscle, or by attenuation of the electrical field at the surface. Thus, for example, small complexes are seen in animals with intrathoracic

fluid (pleural or pericardial effusion). In these cases, it is usually noticeable that all parts of the trace are reduced in amplitude, i.e. the P waves as well as the QRS complex. Increases in height of the waves are usually attributable to an increase in the size of the chamber responsible for that wave; for example, P wave height increases with right atrial enlargement and R wave height with left ventricular enlargement. The ECG does not distinguish between dilation and hypertrophy of a chamber. In addition, since the waves reflect electrical activity of the heart muscle, changes in the electrolyte balance around or within the heart muscle will also produce changes. These are harder to predict from principles but are well established. In these cases, the diagnosis suggested on the ECG can usually be confirmed by blood analysis. A typical example is the changes associated with hyperkalaemia (see below). Normal ranges of wave height and duration (measured in lead II) in the dog and cat are well established and are given in Table 4.14, with a guide to interpretation of abnormalities.

Table 4.14 Normal ranges of wave height and duration

	Normal height	Normal width	Common changes in height	Common changes in width
P wave	Up to 0.4 mV (dog) Up to 0.2 mV (cat)	Up to 0.04 s (dog and cat)	Increase: right atrial enlargement	Increase: left atrial enlargement
PR interval	–	0.06–0.13 s (dog) 0.05–0.09 s (cat)	–	Increased duration: atrioventricular block
QRS complex	R wave height 0.5–2.5 mV (dog) Less than 0.9 mV (cat)	Up to 0.05 s (small dog) Up to 0.06 s (large dog) Up to 0.04 s (cat)	Increase: left ventricular enlargement	Increase: left ventricular enlargement, bundle branch block, severe right ventricular enlargement
T wave	Less than 25% of R wave amplitude but may be negative, positive or biphasic	–	Left ventricular enlargement	–
QT interval at normal rate	–	0.15–0.25 s (dog) 0.12–0.18 s (cat)	–	Electrolyte abnormalities
Normal mean electrical axis (MEA)	+40 to +100 degrees (dog) +0 to +180 degrees (cats) (rarely useful in cats)			
Heart rate	60–160 beats/min (dogs) 90–240 beats/min (cats)			

Changes in the mean electrical axis

Since the QRS complex is the result of the electrical depolarisation of the ventricular myocardium and the lead system of the ECG recording examines the heart in several directions, the ECG can be used to assess the position of the bulk of the ventricular myocardium within the thorax. This is one way in which hypertrophy or dilation of the ventricles can be assessed, although this is more usefully done by ultrasonography when this is available.

In principle, an ECG is taken using the standard three-limb leads or the six-lead system. Using two leads from either the standard or augmented limb leads, the sum of electrical deviation in the QRS complex is calculated for each lead, i.e. count the deflection of the Q wave below the baseline as negative, the R wave above the baseline as positive and the S wave below the baseline as negative. The total for each lead (which may be negative or positive) is plotted on a diagram and then the intersection of the two lines drawn. The angle from the centre to the intersection is the MEA and can be compared to published normal values. A useful rule of thumb is that the MEA is normal if the sum of the QRS complex is most positive in lead II.

A worked example is shown in Figure 4.45 to illustrate the method.

Similarly, the MEA can be considered to be approximately in the same direction as the lead with the most positive deviation.

The MEA can be precisely calculated using the sum of the deviations of the QRS complexes and comparing two leads. Although this can be a useful exercise, a useful rule of thumb is that if the QRS complex is most positive in lead II, then the MEA is normal.

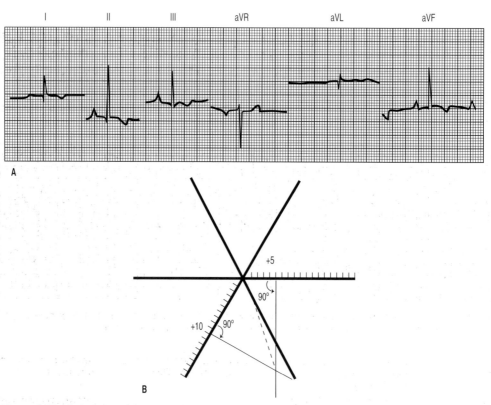

Figure 4.45 Calculation of the mean electrical axis. (Reproduced with permission from Ettinger and Suter 1970.)

The MEA will be altered artefactually if the wave of depolarisation through the ventricles is abnormal: for example, if one of the bundle branches is not conducting normally (bundle branch block). In these cases, the QRS complexes are often also wide and bizarre in form. If the MEA is abnormal, then the sizes of the waves (below) cannot be interpreted in the normal fashion.

Assessment of MEA is of less importance in cats than in dogs. The normal range is wider in this species and it is uncommon for the MEA to be outside this range.

Changes in heart rhythm

The second major finding from the ECG is changes in heart rhythm. In contrast to information on heart size, which radiography or ultrasonography can often confirm, and on electrolyte status, which blood analysis can confirm, the ECG is the most important diagnostic tool in these cases. Since an accurate diagnosis of dysrhythmia cannot be made on clinical examination, one of the common indications for electrocardiography is the investigation of suspected dysrhythmia. Knowledge of the way in which the waves are produced gives a guide to interpretation of changes in rhythm. For example, since P waves are produced by atrial depolarisation, their absence suggests that this is abnormal. For example, the atria may not be electrically active (atrial standstill) or perhaps their depolarisation is very irregular (atrial fibrillation). Similarly, the presence of abnormally large QRS complexes suggests the development of a ventricular tachy-dysrhythmia. The absence of recognisable P–QRS complexes and the presence of a coarse variation in the baseline are suggestive of ventricular fibrillation and the absence of all electrical activity suggests cardiac arrest. The appearance of the common dysrhythmias is given in Table 4.15.

Table 4.15 Appearance of common dysrhythmias

	Appearance	Other features	Clinical significance
Third-degree atrioventricular (AV) block (Fig. 4.46)	P waves present but unrelated to QRS complexes	Slow ventricular rate	Cause of exercise intolerance, syncope and sudden death

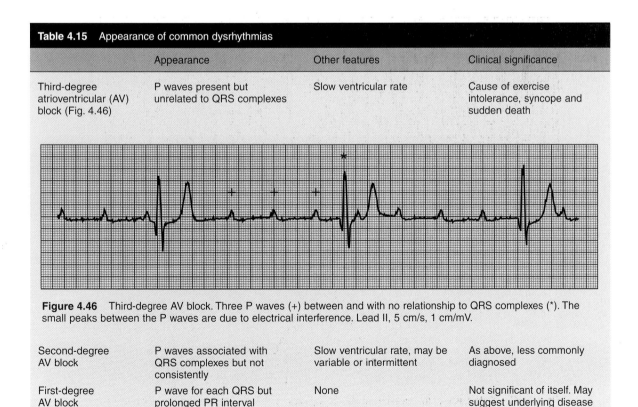

Figure 4.46 Third-degree AV block. Three P waves (+) between and with no relationship to QRS complexes (*). The small peaks between the P waves are due to electrical interference. Lead II, 5 cm/s, 1 cm/mV.

	Appearance	Other features	Clinical significance
Second-degree AV block	P waves associated with QRS complexes but not consistently	Slow ventricular rate, may be variable or intermittent	As above, less commonly diagnosed
First-degree AV block	P wave for each QRS but prolonged PR interval	None	Not significant of itself. May suggest underlying disease

Table 4.15 (*cont'd*)

	Appearance	Other features	Clinical significance
Sinus arrhythmia (Fig. 4.47)	Cyclical variation in P wave interval (and heart rate) Usually related to respiration	Usually disappears with increase in heart rate or atropine administration	Usually not significant in the dog. A sign of heart disease in the cat

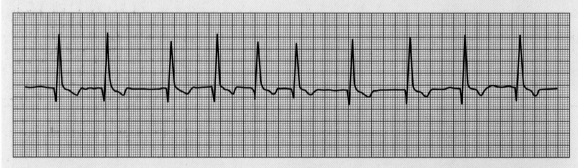

Figure 4.47 Sinus arrhythmia. Note the regular irregularity of the rhythm of the P–QRS complexes and slight variation in P wave height and the heart rate, which is at the low end of the normal range (around 70 beats/min). Lead II, 2.5 cm/s, 1 cm/mV.

Atrial fibrillation (Fig. 4.48)	P waves replaced by fine variations in the baseline (f waves)	Markedly irregular R–R interval. Usually tachycardic, but with pulse deficits	Associated with atrial enlargement. Common in giant breeds of dog with dilated cardiomyopathy

Figure 4.48 Atrial fibrillation. Note the absence of P waves (they were also not present in the other leads), tall R waves and irregular PR interval. Lead II, 5 cm/s, 1 cm/mV.

Single ventricular premature complexes (VPCs) (Fig. 4.49)	Isolated bizarre (tall and wide) QRS complexes, with no preceding P wave	All bizarre complexes may be similar (uniform) or each may be different (multiform). Reset underlying heart rhythm in most cases	Common in various heart diseases and systemic disease (shock, splenic pathology, gastric dilation/volvulus). Sometimes found in normal dogs
Ventricular tachydysrhythmia	VPCs occurring in runs or at greater frequency May be of the same shape (uniform) or of different shapes (multiform)	As above	As above, but not found in normal animals and may reduce cardiac output or progress to more serious dysrhythmias
Ventricular fibrillation	Absence of recognisable P–QRS complexes. Coarse or fine variation in the baseline	Absence of cardiac output (peripheral pulse or apex beat)	Rapidly fatal if not treated by defibrillation

Table 4.15 (*cont'd*)

Appearance	Other features	Clinical significance

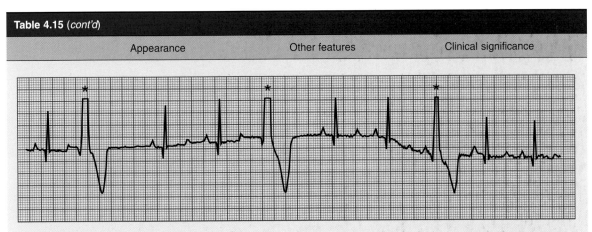

Figure 4.49   Single ventricular premature complexities. The VPCs are indicated by * and are wide, tall and of bizarre configuration compared to the normal QRS complexes. They are not preceded by a P wave and interrupt the underlying rhythm. Lead II, 5 cm/s, 1 cm/mV.

Effects of metabolic changes on the ECG

Changes in the internal environment of the animal affect the depolarisation of the myocardium and hence the ECG. Many metabolic disturbances act in this way and may produce non-specific changes, such as depression of the QT segment. The best described and most specific changes occur with increase in plasma potassium. The classical changes are presented in Table 4.16, but the actual extent of ECG changes in any particular case is rather unpredictable. The changes themselves should not be used to estimate electrolyte changes in the plasma; plasma biochemical analysis is the preferred method since it is more accurate.

Table 4.16   Changes in the electrocardiogram (ECG) described with hyperkalaemia

Serum potassium (mmol/l)	ECG changes
5.5–6.5	Tall peaked T waves, bradycardia
6.5–7.5	Reduced R wave height, widening QRS and PR interval, P wave lower and wider
7.5–8.5	P waves disappear, ST segment deviates from baseline
>11	Ventricular fibrillation/asystole

REFERENCES

Ettinger SJ, Suter PF 1970 Canine cardiology. WB Saunders, Philadelphia

Masters J, Bowden C (eds) 2001 Pre-veterinary nursing textbook. Butterworth-Heinemann in association with BVNA, Oxford, p 58

FURTHER READING

PART 1 EXAMINATION TECHNIQUES

Body fluid collection

Abdominal paracentesis
Kristal O 1997 Veterinary emergency medicine secrets. Abdominal paracentesis. In: Wingfield WE (ed), Hanley and Belfus, Philadelphia, ch 114

Arthrocentesis
Houlton JE 1994 BSAVA Manual of small animal arthrology. BSAVA, Cheltenham
Willard MD, Tvedten H, Turnwald GH (eds) 1999 Small animal clinical diagnosis by laboratory methods. WB Saunders, London

Cerebrospinal fluid collection
1992 Anaesthetic management of patients with neurological abnormalities. Comp Contin Education Practic Vet 14(2): 163–175
Carmichael N 1998 Chapter 13: Nervous system. In: Davidson M (ed) BSAVA Manual of small animal clinical pathology. BSAVA, Cheltenham
Christman C (ed) 1992 Cerebrospinal fluid analysis. Vet Clin North Am: Small Animal Practice 22: 781–808
Oliver JE, Lorenz MD, Kornegay JN (eds) 1997 Handbook of veterinary neurology. WB Saunders, London
Rusbridge C 2001 The nervous system. In: Ramsey I, Tennant B (eds) BSAVA Manual of canine and feline infectious diseases. BSAVA, Cheltenham, ch 15
Wheeler SJ, Sharp NJH (eds) 1994 Small animal spinal disorders: diagnosis and surgery. Mosby-Wolfe, London

Pericardiocentesis
Cobb M 1998 Respiratory tract and cardiovascular system. In: Davidson M (ed) BSAVA Manual of small animal clinical pathology. BSAVA, Cheltenham, ch 10

Prostatic wash and catheter biopsy
Bainbridge J, Elliott J (eds) 1996 BSAVA Manual of canine and feline nephrology and urology. BSAVA, Cheltenham
Holt PE 1994 Colour atlas and text of small animal urology. Mosby-Wolfe, London

Thoracocentesis
Cobb M 1998 Respiratory tract and cardiovascular system. In: Davidson M (ed) BSAVA Manual of small animal clinical pathology. BSAVA, Cheltenham
Luis Fuentes V, Swift S (eds) 1998 BSAVA Manual of small animal cardiorespiratory medicine and surgery. BSAVA, Cheltenham
Taylor N 1997 Thoracic drainage. In: Wingfield WE (ed) Veterinary emergency medicine secrets. Hanley and Belfus, Philadelphia, ch 110

Tracheal wash and bronchoalveolar lavage
Luis Fuentes V, Swift S (eds) 1998 BSAVA Manual of small animal cardiorespiratory medicine and surgery. BSAVA, Cheltenham

Urine collection
Bainbridge J, Elliott J 1996 BSAVA Manual of canine and feline nephrology and urology. BSAVA, Cheltenham
Mensack S, Kristal O (eds) 1997 Urethral catheterisation. In: Wingfield WE (ed) Veterinary emergency medicine secrets. Hanley and Belfus, Philadelphia ch 113
Willard MD, Tvedten H, Turnwald GH (eds) 1999 Small animal clinical diagnosis by laboratory methods. WB Saunders, London

Endocrine and gastrointestinal tests
Feldman EC, Nelson RW (eds) 1996 Canine and feline endocrinology and reproduction. WB Saunders, London
Guilford WG, Center SA, Strombeck DR, Williams DA, Meyer DJ (eds) 1996 Strombeck's small animal gastroenterology, 3rd edn. WB Saunders, London
Thomas D, Simpson JW, Hall EJ (eds) 1996 Manual of canine and feline gastroenterology. BSAVA, Cheltenham
Torrance AG, Mooney CT (eds) 1998 Manual of small animal endocrinology, 2nd edn. BSAVA, Cheltenham
Willard MD, Tvedten H, Turnwald GH (eds) 1999 Small animal clinical diagnosis by laboratory methods. WB Saunders, London.

Neurological and opthalmological examination
King AS 1987 Physiology and clinical anatomy of the domestic mammals, vol. 1. Central nervous system. Oxford Science Publications, Oxford
Oliver JE, Lorenz MD, Kornegay JN 1997 Handbook of veterinary neurology, 3rd edn. WB Saunders, London
Wheeler SJ (ed) 1995 Manual of small animal neurology, 2nd edn. BSAVA, Cheltenham
Wheeler SJ, Sharp NJH 1994 Small animal spinal disorders: diagnosis and surgery. Mosby-Wolfe, London

Tissue biopsy techniques
Davidson M 1998 BSAVA Manual of small animal clinical pathology. BSAVA, Cheltenham
Willard MD, Tvedten H, Turnwald GH (eds) 1999 Small animal clinical diagnosis by laboratory methods. WB Saunders, London
Day MJ, Mackin A, Littlewood J (eds) 2001 BSAVA Manual of canine and feline haematology and transfusion medicine. Collection and interpretation of bone marrow samples. BSAVA, Cheltenham, ch 2

Raskin RE, Meyer DJ (eds) 2001 Atlas of canine and feline cytology. WB Saunders, London

PART 2 ENDOSCOPY
Brearley MJ, Cooper JE, Sullivan M 1991 A colour atlas of small animal endoscopy. Wolfe, London
Cotton P, Williams C 1996 Practical gastrointestinal endoscopy, 4th edn. Blackwell Science, Oxford
Luis Fuentes V, Swift S 1998 Manual of small animal cardiorespiratory medicine and surgery. BSAVA, Cheltenham, ch 5
Roudebush P 1990 Tracheobronchoscopy. Vet Clin North Am: 20 1297

Tams TR 1999 Small animal endoscopy, 2nd edn. Mosby, St Louis

PART 3 ELECTROCARDIOGRAPHY
Edwards NJ (ed) 1987 Bolton's handbook of canine and feline electrocardiology, 2nd edn. WB Saunders, Philadelphia
Luis Fuentes V, Swift S (eds) 1988 BSAVA Manual of small animal cardiorespiratory medicine and surgery. BSAVA, Cheltenham
Tilley LP (ed) 1992 Essentials of canine and feline electrocardiology, 3rd edn. Lea and Febiger, Philadelphia

CHAPTER CONTENTS

5

Laboratory diagnostics

Joan Duncan   Karen Scott

The fundamental aim of the diagnostic laboratory, whether in a veterinary practice, or an external referral laboratory, is to produce quality data, to aid in the diagnosis of clinical disease, and to provide baseline information for the purposes of patient health screening. Clinical pathology is used in veterinary practices on a daily basis, and many tests are performed in the practice laboratory. Although this has made a dramatic impact on veterinary medicine, it has also increased the responsibilities of the veterinary practice. The practice staff are responsible for the provision of reliable results, documentation of quality control and adherence to health and safety (H&S) guidelines. This chapter outlines the H&S issues, quality control techniques and equipment maintenance relevant to the veterinary practice laboratory. The second part of the chapter details the clinical pathology tests commonly used in veterinary medicine, with emphasis on appropriate test selection, technique and interpretation of results.

LABORATORY HEALTH AND SAFETY

Potential hazards in a clinical laboratory generally arise from three main causes: from dangerous chemicals, infected samples, and the use of faulty instruments and apparatus. Carelessness, untidiness, poor hygiene techniques, unsatisfactory facilities and inadequate staff training increase the chances of accidents and resultant injuries occurring.

Aims

As with all other workplaces, there are many Acts and Regulations which must be adhered to within a clinical laboratory. The aims of H&S regulations such as the Health and Safety at Work Act (1974), and Control of Substances Hazardous to Health (COSHH) are to:

- Secure the health, safety and welfare of employees and visitors at work.
- Control the stocking and use of explosive or highly flammable or otherwise dangerous substances, and to prevent people from unlawfully having and using such substances.
- Control the atmospheric release of toxic or offensive substances from the work place – this also comes within the scope of the environmental protection legislation.
- Identify hazards within the workplace, carry out appropriate risk assessments, and introduce control measures to minimise the risks of these hazards.

Regulations

The following legislation is applicable to a clinical laboratory:

- Health and Safety at Work Act (1974)
- Control of Substances Hazardous to Health (COSHH) (1988)
- Control of Pollution Act (1974) and Environment Protection Act (1990)
- Collection and Disposal of Waste Regulations (1992)
- Reporting of Diseases and Dangerous Occurrence Regulations (RIDDOR) (1995)
- First Aid at Work Act.

The Health and Safety at Work Act (1974) was passed to promote and encourage high standards of H&S at work.

Responsibility and compliance

- The first consideration is that H&S is the responsibility of both the employer and employee. All individuals have a responsibility for their own safety as well as that of their colleagues.
- Unless employers are exempt from certain provisions, they require a written statement, including a General Policy on Health and Safety, and a statement of intent of protection of employees (and others who may be affected by the business's working practices). A suggested outline for an H&S policy and procedure is detailed in Table 5.1.
- Employers are required, by law, to report to the Health and Safety Executive (HSE) any 3-day injury or dangerous occurrences/near misses.

Table 5.1 Health and safety (H&S) documentation and major contents

Policy type/documentation	Contents
General policy	H&S general policy
Responsibility	Management structure for implementing H&S Management responsibilities Individual responsibilities
Assessment of risk	Working environment Personal protective equipment Manual handling of loads Display screen equipment Hazardous substances (COSHH) Fire prevention
Safety records and registers	Plant and equipment Electrical equipment Personal protective equipment Display screen equipment Accident, disease or dangerous occurrences Hazard reporting H&S training record Fire prevention and control record
Employee safety handbook	Employees' responsibilities Safety rules Hazard reporting Occupational health First aid Training

COSHH, Control of Substances Hazardous to Health.

- The Health and Safety Inspectorate is responsible for ensuring that H&S regulations are adhered to.

H&S IN THE PRACTICE LABORATORY

Code of conduct

Staff members must be familiar with the local and general safety rules. All staff should set a good example of cleanliness, tidiness and responsible behaviour, and all employees have a duty to ensure that all other employees in their laboratories are adequately trained, in both routine and emergency circumstances. General safety rules include the following:

- Food or drink should never be consumed or stored in the laboratory or laboratory refrigerator.
- Smoking should not be permitted in the laboratory.
- Mouth pipetting should be forbidden and nothing should be placed in the mouth, e.g. pens, pencils.
- The application of cosmetics should be discouraged, although the application of hand/barrier cream is permissible.
- Chemicals should be stored correctly and the provision of a flammables cupboard may be required.

Protective clothing

Laboratory overalls

These are generally accepted as the most suitable protective garment for all kinds of clinical and biomedical laboratory work. The coat should be buttoned to the top, have elasticated cuffs, and, ideally, fall below the knee. A sufficient supply of clean overalls must be made available for all workers as and when required. These must be removed when leaving the laboratory.

Latex disposable gloves

These are recommended for work with blood and other pathogens. Solvent-resistant gloves can be used when working with chemicals and heat-resistant gloves are available for work with hot materials, e.g. hot air ovens and autoclaves.

Disposable aprons

Plastic disposable aprons should be worn over laboratory coats for work with blood and group 3 pathogens.

Safety spectacles/goggles/visors

These are recommended to be worn when dealing with hazardous or corrosive chemicals.

Clothing and hair

Open-toed sandals should not be worn in the laboratory since they increase the risk of trip hazards, breakages and spillages. Long hair should be tied back to ensure that it could not become entangled in apparatus, equipment or chemicals.

Laboratory waste disposal

Chemical waste

There are specific legal requirements about the disposal of waste chemicals into public sewers. The local water authority must be informed and must consent before trade effluents are discharged into sewers (Public Health Act, 1961). Other legislation that may affect the disposal of chemicals includes the Control of Pollution Act (1974), the Deposit of Poisons Act (1972), and the Control of Pollution (Special Waste) regulations (1980).

All chemical reagents used in the laboratory are subject to COSHH regulations and every chemical used within the laboratory must be identified and the hazards and risks associated with its use assessed. Part of this COSHH risk assessment includes the disposal procedures for waste products.

Clinical waste

This is defined as waste that consists wholly or partly of animal tissue, body fluids, drugs or pharmaceutical products. The employer must provide instruction in the safe handling of clinical waste and segregation of waste into colour-coded containers is recommended. Infected or potentially infected material must be made safe by autoclaving before leaving the laboratory. **NB** clinical waste that has been autoclaved must still be disposed of as clinical waste. The following guidelines apply to waste disposal in laboratories:

- Information on colour coding for containers for clinical waste is contained in Table 5.2.
- Plastic bags should be of the appropriate colour (Table 5.2).
- Different types of clinical waste must be carefully segregated. Disposal containers in each laboratory should be clearly marked and, preferably, colour coded to help ensure against mistakes occurring. Procedures for the handling of waste disposal containers must be clearly defined.
- Items for incineration must be securely packaged and transported to an incinerator under the supervision of an appropriately

Table 5.2 Colour coding for containers of clinical waste. Strict adherence to a colour code system will help to ensure against clinical waste finding its way into the general refuse stream. Recommended colours to British Standard BS381C:1980: Yellow – Standard colour ref.: No 309; Light blue – Standard colour ref.: No 175 (Safety in Health Service Laboratories – safe working and the prevention of infection in clinical laboratories. Health Services Advisory Committee, 1991)

Colour of bag	Type of waste
Black	Normal household waste: not to be used to store or transport clinical waste
Yellow	All waste destined for incineration
Yellow with black banding	Waste (e.g. home nursing waste) which preferably should be disposed of by incineration but may be disposed of by landfill when separate collection and disposal arrangements are made
Light blue or transparent with light blue inscriptions	Waste for autoclaving (or equivalent treatment) before ultimate disposal

licensed operator who is fully conversant with appropriate safe working procedures for handling contaminated waste.

Accident and emergency plan

An emergency laboratory plan should be set detailing the procedures for:

- simple breakages
- spillage of chemicals
- spillage of biological substances
- major breakages/release of aerosols.

In the event of an accident or spillage, a senior member of staff should be informed immediately, and suitable precautions must be taken, depending on the chemical involved. The method for clearing up spillages of specific chemicals should be detailed in the COSHH information for that chemical. Protective clothing may be required, e.g. plastic or rubber aprons, heavy-duty rubber and light plastic gloves, and in some cases respirators may be needed. In some cases neutralising agents may be required depending on the chemicals involved. Readily accessible emergency kits containing the following should be readily available:

- Sterile eye wash solutions.
- Bottles of different kinds of undiluted disinfectants and empty bottles for preparing dilutions.
- Paper towels and pieces of strong cardboard about 25 × 10 cm.
- Forceps for picking up broken glass.
- Dustpan and brush capable of being autoclaved.
- Boxes to hold glass or other waste.
- A pack containing disposable gowns, overshoes, face masks, head covers and goggles.
- Rubber shoes (Wellingtons).

Making information available

The practice should have an H&S standard operating procedure, which details H&S policies, personnel responsibilities, review procedures and problem action protocols and lists the location of information and record sheets. H&S information should be made readily available to all staff, although generally a trained safety officer or senior member of staff will be appointed for keeping the necessary records correct and up to date.

COSHH assessments

COSHH assessments (Fig. 5.1) should be made for all hazardous procedures and chemicals. The preparation of assessment sheets has been detailed elsewhere (Butcher 1999). However, the information required includes:

- Route(s) of exposure of the operator to the substance.
- Preventative measures, e.g. use of protective clothing or an alternative substance.
- Specific first aid requirements.
- Chemicals – storage, spillage and disposal procedures.
- Identify high-risk staff.
- Records of the level of exposure (dependent on requirements).

An appropriately stocked first aid box should be kept in the practice, its location and the name(s) of trained first aiders posted on the wall and a RIDDOR-approved accident log kept (Fig. 5.2).

LABORATORY EQUIPMENT

Pipettes

Pipettes are used to measure and dispense designated volumes of reagents and/or samples. The type of pipette used should be appropriate to the volume of fluid being measured (Table 5.3). If pipette tips are used they should be clean and securely fitted. To ensure the optimum performance and accuracy it is essential that pipettes be cleaned, maintained, and their dispensing volumes checked at regular intervals.

Volumetric pipettes

- Ensure they are clean before use.
- Rinse after use, with water, followed by a dilute solution of alkaline detergent. Flush again with water, followed by an alcohol (methanol) rinse to ensure that the inside of the pipette is clean and dry.
- Store clean pipettes upright in a dust-free area.
- Discard pipettes if they are badly etched or have broken tips.

Table 5.3 Types of pipette

Type	Description	Volume range	Use
Graduated	Glass (usually borosilicate) tube that is drawn out to a tip and graduated uniformly along its length Two types – Mohr and serological	Various, from 1 ml to 10 ml	Variable dispensing within the volume range of the pipette Measurement of reagents
Volumetric	Glass (usually borosilicate) cylindrical bulb joined at both ends to a narrower glass tube	Various, from 1 ml to 100 ml	Fixed dispensing volume Measurement of reagents
Volumetric (Oswald-Folin)	Glass (usually borosilicate) cylindrical bulb joined to a narrower glass tube	0.5–3 ml	Viscous fluids, blood, serum
Micropipettes	When the plunger is moved through a complete cycle a predefined volume of liquid is drawn up and then dispensed Requires disposable plastic pipette tips	0.5 µl to 20 ml	Accurate delivery of smaller volumes
Automatic pipettes	Programmable electronic micropipettes	0.5 µl to 20 ml	Multiple delivery of multiple aliquots
Pasteur pipettes	Plastic disposable pipettes with graduated markings	1–5 ml	Transfer of serum or plasma from the cells to another tube

Compiled by: Practice manager **Date:**	**Product:** Domestic bleach
Very toxic ☐ Toxic ☐ Irritant ☒ Harmful ☐ Corrosive ☒	

Physical properties	**First aid action**
Appearance: pale yellow liquid Odour: chlorine (mild form)	Inhalation: remove to fresh air – seek medical aid Skin contact: wash thoroughly, remove contaminated clothing Eye contact: irrigate thoroughly for 15 minutes with sterile eyewash – seek medical aid Ingestion: give plenty of water to drink, do not induce vomiting – seek medical aid

Hazards through	**Fire action**
Inhalation: irritation ☒ Absorption: irritation ☒ Ingestion: irritation ☒ Injection ☐	Extinguish with CO_2, water, foam and other dry chemicals

Precautions	**Spillage/Disposal**
Inhalation: open doors and windows Absorption: wear rubber gloves Ingestion: if ingested, avoid inducing vomiting	Mop up with plenty of water – flush away with plenty of water, open windows and ensure good ventilation

Health effects	**Storage**
Inhalation: Possible dizziness and/or nausea Skin contact: after long exposure, may cause soreness or rash over time Eye contact: may damage eyes if not rinsed immediately Ingestion	Cool, well-ventilated space, keep out of direct sunlight Store away from acids

Figure 5.1 Example of Control of Substances Hazardous to Health assessment sheet.

ACCIDENT BOOK	For use at my work premises		
1. About the person who had the accident	**2. About you, the person filling in this book**	**3. About the accident**	**4. About the accident – what happened**
• Give the full name • Give the home address • Give the occupation	• Please sign the book and date it • If you did not have the accident, write your address and occupation	• When it happened • Where it happened	• Say how the accident happened. Give the cause if you can • If any personal injury, say what it is
Name: Address: Postcode: Occupation:	Your signature: Date: Address: Postcode: Occupation:	Date: Time: In what room or place did the accident happen?	How did the accident happen? Employer's initials:
Name: Address: Postcode: Occupation:	Your signature: Date: Address: Postcode: Occupation:	Date: Time: In what room or place did the accident happen?	How did the accident happen? Employer's initials:

Figure 5.2 Example of an accident book.

Micropipettes and automatic pipettes

- Dismantle the pipette regularly (at least once a month), clean and lubricate the barrel.
- Ensure that the action moves smoothly.
- Ensure the pipette bore is not blocked.
- Test the pipette on a monthly basis to check the dispensing volume
  — Pipette a set volume of water into a weigh boat.
  — Weigh the weigh boat on an accurate balance, which has previously been tared to the weight of the empty weigh boat.
  — The weight will correspond to the volume dispensed, i.e. 1 μg equals 1 μl.
  — Repeat this procedure 10 times.
  — Calculate the mean volume.
  — Ensure the mean volume dispensed is within the defined limits at that volume.
  — If outside limits, refer to manufacturer.

Microscope

A microscope is an essential piece of equipment in both the laboratory and the veterinary practice. Binocular microscopes, i.e. those with two eyepieces, are the preferred type, and usually have the light source built into the base (Fig. 5.3). Each part of the microscope serves a specific function:

1. Eyepieces: contain the ocular objective lenses which magnify the real image to form a virtual magnified image, i.e. they act as a magnifying glass, further magnifying the inverted image formed by the objective (usually ×10).
2. Objective lens system: forms a real, inverted, magnified image of the object within the tube of the microscope, i.e. the image is upside down and reversed. There are usually 3 or 4 objective lenses, commonly 4× (scanning), 10× (low power), 40× (high power dry) and 100× (oil immersion). They are carried on a rotating nosepiece.

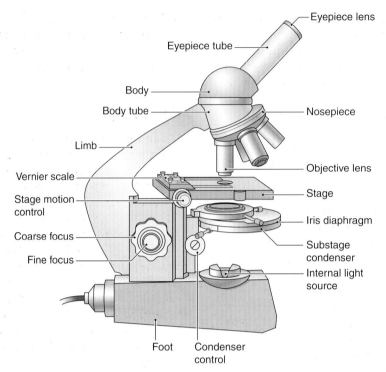

Figure 5.3   Parts of a microscope. (From *Pre-Veterinary Nursing Textbook* by Masters and Bowden (2001). Reprinted by permission of Elsevier Science.)

3. Stage: the device that supports the material under examination, e.g. the glass slide. There are usually clips attached to the stage, which hold the slide down, preventing movement during examination.

4. Sub-stage condenser: forms a perfect image of the light source in the plane of the object being viewed. The condenser is adjustable so that it may have the same numerical aperture as the objective being used, i.e. the cone of light transmitted upwards from the object exactly fills the aperture of the objective allowing full use of the objective's numeric aperture.

5. Light source: built-in. In modern microscopes it is positioned below the condenser. In older microscopes, a mirror and external light source may be used.

6. Limb: forms the main support at the back of the microscope and is used to carry the instrument.

7. Vernier scales: graduated measuring devices attached to the stage, which allow the position of an object on the slide under examination to be accurately recorded. One scale is positioned vertically and the other horizontally, providing, in essence, a grid reference for the object under examination.

8. Coarse and fine focusing controls: move the stage up and down. The coarse focusing control allows large adjustments in the height of the stage to permit slides etc. to be placed on the stage and brought into line with the objective. The fine focusing control allows small adjustments in the focus to be made.

9. Foot: the support plate at the base of the microscope, which provides the instrument with stability.

The microscope is prepared for use as follows:

• Rotate nosepiece until the 10× objective is in the optical path.
• Clean the eyepieces, condenser and objective lenses with a lens tissue.

- Turn down the light control to minimum and switch on the microscope.
- Turn up the light and adjust the distance between the two eyepieces so that each field appears identical, and both fields are viewed as one.
- Nearly close the lamp-lens diaphragm mounted on the base of the microscope controlled by a ring surrounding the lens (clockwise rotation makes the diaphragm smaller).
- Adjust the condenser until the edge of the diaphragm is seen as a sharp image.
- Centralise the disc of light using the two knobs on the front of the condenser body.
- Open the diaphragm until the light fills the whole field.
- Place the slide to be examined on the stage and fasten down with the clips.
- Examine the slide under the 10× objective focusing with the coarse and fine focus (always focus upwards away from the slide, to prevent accidental damage to the objectives). The slide can then be examined on a higher power objective.
- If an oil immersion lens is required, place immersion oil on the slide and rotate the nosepiece until the 100× objective is positioned in the optical path. Focus on to the slide using the fine focus control, and adjust the light intensity.
- After use, reduce the light, rotate the lenses so the lowest power objective is in position and switch off. Remove all oil from the lenses using a lens tissue.

Maintenance

Microscopes are precision instruments requiring regular maintenance:

- Clean after use to prevent the build up of oil and dust on the objective.
- Turn the rheostat down before switching the microscope on or off to prolong the life of the bulb.
- Only clean the lenses with lens tissue or soft gauze moistened with petroleum benzene.

- When not in use, cover the microscope with a vinyl cover and store in a dry place.
- Store the objective lens' eyepieces in a container with desiccant in it.

Centrifuges

Centrifuges accelerate the gravitational separation of substances that differ in mass. Centrifugation is used to separate particles from a solution in which they are suspended, e.g. to separate the cellular elements from blood to provide a cell-free plasma or serum for analysis. Centrifuges contain a rotor or centrifuge head, drive shaft and motor enclosed in the chamber or guard bowl. A timer, speed controller and brake are used to set the time and number of revolutions per minute and slow the centrifuge down. A safety lock should be fitted to stop the lid of the centrifuge being opened whilst the unit is rotating. Three types are available (Table 5.4). The operating guidelines are as follows:

- Use only recommended centrifuge tubes capable of withstanding the centrifugal force – usually polypropylene tubes are used (forces up to 5000 g).
- Fit the tubes securely in the centrifuge rack ensuring the tops of the tubes do not protrude above the bucket and interfere with the rotor action.
- Ensure the rotor is balanced correctly – imbalance will cause vibration and increased wear, and may lead to tube breakage.
- To minimise the risks of aerosol infection do not remove the tops from blood tubes prior to centrifugation.
- If the centrifuge is fitted with bucket lids these should be sealed during centrifugation.
- Ensure that the guard is in place on microhaematocrit centrifuges.
- The breakage of a tube in the centrifuge should be considered an incident and reported to the safety officer. The centrifuge should be kept closed for 30 minutes to allow airborne particles to settle before disinfecting procedures are followed.

Table 5.4 Types of centrifuge		
Type	Description	Common uses
Swing out	The tubes placed in the rotor assume a horizontal position whilst the rotor is in motion and assume a vertical position when the rotor is at rest	Separation of plasma or serum from blood samples
	Following centrifugation the sediment is uniformly distributed against the bottom of the tube and the surface of the sediment stays flat	Preparation of urine or fluid samples for sediment examination
	Allows the supernatant to be removed with a Pasteur pipette	
Angle head	The tubes are held in a fixed position, usually 25–40 degrees from vertical	Separation of plasma or serum from blood samples
	Upon centrifugation the sediment packs against the side of the tube	Preparation of urine or fluid samples for sediment examination
	As the rotor slows, gravity causes the pellet to slide down the tube and so a poorly packed pellet is formed	
	The aerodynamic shape of the rotor allows a much higher centrifugation speed to be achieved	
Microhaematocrit	Tubes held horizontally	Assessment of packed cell volume (PCV) or haematocrit
	The particles are driven outwards, strike the bottom of the tube and pack	
	As the rotor slows, gravity causes the pellet to slide down the tube and so a poorly packed pellet is formed	
	Usually used to centrifuge capillary tubes	

Maintenance

Regular cleaning and maintenance are important to minimise the possible spread of infectious agents. Frequent cleaning will ensure proper operation and prolong the life of the centrifuge. Spills should always be cleaned up when they occur, in order to prevent corrosive or contaminated material from drying on component surfaces.

Swing out and angle head centrifuges

- Daily wipe the bowl with a cloth or paper towel.
- Remove the rotor weekly; clean the bowl, drive shaft and shaft cavity with a mild detergent and then rinse with water.
- Lubricate the drive shaft.
- Remove the air-intake filters and inspect for dust, rinsing with water if necessary.
- Clear the outlet vents of dust.

Microhaematocrit centrifuge

- Daily wipe the centrifuge interior with a damp cloth; clean any leakage from tubes with mild detergent.

- Regularly check the rubber gasket for wear and replace it if necessary.

Haematology analysers

See 'Generating the Haematology Profile,' below.

Biochemistry analysers

Most biochemistry analysers, with the exception of some electrolyte instruments, are photoelectric instruments. These rely on a colour change reaction occurring when a known volume of the test analyte interacts with a known volume of the specific reagent. This colour reaction may take place across a wide range of wavelengths, both within the visible spectrum and beyond. The essential parts of these photoelectric instruments are the light source, sample holders, a means of selecting a monochromatic light of the appropriate wavelength, a series of lenses to focus the emitted light, light detector(s) and a means of displaying the detector output. By comparison with a set of previously run known standards, called the calibration curve, the instrument compares the detected light pattern and determines the absolute analytical value.

Spectrophotometer

A spectrophotometer measures the amount of light absorbed by a coloured solution. Different coloured solutions absorb light of a particular wavelength. Spectrophotometers measure the amount of light passing through a solution and compare it to the amount of light passing through a colourless solution, and from the two readings calculate the amount of light absorbed. The intensity of the colour of the solution is related to the concentration of the analyte in the sample – therefore, if the absorption for an unknown concentration is compared with absorption of a known concentration, it is possible to determine the concentration of the analyte in the unknown solution.

Reflectometer

A reflectometer measures the amount of light reflected by a coloured solution. Reflected light results from illuminating a reaction solution with diffuse light. Reflectometers measure the amount of light reflected by a solution, compare it to the amount of light reflected by a colourless reference solution, and therefore calculate the amount of light absorbed. The intensity of the reflected light is related to the concentration of the analyte in the sample.

Wet and dry chemistry systems

Most biochemistry analysers operated within the veterinary practice are either classed as 'wet' or 'dry' chemistry systems. 'Wet' chemistry systems involve the sample being added to fluid reagent with the resultant colour change being measured on a spectrophotometer system. 'Dry' chemistry systems involve the sample being added to a reagent that has been absorbed on to a membrane and the resultant colour change being measured by reflectometry. Each system has advantages and disadvantages (Table 5.5).

Glucose meters

Glucose meters are 'hand-held' dry-chemistry systems that rely on a colour change reaction occurring. Whole blood samples are used and test results are generally available within 30 seconds. Care should be taken with interpretation of results since most instruments are only available with human reference ranges and glucose results are generally lower in whole blood than in serum.

Refractometers

Refractometers are measuring instruments that rely on the phenomenon of light refraction. Refractometers are based on the principle that as the density of a substance increases (e.g. when sugar is dissolved in water), its refractive index rises proportionately.

- Refractometers utilise a prism which possesses a much greater refractive index than the sample solution to be measured. Measurements are made possible using the refractive phenomena, which arise at the interface of the prism and the sample solution.
- In the case of a weak sample solution, the difference between the refractive index of the solution and that of the prism is large, therefore the angle of refraction is large.
- In the case of a strong sample solution, the difference between the refractive index of the solution and that of the prism is smaller and therefore the angle of refraction is smaller.

QUALITY CONTROL IN THE VETERINARY LABORATORY

Quality data are required to be produced by the most efficient and cost-effective manner to allow the provision of expedient treatment whilst minimising stress to both the patient and the owner. By following a regime of good laboratory practice, laboratories can ensure that accurate, precise results are produced and can minimise errors, repeat tests or inappropriate tests, thus offering peace of mind and cost reduction. Good laboratory practice relies upon the appropriate education and training of laboratory personnel, the standardisation of laboratory procedures, the

Table 5.5 Comparison of the advantages and disadvantages of 'wet' and 'dry' chemistry systems

Dry chemistry analysers	Wet chemistry analysers
Easy to use and maintain – little training required	Higher level of training required to operate and maintain the analyser
Reagent slides are pre-calibrated, so no need for calibration	Reagents need to be calibrated at least at every batch change
Reagent slides generally have a long shelf life and are stable when kept under the recommended storage condition	Reagents are generally less stable and stability depends on the storage conditions. The stability decreases as the storage temperature increases and also when exposed to air and light
Reagent slides are ready to use	Reagents may require reconstitution, therefore it is necessary to purchase distilled water as well as a pipette and pipette tips in order to prepare the reagents
Reagent slides are compact and easy to store	Liquid reagents can be bulky and may require more storage space
No liquid waste for disposal. Disposal of solid waste is generally considered less hazardous	Liquid and solid waste are produced. Liquid waste disposal is generally more hazardous, e.g. picric acid in creatinine reagent is potentially explosive if allowed to dry out
Reaction cells are not necessary – the reaction occurs on the reagent slide itself	Reaction cells are required for analysis
Quality control samples do not need to be run with each sample, as the reagents on the slide are more stable. It is not necessary therefore to batch samples for analysis – they can be analysed as and when required	A quality control sample should be included on each run to ensure reagent viability, so it is more economical to batch samples. Samples should not therefore be analysed individually without a control
Range of tests is limited by the chemistry slides available	The analyser may be programmed to perform different tests as the user requires
Reagent slides available from limited suppliers	Reagents often available from many suppliers
Reagent slides appear more expensive. However, slide usage for calibration is not required and wastage levels are low	Wet reagents appear cheaper. However, reagent usage for priming and calibration is high, as is wastage unless the user has a high throughput
Consumable costs are lower – e.g. only blood collection tubes, pipette tips and paper are generally required	Consumable costs are higher – e.g. blood collection tubes, pipette tips, sample cups, paper, reaction cells, pump tubing, reagent and waste containers, probe-cleaning fluids
Low number of replacement/moving parts – e.g. only one sample probe/syringe and lamp assembly	Higher number of movable/replacement parts – e.g. sample probes, reagent probes, syringes, lamps and filter systems
A separate pipette tip is required for each sample, so there is no carryover of one sample to the next, or problems with blocked sample probes	The sample probe does not use disposable pipette tips, so requires cleaning between samples. This may not eliminate carryover between samples, and the probe may be blocked by fibrin in the samples
The reagents are enclosed on the reagent slides that are individually packaged, so there is no possible carryover of reagents from one slide to the next	The reagent probe requires cleaning between picking up different reagents. If this is not adequate there may be carryover of reagent from one test to the next

maintenance and metrology of laboratory equipment and reagents as well as the use of quality measures. Education and training should include, as a minimum:

- sampling techniques
- sample requirements and quality assessment
- record keeping of patient details
- sample, pre-analytical treatment and dispatch as required
- operation of laboratory equipment in accordance with manufacturers' requirements
- troubleshooting
- H&S

- the recognition of erroneous or incorrect results
- knowledge of species and age reference ranges and degrees of normality.

The standardisation of laboratory techniques is essential to ensure the reproducibility of results, minimise operator bias and reduce operator error. Written standard operating procedures (SOPs) should be provided which should simply and clearly outline the steps involved in the process. As well as assisting with the training of new or inexperienced staff, they ensure that all laboratory operations will take place in a consistent and uniform manner. SOPs should cover all procedures from H&S, through sampling procedures, maintenance of equipment, preparation of reagents, calibration of equipment, use of quality control, operation of laboratory equipment, to troubleshooting. The maintenance and metrology of laboratory equipment are essential for H&S as well as to ensure that the equipment is performing optimally, to maximise its working life and to minimise the chance of failure. Procedures should include:

- cleaning and decontamination
- calibration and standardisation
- temperature control, e.g. incubators, refrigerators
- optical checks, e.g. spectrophotometers, microscopes
- volumetric checks, e.g. volumetric pipettes, sample and reagent dispensers.

Quality measures involve the analysis of both quality control (QC) and quality assessment (QA) materials and a comparison of the results attained against the expected results. Quality control usually involves the measurement of a known QC material and, by ensuring that the results fall within a given range, gives an immediate indication of method acceptability. Quality assessment usually involves the measurement of an unknown sample and a comparison of the results, by an external party, with other similar users, and provides an indication of result accuracy and precision. The use of both QC and QA provides confidence in results, as well as highlighting potential problems, analytical trends, training needs and equipment failure.

Quality control and laboratory error

QC can be defined as the action of detecting errors, and there are many potential errors that can affect the quality of results leaving the laboratory. Errors in analysis can be separated into three groups: pre-analytical, analytical and post-analytical errors.

Pre-analytical errors

These errors occur outside the laboratory but may affect the validity of the results. Considerations include:

- the fasting state of the patient
- prior drug therapy
- appropriate use of correct specimen containers
- suitable sampling procedures
- sample haemolysis
- ethylenediaminetetraacetic acid (EDTA) contamination of serum sample
- correct identification of the tube and request form with patient details.

Analytical errors

These errors occur within the laboratory, and may be caused by:

- incorrect reagent storage
- use of incorrect diluent for diluting samples and reagent preparation
- contamination or improper use of pipettes
- improper use or poor maintenance of equipment
- human error – tiredness, carelessness, lack of training.

QC samples are samples with a known concentration and have a quoted acceptable range of values. QC samples should be analysed in the same manner as patient samples, and their results should fall within two standard deviations of the predetermined mean (Lumsden 1998).

QC samples should be assayed:

- on a regular basis, dependent on manufacturer's recommendation
- following equipment recalibration or maintenance
- following movement of equipment
- to check an unexplained patient result
- following reagent preparation or if reagent stress is suspected.

Post-analytical errors

These errors concern the prompt and correct delivery of the correct report, on the correct patient to the correct physician. May be caused by:

- incorrect or absent sender's information.
- transcription or calculation errors when entering patient information or when reporting results.

In addition, interpretation error, including use of inappropriate reference ranges, is a potential cause of error.

Record keeping

Accurate record keeping is essential in reducing errors and highlighting problems when they occur. The following records should be maintained:

- staff training records
- equipment calibration, maintenance and service records
- QC results for both internal and external schemes
- reagent preparation sheets – detailing preparation, expiry, QC checks, storage requirements and lot numbers
- fridge and freezer temperatures
- patient results
- referral samples.

Assessment

The practice should have a review policy for all QC procedures whereby QC results and records are checked on a regular basis. Any problems should be identified immediately to the designated practice personnel and action taken. A resumé of the QC results should be circulated to all practice staff regularly and should form a point of discussion at practice meetings.

PRINCIPLES OF INTERPRETATION AND TEST SELECTION

Interpretation of results

Clinical pathology is used in a number of circumstances:

- pre-anaesthetic testing
- geriatric screening
- identification of disease
- disease monitoring
- therapeutic monitoring.

In each of these circumstances, interpretation of abnormal results should take into consideration the:

- Degree of abnormality.
- Incidence of disease, e.g. disease is unlikely in a young, healthy patient admitted for elective surgery.
- Clinical signs, history and differential diagnosis list. Abnormalities that were not expected from the clinical presentation should be checked, e.g. marked hypoglycaemia in a patient without accompanying signs.
- Age. Ideally, blood results from young patients should be compared to reference intervals established for this age group. This is often not possible and results have to be compared with adult reference intervals. A number of age-related abnormalities are therefore commonly noted (Table 5.6).
- Breed-related variations are noted in some tests (Table 5.7).
- Formulation of reference intervals (see below).
- Laboratory error (see 'Quality Control and Laboratory Error,' above).

Reference intervals

Patient test results are compared to reference intervals, which, ideally, would be established in a matched population of healthy animals. However, this is not often possible and patients' results

Table 5.6 Age-related changes in laboratory results

Test	Common changes in young patients
PCV, RBC, Hb	High at birth, then low by 4 weeks, and gradually increase to adult values at around 6 months
Total protein	Low in neonates and young animals
Globulins	Low in neonates and young animals
Calcium	Large-breed dogs (<12 months) may have mild increase
Phosphorus	Increase possible in dogs and cats <12 months

PVC, packed cell volume; RBC, red blood cell; Hb, haemoglobin.

Table 5.7 Non-pathological breed-related changes

Test	Abnormality	Breed
PCV, Hb, RBC	Increased	German Shepherd dogs, Greyhound, Doberman
MCV	Increased	Poodles
MCV	Decreased	Akitas
Eosinophils	Increased	German Shepherd dogs
Eosinophils	Vacuolated	Greyhounds
Platelets	Decreased number and/or increased size	Cavalier King Charles Spaniel
Potassium	Increased	Akitas have a high red cell potassium concentration Haemolysis can cause release
Total thyroxine concentration	Decreased	Greyhounds and sight hounds

PVC, packed cell volume; Hb, haemoglobin; RBC, red blood cell; MCV, mean corpuscular volume.

are compared to intervals established using many breeds of adult animals. As a consequence, some breeds will appear to have abnormal test results when compared to these multibreed reference intervals (Table 5.7). In addition, a small percentage of healthy patients (usually around 5% of the population) will have mildly abnormal test results. This reflects the statistical methods used for determination of the reference interval. It has been reported (Lumsden 1998) that in a 20-test profile there is a 64% probability of one or more test results falling outside the reference interval. Abnormal test results, therefore, do *not* automatically indicate disease.

Test selection

Since abnormal test results may be noted in healthy subjects, then it is preferable to select a panel of tests when assessing sick patients. In this way, a number of abnormalities may be noted which could confirm the presence of disease or add further information. The selection of these tests depends upon the:

- possible causes of the clinical signs
- range of conditions to be excluded
- availability of the tests
- cost of tests.

Performing a profile (where finances allow) is a more efficient means of assessing all the possible differentials (Table 5.8). When the clinical signs are vague and a 'general health screen' is required, then it is necessary to select a broad range of analytes, which will reflect a number of common diseases, or pathological states. The inclusion of tests which are not organ-specific, but which provide general information regarding the hydration status and essential body constituents, is worthwhile, e.g. total proteins, albumin, electrolytes and glucose.

COLLECTION OF SAMPLES

Patient preparation

A standardised approach to laboratory testing is essential for comparison of patient results collected on different occasions, or comparison of results with reference intervals. The following are common sources of pre-analytical error:

1. Fasting. In the dog and cat, the absorption of dietary components can affect biochemistry results. The triglyceride concentration is most commonly increased, but glucose, cholesterol and urea may also be affected. The high triglyceride concentration can cause lipaemia, a milky turbidity of the sample, which interferes with many laboratory tests. Lipaemia is most likely in samples collected 2–6 hours after feeding but the increase in triglycerides may persist for longer in

Table 5.8 A selection of profiles for use in small animal practice

Profile	Tests	Indications
Health screen	FBC, TP, albumin, globulin, ALT, ALP, bilirubin, urea, creatinine, calcium, phosphorus, glucose	Routine screening. Add amylase and lipase if canine pancreatitis suspected
Pre-anaesthetic screen	PCV, TP, ALT, ALP, BUN, creatinine, glucose. Examine sample for evidence of icterus	Screen for existing disease prior to routine surgery
Extended health screen	As health screen, plus electrolytes, cholesterol and urinalysis	Gastrointestinal disease, hypoadrenocorticism. Add amylase and lipase if canine pancreatitis suspected
Polydipsia profile	As health screen, plus electrolyte screen, cholesterol, urinalysis (SG, dipstick and sediment examination)	Polydipsia
Seizure profile	FBC, TP, albumin, globulin, ALT, ALP, bile acids, urea, creatinine, glucose, calcium, CK, phosphorus, magnesium, electrolyte screen	Seizures, weakness, episodic collapse
Renal profile	PCV, TP, albumin, globulin, urea, creatinine, sodium, potassium, calcium, phosphorus, urinalysis (SG dipstick and sediment examination)	
Hepatic profile	TP, albumin, globulin, ALT, ALP, AST, GGT, bilirubin, cholesterol and bile acid stimulation test	Monitoring hepatotoxicity

FBC, full blood count; TP, total protein; ALT, alanine aminotransferase; ALP, alkaline phosphatase; PCV, packed cell volume; BUN, blood urea nitrogen; SG, specific gravity; CK, creatinine kinase; AST, aspartate aminotransferase; GGT, gamma glutamyltransferase.

patients with endocrine disease, e.g. canine hypothyroidism. Fasting is not advisable in neonatal patients.

2. Stress. The stress of visiting the veterinary surgeon can cause a leucocytosis in young cats, and hyperglycaemia in both cats and dogs. The hyperglycaemia in cats can be marked and can result in an erroneous diagnosis of diabetes mellitus.

3. Drug therapy. Where possible, all sampling should be performed prior to drug administration, including fluid therapy (Table 5.9).

Sample collection

Before collecting a sample it is essential that the following be confirmed:

* test required
* type of sample to be collected
* ideal method of sample preservation
* quantity of material required
* point of care analysis or referral?
* expected turn around time for client information.

Table 5.9 Possible effects of drug therapy on laboratory results

Drug	Tests commonly affected
Fluid therapy	PCV, proteins
Glucocorticoids	Liver enzymes
	Tests for immune-mediated disease
Anticonvulsants	Liver enzymes
Insulin	Glucose, potassium
Sedation	PCV, glucose
Anaesthesia	PCV

PVC, packed cell volume.

It is important that animals are restrained securely, with minimal stress, and the sample collected in a manner that will minimise haemolysis (Bloxham 1999).

Blood samples

Collection

In the dog and cat, blood is commonly collected from the jugular or cephalic vein. Occasionally, an ear prick technique may be used, e.g. screening for blood-borne parasites. There are advantages

Table 5.10 Jugular venepuncture versus cephalic collection

Jugular	Cephalic
Large quantity blood	Usually small quantity
Shorter collection time	Longer collection time risks onset of clotting in the syringe
Larger-bore needle with less risk of haemolysis	Often smaller-bore needle used with more risk of haemolysis
Requires practice	Vein already commonly used therefore familiarity with technique
Leaves cephalic vein undisturbed for further treatment	May affect subsequent short-term use of vein

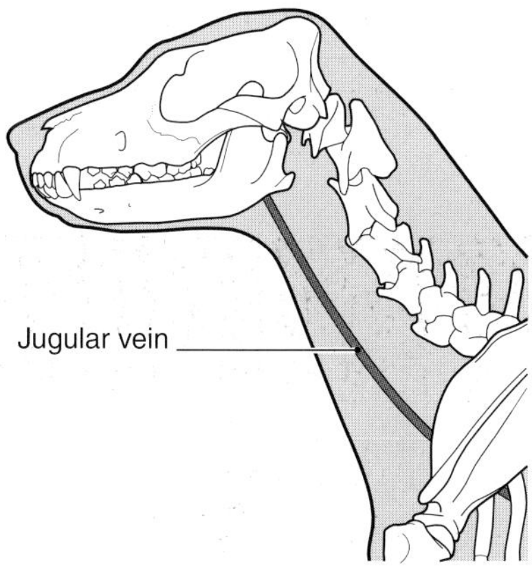

Table 5.11 Sample requirements for blood testing

Tests required	Samples required
Haematology profile*	EDTA and air-dried blood film (check requirements for exotics with referral laboratory – often heparin required)
Biochemistry testing	Heparin plasma or serum
Glucose	Whole blood, heparin plasma or fluoride oxalate plasma, depending on methodology
Coagulation screen	Citrated plasma. Ratio of anticoagulant to blood is critical

*For haematology studies, a blood film, made at the time of sample collection, is essential (Figure 5.10).
EDTA, ethylenediaminetetraacetic acid.

Figure 5.4 Location of the jugular vein. (From *Pre-Veterinary Nursing Textbook* by Masters and Bowden (2001). Reprinted by permission of Elsevier Science.)

to each method (Table 5.10) but the author's preference is for jugular venepuncture. The location of the jugular vein is indicated in Figure 5.4. The details of sample collection have been outlined by Bloxham (1999).

Anticoagulants for routine use

Depending on the analysis required, blood may be collected into samples tubes, with or without anticoagulant. Blood collected without an anticoagulant will clot, extruding serum from the cellular clot. Blood collected into an anticoagulant does not clot, but the cells may be separated from the fluid phase, called plasma, by centrifugation. Anticoagulants have different properties, which make them more suitable for some tests than others (Table 5.11).

Preparation of serum and plasma

Plasma and serum may be separated from the cells by centrifugation. However, if the sample has not been mixed with an anticoagulant then it should not be centrifuged for at least 20 minutes after collection, or until there is evidence of clot formation. Proceed as follows:

- Collect whole blood into a tube containing anticoagulant. Heparin is commonly used for biochemical testing since it has the least detrimental effects in comparison to alternatives.
- Centrifuge sample at 2000–3000 rpm for 10 minutes, or as indicated on practice centrifuge.
- Remove serum or plasma and label.
- Sample should not be exposed to heat or direct sunlight.
- If samples cannot be analysed immediately then the separated serum/plasma can be stored in a refrigerator until analysis. However, delay should always be avoided where possible.

> **Box 5.1** Common causes of haemolysis
>
> Use of too-fine gauge needle
> Use of excessive pressure during sample collection
> Failure to remove needle before ejecting sample into collection tube
> Vigorous shaking of sample
> Failure to separate plasma or serum before posting
> Haemolytic anaemia

Assessing sample quality

A visual appraisal of the sample after centrifugation is an integral part of all analyses. Normal serum/plasma in the dog and cat is pale, often straw-coloured, and clear (i.e. no turbidity). Look out for the following:

- Icterus is a yellow–orange coloration of the sample caused by hyperbilirubinaemia. Hyperbilirubinaemia is detected in the sample at lower bilirubin concentrations than can be detected by visual appraisal of patient.
- Lipaemia is a milky opalescence of the sample, which commonly reflects a failure to fast the patient prior to sampling
- Haemolysis is a red discoloration of the serum caused by leakage of haemoglobin from erythrocytes. It can interfere with biochemical tests and a spun packed cell volume (PCV). Haemolysis may be caused by a poor sample collection technique (Box 5.1).

Urine samples

Urine may be collected by the following means:

1. Voided midstream sample. This type of sample is acceptable for routine screening and chemical analysis. However, cells originating from the genitalia make cytological interpretation difficult and will affect culture results.
2. Catheterisation. Collection of a sample by sterile catheterisation (Chandler 1999) is acceptable for urine culture but a traumatic technique can increase the cellular exfoliation, interfering with cytological interpretation.
3. Cystocentesis may be used by a veterinary surgeon to collect a urine sample for diagnostic testing or to provide relief from increasing pressure within the bladder in cases of urinary tract obstruction (Chandler 1999). In the cat this is often the most practical means of collecting a urine sample for analysis but a full bladder is required for this technique.

Urine should be analysed as soon as possible after collection, especially for cellular assessments and examinations for crystalluria. Where material is to be submitted to an external laboratory for further testing, then additional preservation may be required. Boric acid is a commonly used preservative.

Faecal samples

To avoid environmental contamination, faecal samples must be collected directly from the rectum. A reasonable quantity is required, e.g. one half of a faecal pot, since some bacteria can only be cultured from the poorly oxygenated central region.

Bacteriology and virology

Swabs and viral studies

Material for culture must be transferred immediately into transport media for preservation of the micro-organisms. Transport media provide the nutrients and appropriate oxygen tension for many common pathogens. However, specific transport media are required if you wish to isolate certain pathogens and it is useful to discuss the aims of analysis with a veterinary microbiologist prior to sample collection.

Blood culture

Blood culture is most commonly used in the investigation of pyrexia of unknown origin, septicaemia and inflammatory arthropathies. Blood is collected aseptically into specific media (supplied by a commercial laboratory). It is best if the sample can be incubated within the practice for 24 hours prior to dispatch. Ideally, 2–3 samples should be collected over a 24-hour period.

Skin examinations

The following methods of sample collection are commonly used:

- Hair plucks and brushings: most commonly used to collect material for fungal culture, or for microscopic examination (for fungal elements and superficial parasites). Hairs are plucked in the direction of growth, removing the hair bulb and shaft. Brush the coat of long-haired cats for 10 minutes with a new toothbrush. Submit the whole brush and hair plucking for fungal culture to identify cats infected with *Microsporum canis.*
- Skin scrapes (Fisher 1999): Collect material using a scalpel blade held perpendicular to the skin. The skin should be scraped until there is capillary ooze. The material may then be transferred to a slide for preparation or a sterile container for submission to a referral laboratory.
- Impression smears: provide material from pustules or ulcerated lesions for cytological examination. Pustules are punctured using a sterile needle and the contents 'touched' onto a smear. The smear is stained and examined for evidence of inflammation and organisms. Material is also collected onto a swab for culture.

Samples for cytological examination

Cytology is the study of individual cells and groups of cells aspirated from tissue or body fluids. Smears for examination are prepared by:

- Direct squash preparation (Fig. 5.5).
- Direct wedge/line smear. A line smear is similar to a routine blood smear but the spreader slide is stopped before reaching the end of the smear. The spreader is lifted, creating a line of fluid on the smear.
- Sediment squash smear. Sediment is prepared from a body cavity fluid by centrifugation at 1000–2000 rpm for 5 minutes.

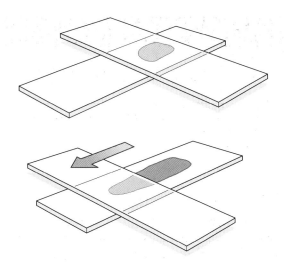

Figure 5.5 Preparation of a squash smear for cytological examination. Only a very small amount of material should be used for each smear. Rapid drying is required and it may be necessary to use a hair dryer (air flow directed on to the back of the slide) for viscous material, i.e. synovial fluid.

The supernatant is removed, leaving a few drops in which the pellet of cells is re-suspended (by gently flicking the bottom of the tube). A squash smear is made from the cellular material.

If the samples are to be referred to a commercial laboratory for analysis, then it is essential to liaise with the pathologist or refer to the laboratory guidelines prior to sampling, since some pathologists prefer to examine fixed material. Table 5.12 outlines the types of samples that might be collected, and the preferred method of sample preparation.

Samples for histological examination

Histology is the study of a section of tissue in which the three-dimensional architecture of the tissue has been maintained. It requires fixation of the sample, commonly using a fixative based on formalin, e.g. 10% formal saline (Bloxham 1999). The material may be collected using small biopsy punches, Tru-Cut biopsy needles, bone marrow core biopsy needles or by surgical methods. The sample should be fixed immediately according to the following guidelines:

Table 5.12 Uses of cytology in veterinary medicine and sample requirements

Type of sample	Sample preparation method
Fine needle aspirate	Direct squash smears
Lymph node aspirate	Direct squash smears
Peritoneal fluid	Sediment, squash or line smears
Pleural fluid	Sediment, squash or line smears
Cerebrospinal fluid	Specialist centrifuge required. Contact laboratory
Prostatic wash	Direct or sediment smears
Urine	Sediment, squash or line smears
Synovial fluid	Direct squash smears
Tracheal wash	Direct squash smears of mucus. Sediment smears of remaining fluid

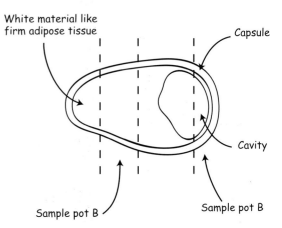

8 cm x 6 cm soft mass, lateral aspect, left elbow

Figure 5.6 Example of submission information for histological examination. Details should include the location of the lesion, its size, texture and gross appearance, in addition to a 'map' of the submitted tissue (if the whole mass has not been sent).

- Thick material must be divided so that the maximum width of any portion is not greater than 1 cm. This allows adequate and rapid penetration of the fixative.
- The volume of fixative should be at least 10 times greater than the volume of tissue to be fixed.
- The use of card to flatten biopsy specimens, e.g. intestinal samples, is not recommended by many pathologists. Practices should contact their own pathologist for advice.
- Details must be submitted to the pathologist (Fig. 5.6).

Dispatch of samples

The postal regulations for packaging pathological material have been reviewed elsewhere (Bloxham 1999, Duncan and Broadley 1999). Commercial laboratories provide specific containers, which should always be used when posting samples.

HAEMATOLOGY

CELL DEVELOPMENT

The cells of the blood include erythrocytes, leucocytes and platelets. Each has a specific function in the maintenance of health. The cells develop from the pluripotent stem cell in the bone marrow (Fig. 5.7). The mitotic divisions facilitate production of many mature cells from a small population of stem cells (Fig. 5.8). Neoplastic transformation of the stem cells can result in leukaemia.

GENERATING THE HAEMATOLOGY PROFILE

The haematology profile is an essential part of the assessment of many sick patients and can be expected to provide information regarding the nature (although not usually the location) of the pathological process. The analysis includes two components:

1. Quantitative analysis provides a numerical assessment of the red cell mass, a statistical description of the appearance of the red cells, e.g. mean cell size and variation in cell size, the number of leucocytes, and a platelet count.
2. Qualitative analysis allows a microscopic examination for morphological changes in the cells, which cannot be appreciated by numerical means.

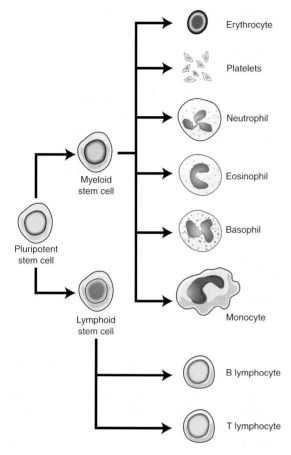

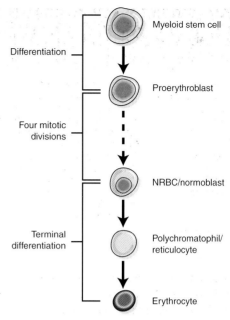

Figure 5.8 Terminal differentiation of erythroid cells produces nucleated red blood cells (NRBCs or normoblasts), polychromatophilic cells (or reticulocytes) and mature erythrocytes. Mitotic divisions produce 16 mature cells from each erythroid precursor.

Figure 5.7 Differentiation of the pluripotent stem cell into myeloid and lymphatic cells. The myeloid stem cell develops into platelets, erythrocytes, neutrophils, eosinophils, basophils and monocytes.

Quantitative analysis

In recent years there has been an increase in the number of patient-side or in-clinic analysers which provide a quantitative haematological analysis. The number of parameters produced by each analyser depends upon the method of analysis and the individual analyser (Box 5.2).

The total nucleated count generated by automated cell counters includes any nucleated red blood cells (NRBCs/normoblasts) which were present. Since these are not part of the leucocyte profile and should be counted separately, the total nucleated count must be corrected for this error. The corrected total leucocyte count is calculated by the haematologist/clinician performing the

---

Box 5.2 Erythrocyte, leucocyte and platelet parameters generated by haematology analysers

Erythrocytes

RBC	red blood cells ($\times10^{12}$/l)
Hb	haemoglobin (g/dl)
PCV	an estimate of the red cell volume measured by microhaematocrit tube (%)
Hct	calculated measurement using the MCV and red cell count (l/l)
MCV	the average size of the erythrocytes (fl)
MCH	the Hb per average erythrocyte (pg)
MCHC	mean concentration of Hb in the erythrocytes (g/dl)
RDW	red cell distribution width, which describes the variability of red cell size (%)

Leucocytes

Total nucleated cell count: includes leucocytes and nucleated red blood cells ($\times10^9$/l)
Total white cell count: total leucocytes ($\times10^9$/l)
Differential white cell count (2, 3 or 5 part differential)

Platelets

Plateletcount ($\times10^9$/l)
Mean platelet volume (fl)

Box 5.3 Calculating the total white cell count

Correcting the total nucleated cell count:
1. Include the NRBCs in the 100 cell differnetial
2. Calculate the absolute number of NRBCs (from the total nucleated cell count and % of NRBCs in the differential)
3. Subtract the absolute NRBC count from the total nucleated cell count

NRBC, nucleated red blood cell.

---

differential count (Box 5.3). The results of automated counters should be validated by performing a manual differential count on a minimum of 100 nucleated cells. The percentage of each cell type present is converted to an absolute number using the corrected total white cell count. The absolute cell counts, rather than the relative percentages, must be used when assessing the significance of quantitative abnormalities.

Three types of analyser are routinely used in veterinary medicine.

Impedance/electronic cell counters

These measure the electrical resistance as cells pass through a small aperture. Cells passing through the aperture are poor conductors and disrupt this current. A number of analysers are marketed for veterinary use and recent equipment gives a differential white cell count.

Laser counter

These use laser systems to detect the light scatter as the cells pass through a light beam. They provide the largest number of parameters and draw histograms to illustrate the cell populations. These analysers are primarily used in commercial laboratories.

Quantitative buffy coat analyser

One analyser for use in veterinary practice uses this technique. This form of analysis relies upon two principles:

1. Addition of a 'float' to a microhaematocrit tube spreads the cells in a thin layer between

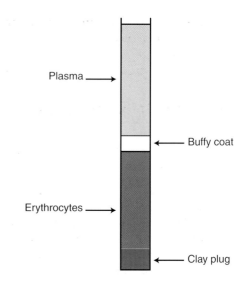

Figure 5.9 Diagrammatic representation of a centrifuged microhaematocrit tube and the estimation of the total leucocyte count.

the tube walls and the float, producing expansion of the buffy coat (Fig. 5.9).
2. The inside of the microhaematocrit tube is coated with a stain, which is taken up by cellular components. Cellular DNA and RNA display characteristic fluorescence, which allows differentiation of cell populations.

Microhaematocrit centrifuge method

An estimate of the number of erythrocytes and leucocytes can be easily obtained by measuring the PCV (Bloxham 1999) and the height of the buffy coat in a microhaematocrit tube (Villiers and Dunn 1998). The height of the buffy coat can be used as an approximate guide to the total leucocyte count (Fig. 5.9). The following may affect the accuracy of results using this method:

- failure to mix the sample adequately
- haemolysis
- incomplete centrifugation, either too short duration of centrifugation or failure of centrifuge to reach adequate speed.

Manual cell counts

Haematology profiles are generally produced by automated analysers. Manual counts using an improved Neubauer haemocytometer were previously used for whole blood and are still used for other fluids, e.g. joint fluid. Manual cell counts are still used in avian and reptilian haematology.

Sources of error in haematology profiles

The following features may produce erroneous haematology results:

1. Haemolysis more commonly occurs as a sample artefact rather than an in vivo change. Loss of intact cells results in inaccuracy of the PCV and red cell count. The measurement of haemoglobin is the only reliable red cell parameter. Multiplication of the haemoglobin by a factor of 3 gives a useful approximation of the PCV.
2. Lipaemia causes a spurious increase in haemoglobin concentration (measured by spectrophotometric methods). In these samples, the PCV and red cell count are more reliable indicators of the red cell mass. Lipaemia may predispose the red cells to lysis, therefore many lipaemic samples are also haemolysed. If the artefacts are marked then there is no reliable indicator of red cell mass.
3. Raised mean corpuscular haemoglobin concentration (MCHC) is always an erroneous finding and indicates the presence of interfering substances. Most commonly, the false increase is associated with lipaemia and haemoglobinaemia (from haemolysis), but the presence of Heinz bodies will also cause a spurious increase.
4. Auto-agglutination of red cells (see Haemolytic anaemia, below) falsely decreases the red cell count and the haematocrit on automated analysers and falsely increases the mean corpuscular volume (MCV). In these cases, measurement of the PCV using a microhaematocrit centrifuge, and the haemoglobin concentration, are the most reliable parameters.
5. Prolonged contact of the red cells with EDTA results in swelling which produces a falsely increased MCV.
6. Inadequate restraint of a patient during

sample collection, resulting in excessive 'probing' of the subcutaneous tissues and muscles, can cause a decrease in the platelet count and release of tissue clotting factors. In the latter, the activation of the clotting cascade produces shortened coagulation times.

Qualitative assessment

The examination of a blood film is an essential part of all haematological profiles. A large amount of information is available on a blood film, which cannot be provided by many haematology analysers (Table 5.13). It is important to remember that the red cell indices, i.e. MCV,

Table 5.13 Abnormalities which may be identified on a blood film, but not reflected in the profile results

Abnormality	Comments
Mild anisocytosis	Variation in red cell size can be assessed using the red cell distribution width (RDW) in more sophisticated analysers
Mild hypochromasia	
Polychromasia	Identification of polychromatophilic cells is an essential step in the assessment of anaemic patients. These are immature erythrocytes which have a bluish tint on Romanowsky-stained films
Rouleaux formation	Increased rouleaux support inflammation
Auto-agglutination	Associated with auto-immune haemolytic anaemia
Poikilocytosis	Changes in red cell shape which can help to direct further investigation, e.g. schistocytes, spherocytes
Identify band neutrophils	Increased numbers of band cells commonly reflect inflammation but analysers do not differentiate these cells from mature cells
Identify toxic change in neutrophils	Commonly noted with bacterial infection and toxaemia
Identify atypical cells	Identification of blast cells, e.g. lymphoblasts
Identification of platelet clumping	Platelet clumping can produce an erroneous thrombocytopenia. Examination of a blood film is essential to confirm this abnormality

mean corpuscular haemoglobin and MCHC, are average figures. It may take many large or small cells to change the MCV, but occasional large or small cells would be detected on microscopy.

Making a blood smear

Preparation of good-quality blood smears (Bloxham 1999) requires practice. The aim is to produce a monolayer of cells for examination (Fig. 5.10). Some common problems are associated with the use of poor-quality slides while others are a reflection of operator technique (Table 5.14).

Staining blood films for routine examination

Romanowsky stains are most commonly used for routine haematological examination, e.g. Wright's stain, Leishman's stain. Rapid stains, e.g. Diff-Quik®, are most commonly used in veterinary practice. For fresh stain, it is usually sufficient to dip the slide in each stain five times. However, for thicker smears or older stain, the staining time must be increased. With the rapid stains, a number of problems may be encountered (Table 5.15). It is always preferable to make at least two blood films from each patient sample so that any staining problems can be corrected.

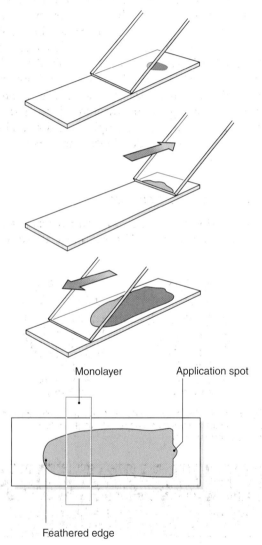

Figure 5.10 Preparation of a blood smear. The monolayer is the region in which approximately half of the erythrocytes are in contact. It is the best area of the smear in which to identify changes in the erythrocyte appearance and to perform a differential white cell count.

Monolayer   Application spot

Feathered edge

Table 5.14   Common problems in blood smear preparation

Smear appearance	Cause
Ragged smear edge	Spreader edge too dirty or rough
Blood extends over end of slide	Too much blood applied
Irregular cell distribution	Rough or dirty spreader or uneven pressure
Smear cracked and flaking	Too much blood and/or too thickly applied

Table 5.15   Common staining problems

Problem	Possible cause
Too blue (erythrocytes often blue/green)	Too long in blue stain Inadequate wash Exposure to formalin vapours
Too pink	Too long in red stain Inadequate time in blue stain
Weak staining	Poor contact with stains (ensure slide is well coated) Exhausted stains
Precipitate	Inadequate washing Dirty slides Bacteria and contaminants present

Staining for reticulocyte counts

In addition to the stains used for a routine blood film examination, it is often necessary to perform a reticulocyte count in anaemic patients. This allows differentiation between a regenerative and non-regenerative anaemia. A regenerative anaemia is one in which there is a bone marrow response with production and release of immature cells. Immature, RNA-rich erythrocytes are recognised as polychromatophilic cells (cells which stain bluish) on Romanowsky stains. Unfortunately, it can be difficult to appreciate this polychromasia (variation in red cell colour) using rapid stains, but the presence of immature cells can be confirmed using a supravital stain, e.g. new methylene blue (NMB). NMB causes precipitation of the intracellular ribosomal RNA protein, with the formation of dense blue aggregates in the immature cells. When identified using this staining technique, the immature cells are called reticulocytes (Fig. 5.11) and their presence indicates production and release of cells by the bone marrow. Canine reticulocytes contain a large amount of precipitated material in dense aggregates (aggregate reticulocytes). In the cat, two forms are noted: aggregate and punctate (Fig. 5.11). The former are similar to the canine form and rapidly mature into punctate reticulocytes. Punctate reticulocytes have 1–8 single 'dots' of precipitated material and a long survival time in the circulation (3–4 weeks). Routinely, only the aggregate reticulocytes are counted when performing a reticulocyte count in a cat. Reticulocyte count method is as follows:

- Equal quantities of *fresh* EDTA blood and 0.5% NMB in normal saline are placed in a tube and labelled. Mix contents.
- Incubate the contents of the tube at room temperature for 10–20 minutes.
- Mix contents.
- Make wedge smears of the NMB/blood mixture using the technique for a routine blood film.
- Observed reticulocyte count (%) = percentage of total red cells which are reticulocytes (count 500 cells).

- Calculate the absolute reticulocyte count:
  Absolute reticulocyte count = Observed reticulocyte % × RBC ($\times 10^{12}$/l) × 10.

The observed reticulocyte count is affected by the total number of red cells present, i.e. the same absolute number of reticulocytes will appear as a greater percentage of the red cell total if there is a severe anaemia versus a mild anaemia. Calculation of the absolute reticulocyte count takes into account the total number of red cells present and is the preferred method of recording reticulocyte data. Guidelines for interpretation of the absolute reticulocyte count in dogs and cats (Thrall 1997) are provided in Table 5.16. The manual count of reticulocytes is an imprecise method, due to the small number of cells counted, and can have significant variation if repeated on the same sample on multiple occasions. Flow cytometry may provide a better measurement in the future.

Examination of a blood film

Examination of a blood film requires practice but is made much easier if a routine procedure is

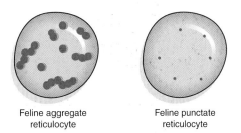

Figure 5.11 Feline aggregate and punctate reticulocytes. The punctate reticulocytes have 1–8 single 'dots' of precipitated material.

Table 5.16 Absolute reticulocyte numbers in dogs and cats	
Classification	Absolute reticulocyte count ($\times 10^9$/l)
Normal	>60
Non-regenerative anaemia	<60
Moderate regeneration	100–200
Marked regeneration	>300

applied (Table 5.17) and the aims of the examination initially limited to specific questions (Box 5.4). However, irrespective of the experience of the operator, there will always be occasions when a second opinion is desirable, if not essential.

Table 5.17	Routine examination of a blood film
Low-power examination	
Platelets	Check the tail for platelet clumping which will lower the count, especially in cats
Erythrocytes	Identify the monolayer
Leucocytes	General assessment of numbers and distribution. Large cells often travel to the feathered edge or the edges of the smear
High power examination (100× oil for most operators but experienced technicians may use 40×)	
Erythrocytes	Anisocytosis, polychromasia, variations in red cell shape (may be film artefacts or pathological)
Nucleated cells	Differential count is performed on 200 cells
Neutrophils	Band cells, toxic changes
Lymphocytes	Size, chromatin pattern and the presence of nucleoli. Referral indicated if abnormal cells are identified
Normoblasts	Included in the differential and then the total nucleated cell count is corrected. Degree of maturity should be noted
Monocytes	Excessive vacuolation?
Eosinophils	May be vacuolated in Greyhounds
Atypical cells	Referral is indicated
Platelets	Platelet size, anisocytosis and number. Each platelet per high power field = approximately 12–15 platelets × 10^9/l

HAEMATOLOGY: CELL IDENTIFICATION AND EFFECT OF DISEASE

Erythrocytes

Mature erythrocytes

The erythrocytes are biconcave discs, which are produced from precursors in the bone marrow. When viewed in a blood film, the biconcave structure produces the appearance of a dense outer rim with a pale centre. The red cells of the cat are smaller than those of the dog and the area of central pallor is less pronounced.

Immature erythrocytes

The NRBC or normoblast (Fig. 5.12) is the most immature erythroid cell commonly recognised in blood. It still contains a nuclear remnant, which is subsequently removed in the spleen. Identification of these cells may reflect:

1. regenerative anaemia (there should also be increased numbers of reticulocytes)
2. feline leukaemia virus (FeLV) infection
3. splenic disease
4. lead toxicity
5. bone marrow disease.

Loss of the nucleus from the NRBC produces a polychromatophilic cell (reticulocyte). These cells are larger than mature cells and appear bluish in Romanowsky-stained films. Polychromasia is the term given to the variation in cell colour noted

Box 5.4	Aims of blood film examination depending upon experience of operator	
Beginner	**Intermediate**	**Advanced**
Identify platelet clumps Perform manual platelet count Identify rouleaux Identify auto-agglutination Grade polychromasia Perform differential white cell count Identify band neutrophils Recognise atypical cells Perform reticulocyte count on new methylene blue preparation	As for beginner plus: Identify toxic change Identify reactive lymphocytes Recognise atypical cells Identify spherocytes and schistocytes Recognise the presence of intracellular parasites	As for intermediate plus: Recognise less common red cell changes Identify intracellular red cell parasites Identify subtle leucocyte morphological changes including alterations of granulation Discuss possible lineage and significance of blast cells present

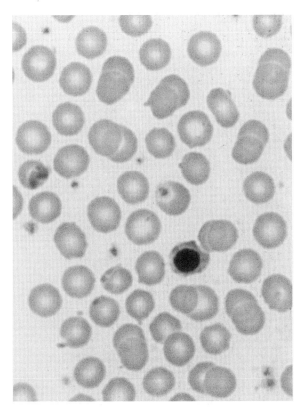

Figure 5.12 Nucleated red blood cells still contain nuclear remnant, which should be removed during the subsequent maturation process.

when immature erythrocytes are present. These cells can be difficult to recognise with the rapid haematology stains but are easy to identify if the blood is first mixed with NMB. If necessary, the number of immature cells can be quantified using a reticulocyte count.

Erythrocyte changes associated with disease

Changes in red cell number, size and appearance may direct the clinician towards specific disease processes. Information obtained from the blood analysis and smear examination (Table 5.17) is considered. The red cells are classified according to their size (macrocytic, normocytic and microcytic) and their density of staining (normochromic or hypochromic).

Changes in red cell size

- **Macrocytosis:** the presence of large erythrocytes. These are usually immature polychromatophilic cells. Less commonly, macrocytic normochromic cells are noted. These are an incidental finding in Poodle macrocytosis but are also associated with FeLV infection.
- **Microcytosis:** the presence of small cells. Commonly noted with iron deficiency or congenital portosystemic shunts. The cells are usually hypochromic.
- **Anisocytosis:** variation in erythrocyte size due to the presence of macrocytic or microcytic cells. The red cell distribution width is a measure of variation in cell size and is increased with anisocytosis.

Changes in red cell colour

- **Hypochromasia:** the presence of paler erythrocytes with a thin haemoglobinised rim and increased area of central pallor. Hypochromic, microcytic cells are commonly noted in iron deficiency and with portosystemic shunts.
- **Polychromasia:** variation in erythrocyte colour noted in Romanowsky stains due to the presence of immature erythrocytes. A semi-quantitative grading scheme is useful to ensure a standardised approach to recording polychromasia (Table 5.18).

Changes in red cell shape

- **Poikilocytosis:** a general term used to describe abnormalities of erythrocyte shape. More specific descriptions should be applied

Table 5.18 Semi-quantitative scheme for recording polychromasia based on the number of polychromatophilic cells per field using the oil immersion lens (Reagan et al 1998)

	1+	2+	3+	4+
Dog	2–7	8–14	15–29	>30
Cat	1–2	3–8	9–15	>15

where possible since the more specific terms may provide a clue to the underlying disease.

- **Echinocytes:** erythrocytes with uniform, short, evenly spaced, sharp to blunt cytoplasmic projections. They are commonly noted as an artefact associated with slow drying of blood films (also known as crenated cells) but can be secondary to uraemia or lymphoma in dogs.
- **Acanthocytes:** the cell membrane forms spicules of uneven distribution and variable length/diameter. Noted in dogs with liver disease, portosystemic shunts and vascular neoplasia (haemangioma/haemangiosarcoma).
- **Spherocytes:** appear as small spherical cells, which lack central pallor and appear darker than surrounding normal or immature erythrocytes. They are formed by removal of part of the cell membrane by macrophage activity triggered during haemolytic anaemia. These cells are difficult to recognise in the cat because of the small size of normal erythrocytes, and their presence should be confirmed by an experienced haematologist.
- **Schistocytes:** an irregular red cell fragment. Present in dogs with haemangiosarcoma, disseminated intravascular coagulation (DIC), cardiac disease and glomerulonephritis.
- **Target cells/leptocytes:** these cells have a dense central area surrounded by a clear zone and an outer haemoglobinised rim. Target cells are often present in dogs with liver disease, iron deficiency anaemia and post-splenectomy but are not specific for these disease processes.

Red cell inclusions

- **NRBCs/normoblasts:** the presence of NRBCs may reflect a regenerative response but is also associated with splenic disease and FeLV infection.
- **Howell–Jolly bodies:** small, dense nuclear remnants resulting from incomplete extrusion of the nucleus. These are generally removed by the spleen and are therefore commonly identified in splenectomised patients and in immature red cells during a regenerative response.

- **Basophilic stippling:** fine dark-blue staining in the red cells (Wright's stained films). They are recognised in cats with a regenerative response but if they are identified in the dog then consideration should be given to lead toxicity.
- *Haemobartonella: H. felis* appears as dark purple, coccoid, rod-shaped or ring-like structures at the edge of the cell. The parasites 'fall off' the cells when blood is mixed with an anticoagulant and smears should be made immediately after collection and straight from the hub of the collection syringe. It can be difficult to differentiate the parasite from stain precipitate. The parasitaemia may be cyclical and multiple examinations or trial treatments are advisable before excluding this diagnosis. *H. canis* is rarely recognised except in splenectomised dogs, where it may be an incidental finding.
- *Babesia canis:* teardrop shaped organisms present inside, and occasionally, outside, the erythrocytes. They are often noted in pairs. Infected red cells commonly migrate to the tail of the blood film (Fig. 5. 13).
- **Heinz bodies:** single refractile, or pale-staining projections from the erythrocyte. They are a consequence of haemoglobin denaturation secondary to oxidant injuries and are noted especially in cats. They are found in normal cats although there is marked variation in the percentage noted as an incidental finding (5–45%). Both hyperthyroidism and diabetes mellitus in the cat are particularly associated with their formation (see Haemolytic anaemia, below).

Changes in red cell arrangement

- **Rouleaux formation:** the formation of 'stacks' of red cells. A mild degree of rouleaux is normal in the cat, but an increase is associated with increased plasma proteins and inflammatory disease.
- **Auto-agglutination** is identified by microscopic examination as clumps of red cells, which appear similar to a bunch of grapes. Agglutination must be differentiated from rouleaux. The latter usually disperses

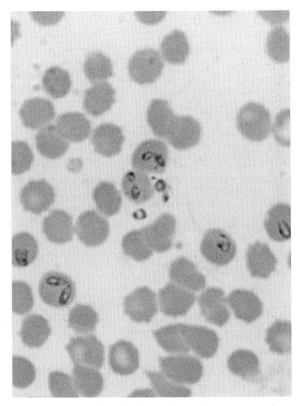

Figure 5.13 *Babesia canis* often appears as paired intracellular organisms.

Table 5.19 Guidelines to the classification of the severity of anaemia on the basis of packed cell volume (%)		
Degree of anaemia	Dog	Cat
Mild	30–37	20–26
Moderate	20–29	14–19
Severe	13–19	10–13
Very severe	<13	<10

consideration should be given to breed variation when assessing the degree of anaemia, e.g. normal Greyhounds, German Shepherd dogs and Boxers have raised PCVs. In addition, the PCV may take 12–24 hours to decrease after an acute blood loss. In these cases, the PCV may appear relatively normal but the patient shows signs of circulatory collapse and haemorrhage may be evident. In general, persistent, mild anaemias are secondary to metabolic or inflammatory disease, while moderate to severe anaemia reflects haemorrhage, red cell destruction or suppression of production.

Erythrocyte statistics

Erythrocytes are classified according to their size (macrocytic, normocytic and microcytic) and their density of staining (normochromic or hypochromic) (Fig. 5.14).

when the sample is diluted (1:1) with saline. Auto-agglutination is associated with haemolytic anaemia.

THE INVESTIGATION OF ANAEMIA

Anaemia is defined as a decrease in the red cell mass, which may be classified according to the following:

- severity of anaemia
- erythrocyte statistics, i.e. erythrocyte volume and density of haemoglobin per cell
- regenerative versus non-regenerative according to the degree of marrow response.

Severity of anaemia

The PCV is generally used to provide a guide to the degree of anaemia (Table 5.19). However,

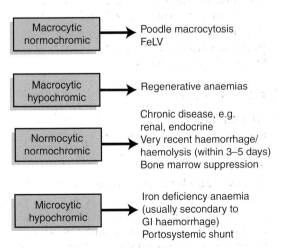

Figure 5.14 Possible causes of anaemia, with regard to red cell statistics. FeLV, feline leukaemia virus; GI, gastrointestinal.

Degree of regeneration

Anaemia may be classified by the degree of regeneration present. A regenerative anaemia is one in which there is an appropriate increase in red cell production. It may be necessary to perform a reticulocyte count to classify the degree of regeneration present (Table 5.16). The classification of an anaemia as regenerative or non-regenerative can help to identify possible underlying causes (Box 5.5).

Regenerative anaemia

Acute haemorrhage

Acute, recent haemorrhage is not reflected in the PCV until the fluid volume has been restored. Without fluid therapy this may take 12–24 hours. During this time there may be a decline in the PCV and often the plasma proteins (Box 5.6). The measurement of plasma proteins and a platelet count are essential in assessing an anaemic patient. Evidence of regeneration is not noted until 3–5 days after the initial incident. If there is continued blood loss then there may be a decline in PCV despite a moderate to marked increase in production and release of immature erythrocytes.

Chronic haemorrhage

Chronic external haemorrhage is most commonly associated with parasitism in young animals and intestinal disease in adults. A regenerative response is noted after the first 3–5 days, but prolonged blood loss (weeks/months) results in depletion of the body iron stores and iron deficiency anaemia. Morphologically, iron deficiency anaemia is characterised by microcytic, hypochromic red cells (Box 5.7). Iron deficiency anaemia is rare in cats but may occur in young kittens secondary to flea infestation. Canine iron deficiency anaemia is commonly a consequence of chronic gastrointestinal (GI) haemorrhage associated with neoplasia, ulceration or, in young animals, parasitic disease. The morphological features of the anaemia are usually sufficient to support iron deficiency. In early cases, measurement of serum iron may reveal a reduced concen-

Box 5.5	Causes of anaemia in the dog and cat	
Regenerative anaemia	**Non-regenerative anaemia**
Haemorrhage	Very recent haemorrhage or
Haemolytic anaemia	haemolysis (within 3–5 days)
	Bone marrow suppression
	Iron deficiency anaemia
	(late-stage)

Box 5.6	Features of acute haemorrhage
PCV/Hb only reduced after 12–24 hours	
Normocytic, non-regenerative until 3–5 days	
Macrocytic after 3–5 days due to release of immature cells from marrow	
Decreased plasma proteins after 12 hours for external blood loss. Proteins may be normal for intracavity haemorrhage	
Thrombocytopenia followed by thrombocytosis	

PCV, packed cell volume; Hb, haemoglobin.

Box 5.7	Features of iron-deficiency anaemia
Features of chronic haemorrhage	
Microcytosis	
Hypochromasia	
Usually mild to moderate regeneration at the time of presentation but progresses to non-regenerative	
Thrombocytosis	

tration but this is also a feature of inflammatory disease and is not specific for a depletion of body stores. Absence of stainable bone marrow iron provides confirmation but is not commonly used clinically. A faecal occult blood test can be used to confirm GI haemorrhage but false positive results are noted in dogs fed commercial foods and the diet should be meat free for 3–5 days prior to sampling.

Haemolytic anaemia

Haemolytic anaemia results from an increased rate of red cell destruction. Most commonly, the cells are phagocytosed in the spleen, liver or bone marrow (extravascular haemolysis). Rarely, red cells may be lysed and release haemoglobin in the circulation (intravascular haemolysis). Haemolytic disease (>4 days' duration) is generally accompanied by evidence of marked erythropoiesis, including the presence of an increase in reticulocytes, nucleated red cells and Howell–Jolly bodies. Other classical changes are noted in Box 5.8. Most cases of haemolytic anaemia in the dog are primary immune-mediated haemolytic anaemia. Other causes are listed in Table 5.20.

NON-REGENERATIVE ANAEMIAS

Diagnostic considerations

Non-regenerative anaemia could be caused by bone marrow suppression or by very recent haemorrhage or haemolysis (prior to the onset of a marrow response). The following factors are considered when investigating a non-regenerative anaemia:

1. Onset and nature of signs. Animals with recent onset haemolytic disease or haemorrhage often show significant clinical signs at PCV >20%. Signs include collapse, lethargy, tachypnoea and fever. Patients (especially cats) with non-regenerative anaemia may not present until the PCV is very low (even <10%).
2. Persistent? If there is no evidence of regeneration then further testing in 3–5 days can be useful to confirm a poor marrow response.

3. Severity of anaemia. Mild/moderate, persistent, non-regenerative anaemia is usually associated with systemic or inflammatory disease (Box 5.7). Diagnostic efforts should be directed toward identifying the underlying cause.
4. Red cell morphology changes? Iron deficiency, lead toxicity and FeLV infection may all cause non-regenerative anaemia but would commonly produce changes in red

---

Box 5.8 Features of haemolytic disease

Highly regenerative with marked polychromasia*
High reticulocyte count*
Normal plasma proteins
Spherocytosis
Coombs test positive in approximately two thirds of cases
Auto-agglutination
Platelet count normal except where there is concurrent immune-mediated thrombocytopenia

* Non-regenerative form of disease caused by destruction of marrow precursors.

Table 5.20 Causes of haemolytic anaemia in the dog and cat

Causes of haemolytic anaemia	Comment
Auto-immune haemolytic anaemia	
Secondary immune-mediated haemolytic anaemia	Associated with SLE, neoplasia, inflammatory disease
Cold agglutinin disease	Antibody attaches to red cells in cooler regions of the body, i.e. ear tips, tail tips and paws, resulting in ischaemic necrosis
Transfusion reactions	Blood type and cross-match essential for any cat transfusion and second and subsequent dog transfusions
Neonatal isoerythrolysis	
Haemobartonella felis and *canis*	
Babesia canis	
Heinz body anaemia	Heinz body production in cats with diabetes mellitus, lymphoma and hyperthyroidism. Onion toxicity in dogs
Microangiopathic haemolytic anaemia	Red cells damaged while passing through vascular neoplasms and fibrin mesh, e.g. disseminated intravascular coagulation
Pyruvate kinase deficiency	Inadequate provision of energy for red cell function. Seen in the Basenji and Beagle
Phosphofructokinase deficiency	English Springer Spaniel

SLE, systemic lupus erythematosus.

Box 5.7 Causes of mild non-regenerative anaemia in the dog and cat

Anaemia of chronic or inflammatory disease
Renal disease
Endocrine disease, e.g. hypothyroidism
Liver disease

cell morphology, e.g. microcytic, hypochromic erythrocytes associated with iron deficiency.
5. Leucopenia and/or thrombocytopenia? If suppression of multiple cell lines is noted then bone marrow suppression is likely to be a consequence of drug therapy, oestrogen excess (Sertoli cell neoplasia of the testicles), FeLV infection or neoplasia.
6. Abnormal cells present? The presence of atypical cells in the peripheral blood could reflect neoplasia
7. None of the above? Where no morphological changes of the red cells are noted, or where there is no other evidence of bone marrow suppression then immune-mediated destruction of the red cell precursors in the bone marrow is most likely. FeLV is a possible cause.

The observations help to formulate a differential diagnosis list and select further tests. However, in most cases of non-regenerative anaemia, examination of a bone marrow aspirate or core biopsy is likely to be required.

Reaching a definitive diagnosis

Bone marrow examination is necessary for the investigation of moderate/severe, non-regenerative anaemia, where the initial haematology screen and biochemistry panel has failed to provide a diagnosis. It is essential in the investigation of bicytopenia, pancytopenia and when abnormal cells have been identified in the peripheral circulation. An EDTA sample for a haematology profile should be collected at the same time as the marrow. The sites for bone marrow collection are indicated in Figure 5.15. A bone marrow aspirate needle and core biopsy needle are essential for collection of a marrow aspirate and biopsy, respectively. Only a small amount of material is aspirated, and squash smears are made immediately (Villiers and Dunn 1998).

BLOOD TYPING AND CROSSMATCHING

Canine blood types

The canine blood-typing system has been described extensively elsewhere (see Further Reading) and classification is according to the surface antigens on the red cells. The presence of eight dog erythrocyte antigens is commonly accepted but laboratory testing is not available for all antigens and is only routinely available for DEA1.1. DEA1.1 is the most antigenic blood type. When DEA1.1-positive blood is transfused into a DEA1.1-negative individual, it produces a strong antibody reaction, which, in turn, causes a haemolytic reaction if transfusion of this patient with DEA1.1 is repeated. The transfusion reaction may start within minutes of blood administration and results in rapid removal/destruction of transfused red cells. Clinical signs include tachycardia, hypotension, dyspnoea and tremors. Canine blood grouping is most commonly used to identify suitable blood donors within a veterinary practice. Donors should be DEA 1.1-negative.

Feline blood types

There are three blood types in the cat: A, B and AB. A recent study has shown that type A is more common in the UK than type B or type AB (Knottenbelt et al 1999). However, in some breeds, especially the British shorthaired, Rex and Birman, the frequency of type B is much higher. Unlike dogs, cats have naturally occurring antibodies to other blood types. Type B cats over 3 months of age have high titres of anti-A antibodies, which act as haemolysins and haemagglutinins. Type B cats, transfused with type A blood, develop rapid, and often fatal, transfusion reactions, while type A or AB kittens born to type B queens develop neonatal isoerythrolysis. All

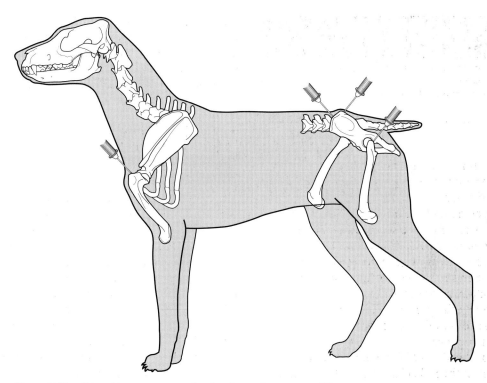

Figure 5.15 Sites of bone marrow collection: femur, humerus and iliac crest.

cats and potential donors should be cross-matched prior to transfusion

POLYCYTHAEMIA

Polycythaemia is an increase in the PCV, red blood cell count and haemoglobin.

Relative polycythaemia

Polycythaemia commonly reflects dehydration, which causes a concurrent increase in plasma protein concentration. Relative polycythaemia responds well to fluid therapy. Splenic contraction may transiently increase in the PCV in some breeds, e.g. Greyhounds.

Secondary polycythaemia

Polycythaemia may develop secondary to chronic hypoxic states, e.g. cardiac disease and severe pulmonary disease. Neoplastic processes, which produce increased quantities of erythropoietin,

also cause secondary polycythaemia. These include renal carcinoma and renal lymphoma.

Primary polycythaemia

This is an absolute increase in red cell mass without evidence of haemoconcentration. Primary polycythaemia is characterised by a persistently high PCV in the absence of causes of secondary polycythaemia. The clinical signs include central nervous system (CNS) disturbances, brick red mucous membranes and weakness. Primary polycythaemia has only been reported in small numbers of cats and dogs but the condition has been successfully managed by repeated removal of blood or the use of hydroxyurea.

LEUCOCYTES: CELL MORPHOLOGY
Neutrophils

Mature/segmented neutrophils possess a nucleus with darkly stained clumped chromatin and 3–5 nuclear lobes (Fig. 5.16). The cytoplasm of the cell is clear/pale pink and contains indistinct granules.

Band neutrophils are approximately the size of mature cells but the nucleus has parallel sides with no lobulation (Fig. 5.17). Small numbers of band cells can be noted in normal peripheral blood, but an increase in numbers is called a 'left shift'.

Toxic changes in neutrophils are usually a consequence of bacterial infection or toxaemia. The presence of these changes in a blood film should always be noted (Box 5.10).

Hypersegmented neutrophils (>5 nuclear lobes) are found in dogs on corticosteroid therapy and may be associated with uraemia (increased blood urea concentration). In addition, they can be recognised in Poodles as an incidental finding.

Eosinophils

The nucleus of an eosinophil is less segmented than a neutrophil and is often bilobed. They possess cytoplasmic granules, which are generally orange–red and loosely pack the cell but have a variable appearance depending on the species. The granules in the dog are approximately round

Box 5.10   Toxic changes in neutrophils
Chromatin less condensed (and therefore paler) and the nuclear lobes wider than normal cells
Cytoplasmic basophilia (light blue or grey hue rather than the normal pink)
Döhle bodies present. These are small blue round or angular inclusions in the cytoplasm
Cytoplasmic vacuolation is noted in severe toxaemia

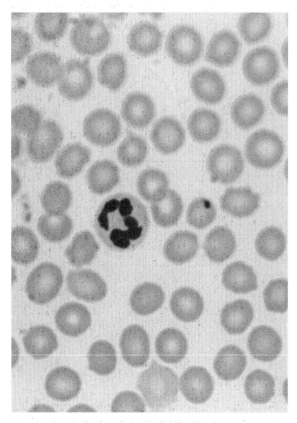

Figure 5.16 Mature neutrophil with darkly stained nuclear chromatin and nuclear lobes.

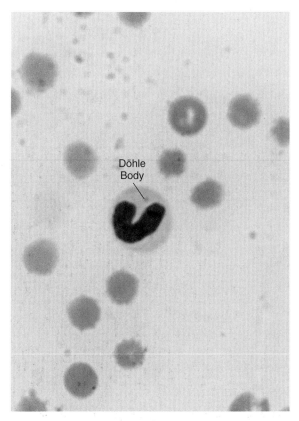

Döhle Body

Figure 5.17 Band neutrophil with parallel sides. This cell contains a Döhle body.

while those of the cat are rod-shaped. Canine eosinophils can display some vacuolation, but in the Greyhound they are highly vacuolated.

Basophils

These cells are rare in normal blood but have a ribbon-like nucleus in the dog, with red-violet granules, which can obscure the nucleus. In the cat, the granules are orange/lavender on a grey cytoplasmic background.

Monocytes

On average, these are the largest circulating cells in normal blood (Fig. 5.18) and have a very variable nuclear appearance with relatively abundant grey/blue cytoplasm, which has a ground-glass

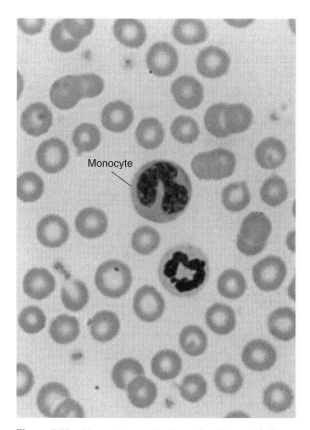

Figure 5.18 Monocytes are the largest cells in normal peripheral blood. A monocyte is present at the top with mature neutrophil below.

appearance. The cytoplasm may contain vacuoles. The nuclei of some cells resemble those of immature neutrophils (bands, metamyelocytes) and differentiation can be difficult. The monocyte nuclei have a lacy chromatin pattern with some areas of condensation. The chromatin is less clumped than neutrophil nuclear chromatin.

Lymphocytes

Small mature lymphocytes are smaller than neutrophils. In the dog, the nucleus is similar in size to an erythrocyte. They possess round nuclei (occasionally oval or indented) with dark, condensed chromatin and a narrow rim of pale blue cytoplasm, which is often not clearly visible.

Reactive lymphocytes are larger cells with basophilic cytoplasm. The nuclear chromatin is still mature in appearance. The nucleus may be larger and more convoluted.

Lymphoblasts are larger cells (2–3 × red cells) with a smooth nuclear chromatin pattern and prominent nucleoli or nucleolar rings. The nucleolus is a round, pale blue structure surrounded by a denser ring of chromatin.

Mast cells

This is a large cell with a round nucleus and deeply staining reddish-purple granules, which obscure the nucleus. These cells are rarely found in peripheral blood.

LEUCOCYTES IN DISEASE

Abnormalities of the white blood cells may be noted in disease. The abnormalities include changes in the number of cells present (Table 5.21) and changes in their appearance or function. Alterations in appearance (morphological changes) can only be identified by microscopic examination.

Neutrophilia

Neutrophilia is a commonly noted abnormality, which can be associated with physiological or pathological conditions (Table 5.22).

Inflammation

The leucocyte patterns associated with inflammation depend on the duration and nature of the inflammatory focus, and the patient's ability to mount a response. The differentiation between a corticosteroid-mediated stress response and an inflammatory response can only be made if there is evidence of a left shift, toxic change of the neutrophils, or a very marked increase in the total white cell count (Fig. 5.19). The absence of leucogram changes does not completely exclude the possibility of inflammatory disease. Measurement of serum proteins, serum protein electrophoresis (SPE), survey radiography and complete urinalysis may all provide helpful information, depending on the initial presenting signs. Measurement of total proteins and SPE can provide evidence of inflammatory disease where the leucogram does not show significant changes.

Degenerative left shift

A 'degenerative left shift' indicates that the number of immature neutrophils is greater than or equal to the number of segmented cells. This pattern is most common in the early stages of Gram-negative sepsis and where there is inflammation affecting a large surface area, e.g. peritonitis. There may be a left shift or degenerative left shift without a change in total leucocyte count. In these cases, examination of a blood film will give the only indication of the presence of an inflam-

Table 5.21 Quantitative leucocyte changes noted in physiological and pathological conditions

Abnormality	Definition	Common causes
Neutrophilia	Increased number of neutrophils	Inflammation, glucocorticoids, adrenaline (epinephrine), hyperadrenocorticism
Neutropenia	Decreased number of neutrophils	Severe infection, bone marrow suppression, chemotherapy
Lymphocytosis	Increased number of lymphocytes	Viral infection, leukaemia, adrenaline (epinephrine) (especially young cats)
Lymphopenia	Decreased number of lymphocytes	Viral infection, neoplasia, stress, glucocorticoids
Monocytosis	Increased number of monocytes	Inflammation including tissue necrosis, glucocorticoids (dogs)
Eosinophilia	Increased number of eosinophils	Parasite burden or allergic disease of the intestinal or respiratory tract, or skin
Eosinopenia	Reduced number of eosinophils	Glucocorticoid therapy, hyperadrenocorticism

Table 5.22 Common causes of neutrophilia

Causes of neutrophilia	Characteristics	Comment
Adrenaline (epinephrine)-mediated leucocytosis	Neutrophilia Normal/increased lymphocytes Normal/increased eosinophils	Common in young excited cats
Corticosteroid-mediated leucocytosis	Total white cell count can be as high as 30×10^9/l Neutrophilia (no left shift) Eosinopenia Lymphopenia (or low–normal count) Monocytosis (dog only)	Associated with drug therapy, chronic illness and hyperadrenocorticism
Inflammation	Neutrophilia +/– Left shift +/– Toxic change +/– Increased rouleaux +/– Abnormal serum protein electrophotesis	It can be impossible to differentiate between inflammation and corticosteroid-mediated (see text)
Leukaemoid reaction	Neutrophilia $> 50 \times 10^9$/l	Severe localised inflammation, e.g. closed pyometra, and haemolytic anaemia

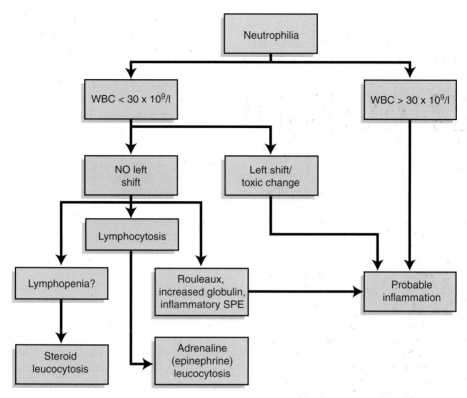

Figure 5.19 Identification of the causes of neutrophilia in the dog and cat. WBC, white blood cell; NO, nitric oxide; SPE, serum protein electrophoresis.

matory response and may also reveal evidence of toxic change of the neutrophils.

NEOPLASIA
Lymphoid neoplasia

Lymphoid neoplasia results from the neoplastic transformation of a single lymphocyte (T or B cell).

Canine lymphoma (lymphosarcoma)

Neoplasia arises in tissues other than the bone marrow, e.g. spleen, liver, lymph nodes and intestinal tract, but the skin, eye and nervous tissue may also be affected. The marrow becomes infiltrated in some cases resulting in suppression of bone marrow function. Neoplastic cells may

be identified in the peripheral blood of affected patients. In most cases these cells have the appearance of immature lymphoid cells, which are larger than mature lymphocytes, with deeply basophilic cytoplasm. The nuclear chromatin pattern is paler and less clumped than a mature cell. A veterinary haematologist should confirm the identity of these cells. Examination of a blood smear does not allow confirmation of lymphoma and fine needle aspirate or biopsy of lymph nodes or affected tissue is required.

Feline lymphoma

FeLV causes the majority of lymphoid and myeloid tumours in the cat. Lymphoma in the cat is also classed by the anatomic location, i.e. mediastinal, alimentary, renal, multicentric and extranodal, and the clinical signs vary depending on the location of the neoplastic infiltrate.

Acute lymphoblastic leukaemia (ALL)

This neoplasm arises in the marrow and extends to the liver and spleen (occasionally lymph nodes). In ALL the neoplastic cells are immature lymphoid cells, which are often present in large numbers in the circulating blood and marrow. In some cases it is difficult to differentiate between immature lymphoid cells and blast cells of the granulocyte line. In these cases, cytochemical staining is necessary to differentiate between ALL and acute myeloid leukaemia. The marrow is replaced to such an extent that there is concurrent thrombocytopenia and neutropenia (moderate to severe). Anaemia (to varying degrees) may also be present. ALL has a rapid clinical progression.

Chronic lymphocytic leukaemia (CLL)

This form of leukaemia is characterised by a moderate to marked lymphocytosis in peripheral blood. The cells have the appearance of small mature lymphocytes. This form of neoplasia is recognised in older patients and may be identified as an incidental finding during investigation of another disease process. The marrow is infiltrated to varying degrees at the time of diagnosis and the spleen, liver and lymph nodes may be enlarged. When the tumour burden is large and the marrow severely infiltrated then patients also present with signs related to thrombocytopenia and anaemia.

Haematopoietic neoplasia

Leukaemia is a neoplastic process involving one or more of the haematopoietic cell types. They may be classified as acute or chronic, depending on the maturity of the neoplastic cells, the degree of bone marrow infiltration and the clinical course. In acute leukaemia there is a predominance of immature (blast) cells in the circulation and bone marrow, frequently with evidence of concurrent suppression of normal haematopoiesis. Chronic leukaemia is characterised by the presence of mature cells in the peripheral blood and marrow. In cats, haematopoietic neoplasms are often associated with FeLV infection.

Diagnosis of leukaemia is likely to require specialised cytochemical staining techniques on peripheral blood, cytological examination of a bone marrow aspirate and, possibly, biopsy of internal organs. Acute leukaemia in the dog and cat generally carries a poor prognosis and is treated on an individual basis. Large studies of therapeutic protocols have not been carried out.

Myelodysplastic syndrome (MDS)

MDS and 'preleukaemia' are terms used to describe a group of disorders which precede the development of overt leukaemia (usually acute myeloid leukaemia). The disease may progress over a period of months to years. There are many possible manifestations, but MDS is characterised by abnormalities of cell maturation and production resulting in anaemia, neutropenia and thrombocytopenia (singly or in combination). In cats with FeLV, the anaemia of MDS is often non-regenerative and macrocytic–normochromic (although may be normocytic–normochromic).

HAEMOSTASIS

Haemostasis is commonly divided into three stages:

1. Primary haemostasis indicates the initial responses to vascular injury, which include vasoconstriction and the formation of a primary platelet plug. The proteins released during primary haemostasis trigger secondary haemostasis.
2. Secondary haemostasis includes the initiation of the clotting cascade which results in the deposition of fibrin round the platelet plug, forming a clot.
3. Fibrinolysis indicates the mechanisms that limit the clot formation to the localised region, preventing widespread thrombosis.

Investigation of bleeding disorders

Bleeding disorders may be classified as abnormalities of primary or secondary haemostasis and are inherited or acquired (Feldman 1992) (Box 5.11). Diagnosis is based on the results of

> **Box 5.11** Disorders of primary and secondary haemostasis
>
> | Primary haemostasis | Secondary haemostasis |
> | --- | --- |
> | Thrombocytopenia | Rodenticide toxicity |
> | Platelet dysfunction | Liver disease/biliary stasis |
> | Von Willebrand's disease | Haemophilias |
> | Vasculitis | Disseminated intravascular coagulation (DIC) |

> **Table 5.23** Clinical signs associated with bleeding disorders
>
> | Primary haemostasis | Secondary haemostasis |
> | --- | --- |
> | Petechiae common (mucous membranes, skin) | Petechiae rare |
> | Haematomas rare | Haematomas common |
> | Bleeding usually at multiple sites | Bleeding frequently localised |
> | Mucosal haemorrhage: epistaxis, haematuria, melaena | Bleeding into muscles or joints common |
> | Bleeding from cuts (or venepuncture sites) prolonged | Delayed bleeding after venepuncture; initially stops then restarts |
> | | Bleeding associated with shedding teeth in inherited disease |

laboratory testing which is often selected according to the signalment, history and clinical signs.

Spontaneous or excessive bleeding following surgery or trauma is relatively common in the dog but rare in cats. Severe inherited disease usually presents by 6 months of age. Milder forms may only become evident after surgery or trauma. Disorders of primary and secondary haemostasis produce different clinical presentations (Table 5.23).

Haemostatic evaluation

Laboratory tests can be divided into those used to assess primary haemostasis, or secondary haemostasis (Box 5.12). The tests commonly used in practice are described in more detail.

Platelet count

Platelet counts can be derived by automated methods but the presence of thrombocytopenia should be confirmed on examination of a stained blood film. All samples should be checked for evidence of clot formation before analysis. During film examination the presence of platelet clumps, which are identifiable in the tail of the smear, should be recorded since these will result in an erroneous decrease in the platelet count. The platelet count may be estimated from the blood film (using the 100× objective) as follows:

$$\frac{\text{Each platelet per}}{\text{high power field}} = \frac{\text{approximately}}{12\text{–}15 \text{ platelets} \times 10^9/\text{l}}$$

The size and morphology of the platelets should also be noted. In the dog, most platelets are less than a quarter of the diameter of an ery-

> **Box 5.12** Tests used in the investigation of bleeding disorders
>
> | Primary haemostasis | Secondary haemostasis |
> | --- | --- |
> | Platelet count | Cuticle bleeding time: this test has been used for identification of coagulopathies but is also affected by abnormalities in primary haemostasis and is very painful |
> | Buccal mucosal bleeding time | Whole blood clotting time |
> | Clot retraction time | Activated clotting time (ACT) |
> | | Activated partial thromboplastin time (APPT) |
> | | One-stage prothrombin time (OSPT) |
> | | Thrombin time (TT) |

throcyte. Larger platelets are likely to be immature thrombocytes, except in the Cavalier King Charles, where thrombocytopenia and macrothrombocytes are noted as incidental findings. Bizarre platelet shapes can reflect platelet destruction.

Buccal mucosal bleeding time (BMBT)

The BMBT tests the vascular response, platelet numbers and function. The test measures the duration of haemorrhage from a standardised incision in the mucosal surface of the upper lip. The cuts are made by a disposable, spring-loaded device (Simplate–II), which delivers two parallel incisions of equal depth and length. In healthy, anaesthetised patients, the BMBT is usually less than 4–5 minutes.

Activated clotting time (ACT)

Commercially prepared tubes are available and this test can be used as an in-house screening test for disorders of secondary haemostasis. However, only very severe disease produces abnormal ACT results.

Activated partial thromboplastin time (APTT) and one-stage prothrombin time (OSPT)

These tests are usually performed at a commercial laboratory although an in-clinic coagulometer is available. Samples are collected into 3.8% sodium citrate (1:9 ratio of sodium citrate to blood). Blood should be collected with minimal trauma, since poor technique can result in contamination of the sample with tissue thromboplastin, activation of the coagulation cascade and spurious results. Tubes should be filled to the mark to give the correct ratio of anticoagulant to blood. Compression should be maintained over the venepuncture site for 5 minutes. The APTT is far more sensitive than the ACT. The OSPT is very sensitive to vitamin K antagonism and is an essential part of the diagnostic investigation where rodenticide toxicity is suspected.

Fibrin degradation products (FDPs)

FDPs are the end products of fibrinolysis. The plasma concentration is increased where there is excessive clot formation and breakdown, e.g. in DIC.

Disorders of primary haemostasis

Thrombocytopenia

Immune-mediated thrombocytopenia is, perhaps, the most common bleeding disorder encountered in veterinary practice. Patients usually present

Table 5.24 Possible causes of thrombocytopenia

Cause of thrombocytopenia	Underlying processes
Primary immune-mediated	
Secondary immune-mediated	trimethoprim (TMP)-sulphonamides therapy, systemic lupus erythematosus, neoplasia
Consumption/sequestration	Haemorrhage, disseminated intravascular coagulation, splenic torsion /neoplasia
Bone marrow suppression	Neoplasia, aplastic anaemia, drugs, e.g. oestrogens
Incidental finding	Cavalier King Charles Spaniels

with the described clinical signs (Table 5.23) with no evidence of systemic disease. The platelet count can easily be estimated on examination of a blood film. Signs are not usually present unless the count is $<30–50 \times 10^9/l$. Other causes of thrombocytopenia should be considered (Table 5.24).

Platelet function abnormalities

Platelet dysfunction may be suspected when there are clinical signs, which would be compatible with thrombocytopenia, but the platelet count is within the reference range. A BMBT is used to confirm the clinical suspicion. Acquired platelet function defects are most common and causes include drug therapy (aspirin, non-steroidal anti-inflammatory drugs (NSAIDs), dextrans, heparin, antihistamines) and systemic disease (uraemia, liver disease, DIC, gammopathies). Inherited platelet function abnormalities have been described in Otter Hounds, Basset Hounds, Collies and Persian cats.

von Willebrand's disease

This is the most common inherited bleeding disorder of dogs, which is known to affect more than 50 breeds. The disorder results from a deficiency of von Willebrand's Factor (vWF), a protein that links platelets to the subendothelium and assists in platelet to platelet aggregation.

Clinical signs include mucosal bleeding, e.g. epistaxis, gingival haemorrhage and haematuria. Gastrointestinal haemorrhage (with or without diarrhoea) can also be noted. Affected dogs may be prone to excessive haemorrhage at any site of injury or surgery. The vWF antigen test is used to predict the genetic status of individuals.

Disorders of secondary haemostasis

Vitamin K antagonism/deficiency

Rodenticide toxicity is a fairly common cause of vitamin K antagonism in the dog, but less common in the cat. The anticoagulant rodenticides interfere with the synthesis of the vitamin K-dependent clotting factors. This results in a bleeding disorder often characterised by the formation of petechial and ecchymotic haemorrhages, intra-cavity haemorrhage and epistaxis. Usually, by the time the patient presents to the clinician, the partial thromboplastin time and prothrombin time are both prolonged. Diagnosis is made on the basis of clinical signs and history, compatible abnormalities of haemostatic tests and exclusion of liver disease (which can be associated with similar haemostatic test abnormalities).

Liver disease, biliary stasis and feline inflammatory bowel disease can all be associated with bleeding tendencies and a coagulation screen prior to surgery in these cases is warranted.

Haemophilia A and B

Haemophilia A is the result of Factor VIII deficiency and displays an X-linked mode of inheritance, leading to clinical disease in males. Clinical signs are typical (Table 5.23) and investigation may require measurement of APTT and specific factor assays. Haemophilia B (Factor IX deficiency) is less common than haemophilia A but is similar in presentation and inheritance. Most affected individuals have a prolonged APTT.

Disseminated intravascular coagulation

DIC is a syndrome of increased clotting with a concurrent increase in fibrinolysis. This results in utilisation and exhaustion of the clotting factors. Many processes may trigger the onset of DIC including:

- haemangiosarcoma
- sepsis
- immune-mediated haemolytic anaemia
- pancreatitis
- *Angiostrongylus vasorum*
- other malignancies.

Clinical manifestations of DIC include bleeding tendencies with bleeding from multiple sites and the development of ischaemia and organ failure (associated with deposition of fibrin in the vessels). Diagnosis is confirmed if three of five haemostatic parameters (OSPT, APTT, platelets, fibrinogen, FDPs) are abnormal.

BIOCHEMISTRY

EVALUATION OF THE LIVER

The clinical signs associated with liver disease are often vague or mimic many other diseases. Biochemical assessment of the liver is therefore frequently required. Liver disease has an impact on many laboratory parameters but investigation often requires additional radiographic studies, ultrasound examination and biopsy. The biochemical parameters used to assess liver pathology include hepatocellular enzymes, indicators of liver function, and general health screening tests (including haematology and urine analysis). The 'liver enzymes' originate from specific regions within the hepatocyte (Fig. 5.20) and patterns of enzyme change can help to differentiate between pathological processes. The enzymes of particular interest are:

- alanine aminotransferase (ALT)
- aspartate aminotransferase (AST)
- alkaline phosphatase (ALP)
- gamma-glutamyl transferase (GGT).

Bilirubin, serum albumin and serum bile acids are considered to be indicators of hepatic function. Liver enzymes are not function indicators.

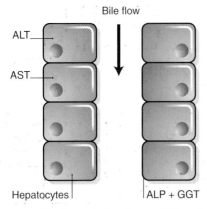

Figure 5.20 Alanine aminotransferase (ALT) and aspartate aminotransferase (AST) are found in the cytoplasm of the hepatocyte, while alkaline phosphatase (ALP) and gamma-glutamyltransferase (GGT) are predominantly membrane-bound.

Leakage enzymes

Alanine aminotransferase

ALT is found in the cytoplasm of hepatocytes and is usually considered to be liver-specific in the dog and cat, although small quantities may originate from muscle. The enzyme is an indicator of increased permeability of the hepatocyte membrane but increases need not reflect cell necrosis or death. The increase in activity roughly parallels the number of cells but does not correlate with the potential reversibility of the pathological process. Raised serum activity may be associated with inflammatory, toxic or neoplastic processes in the dog and cat (Box 5.13). Chronic hepatic disease, e.g. chronic active hepatitis, often only produces a mild to moderate increase in ALT activity but the abnormality is persistent. Liver disease is not always accompanied by increased ALT activity and some pathological processes, e.g. cirrhosis and congenital portosystemic shunts, may produce a negligible increase in serum ALT activity. Although ALT originates from the hepatocytes, other diseases can cause an increased activity (Box 5.13).

Aspartate aminotransferase

AST is present in hepatocytes, erythrocytes, and in muscle. Liver disease, myopathies and muscular trauma (including recumbency) may cause increases. AST is not usually included in screening profiles but may be included where the clinician is monitoring hepatic disease or the effects of a hepatotoxic drug.

Cholestatic enzymes

Alkaline phosphatase

There are three major forms (isoenzymes) of ALP which are important:

1. Hepatic. This activity is increased secondary to biliary stasis, often associated with hepatocyte swelling (Box 5.14). A clinically insignificant, but sometimes marked, increase in ALP is

Box 5.13	Possible causes of increased liver enzyme activity in the dog and cat	
Primary hepatic causes	**Other causes**	**Drugs**
Infectious disease	Intestinal disease	Glucocorticoid therapy
Toxin- or drug-related hepatic insult	Hyperthyroidism	Anticonvulsants
Trauma	Cardiac disease	Griseofulvin
Cholangitis/cholangiohepatitis	Shock	Ketoconazole
Chronic active hepatitis	Hyperadrenocorticism	Phenylbutazone
Hepatic lipidosis	Diabetes mellitus	
Feline cholangitis/cholangiohepatitis	Hypothyroidism	
Diffuse neoplasia, e.g. lymphoma	Severe dental disease	
	Pyometra	
	Abscessation	

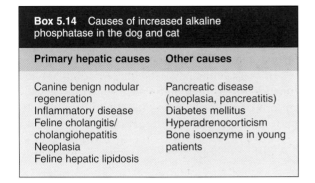

Box 5.14 Causes of increased alkaline phosphatase in the dog and cat

Primary hepatic causes	Other causes
Canine benign nodular regeneration Inflammatory disease Feline cholangitis/ cholangiohepatitis Neoplasia Feline hepatic lipidosis	Pancreatic disease (neoplasia, pancreatitis) Diabetes mellitus Hyperadrenocorticism Bone isoenzyme in young patients

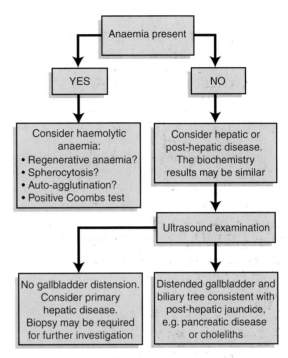

Figure 5.21 Investigation of hyperbilirubinaemia/jaundice.

noted in older dogs as a consequence of benign nodular regeneration of the liver.

2. Bone. The ALP activity is increased in young, growing animals but the increase is rarely more than two to three times greater than the upper limit of the adult reference range.

3. Steroid-induced (dog only). An increase in ALP can be associated with steroid administration. The degree of increase varies depending on the patient, the drug used, and the route of administration. In some individuals, drug administration (oral, parenteral, topical) may cause enzyme increases, which persist for at least 6 weeks. Endogenous glucocorticoids, e.g. hyperadrenocorticism, also cause an increased ALP activity.

Gamma-glutamyltransferase

GGT is found in highest concentrations in the bile duct epithelium. This enzyme is an indicator of cholestasis. The clinical causes are similar to the hepatic isoenzyme of ALP but it is helpful to measure both ALP and GGT where there is a high index of suspicion for hepatic disease, for monitoring recovery, and for drug monitoring.

Hepatic function indicator

Bilirubin

Bilirubin is formed from the catabolism of haemoproteins in the reticuloendothelial system. The newly formed bilirubin is bound to albumin and transported to the liver where it is converted to water-soluble bilirubin and excreted in the bile. Measurement of bilirubin is indicated where there is jaundice on clinical examination, visible icterus of the serum or plasma, or suspected hepatic disease. Clinical jaundice is detected only when the bilirubin is approximately 30 µmol/l but changes in the appearance of the serum are noted at <20 µmol/l.

Jaundice may be classified according to the underlying pathological process:

1. Prehepatic jaundice is the consequence of increased production of bilirubin secondary to haemolytic anaemia or internal haemorrhage. A full haematology profile and blood smear are essential in the investigation of jaundice (Fig. 5.21).

2. Hepatic jaundice. Hyperbilirubinaemia may be the result of a failure of uptake or conjugation of bilirubin and can be noted with acute and chronic hepatopathies.

3. Post-hepatic jaundice is caused by obstruction of the biliary tree which often causes a marked increase in bilirubin, e.g. pancreatic neoplasia, chronic pancreatitis

and, rarely, choleliths. Differentiation between hepatic and post-hepatic jaundice often requires ultrasound examination (Fig. 5.21).

Bile acids

The bile acids are produced in the liver from cholesterol, excreted into the biliary tree, and stored in the gallbladder. Gallbladder contraction (stimulated by ingestion of food) releases the bile acids into the intestines where they facilitate the digestion and absorption of dietary lipid. The bile acids are efficiently re-absorbed in the ileum

resulting in very small faecal loss (Fig. 5.22). The bile acids are sensitive indicators of hepatic function. Bile acids may be measured as a single fasting test, but the bile acid stimulation test provides additional information regarding hepatic function. It is especially useful in the investigations of portosystemic shunts and cirrhosis. To perform the bile acid stimulation test:

- collect basal, fasting blood sample
- give a small feed of high-fat diet
- collect a postprandial sample 2 hours after feeding.

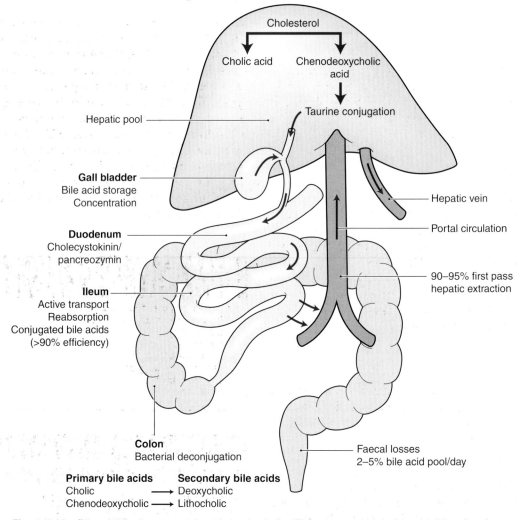

Figure 5.22 Bile acids undergo enterohepatic re-circulation. They are sensitive indicators of liver function but do not provide specific information regarding the nature of the pathological process.

Since systemic diseases, e.g. cardiac disease and hyperadrenocorticism, produce liver changes, they may also produce abnormal bile acid results. Increased bile acids, therefore, need not reflect primary hepatic disease.

Albumin

Hepatic protein synthesis is reduced in severe hepatic dysfunction and hypoalbuminaemia may be noted in chronic hepatic disease. Other causes of hypoalbuminaemia, including renal and intestinal disease, should be excluded where possible. Hypoalbuminaemia may contribute to the development of ascites in liver disease.

Urea

Reduced hepatic production of urea can result in low serum concentration in patients with diffuse liver disease. However, low-protein diets and chronic polydipsia/polyuria will also produce a low blood urea concentration.

Cholesterol

Low cholesterol may be associated with severe hepatic dysfunction, congenital portosystemic anomalies or intestinal disease. Increased concentrations are commonly noted with cholestasis and endocrine disease (diabetes mellitus, hyperadrenocorticism). There is usually notable hyperbilirubinaemia by the time the increased cholesterol concentration develops in patients with cholestatic liver disease.

Glucose

Hypoglycaemia may be noted in severe hepatic insufficiency, e.g. cirrhosis, and, occasionally, with hepatic neoplasia.

Urinalysis

Many animals with hepatic disease are unable to concentrate their urine maximally and urine specific gravity (SG) is frequently <1.030. Bilirubinuria can be an incidental finding in canine urine, especially where the urine is concentrated (SG >1.020). However, bilirubinuria in the cat is considered significant and precedes hyperbilirubinaemia. The formation of ammonium biurate crystals is often noted in dogs with congenital portosystemic anomalies but they are not commonly noted in the urine of affected cats.

Haematology abnormalities

A number of haematological abnormalities may be noted with liver disease (Box 5.15).

Ascitic fluid

The formation of ascites in association with liver disease can be a reflection of severe hypoalbuminaemia (<15 g/l) but is more commonly a consequence of portal hypertension. Sodium retention and alterations in hepatic and intestinal lymph flow also play a role in the development of ascites. The fluid may be a true transudate or a modified transudate (Table 5.25) depending upon the total protein concentration (measured by refractometer) and cell counts. Fluid with a high protein concentration (>38 g/l) is commonly noted in cats with FIP and chronic lymphocytic cholangiohepatitis.

Box 5.15 Haematological abnormalities which may be associated with liver disease

Mild, non-regenerative anaemia
Microcytosis and hypochromasia
Acanthocytes
Schistocytes
Poikilocytosis
Inflammatory leucogram
Platelet dysfunction
Coagulopathy

Table 5.25 Classification of abdominal fluids

Classification	Protein (g/l)	Cell count (cells/μl)
True transudate	<25	<1500
Modified transudate	25–75	<5000
Exudate	>30	<5000

Further investigations

Routine profiles and pre-anaesthetic screens frequently include leakage enzymes, cholestatic enzymes and function indicators. The following tests are also included in a diagnostic plan where there is a suspicion of hepatic disease or where the initial blood screen has produced abnormal liver test results:

1. Bile acid stimulation test: a sensitive indicator of hepatic function.
2. Screen for other diseases which might affect the liver, e.g. cardiac disease, intestinal disease, endocrine disease.
3. Radiography for liver size and shape, e.g. solitary hepatic mass, which might reflect neoplasia. Contrast radiography is used in the diagnosis of congenital portosystemic shunts.
4. Ultrasound examination: for focal lesions, changes in density and distension of the bile ducts/gallbladder.
5. Liver biopsy: for a definitive diagnosis.

Biopsy

Definitive diagnosis of liver disease usually requires histological examination of a biopsy although portosystemic shunts are more commonly confirmed by ultrasound or radiographic studies. For some conditions, e.g. hepatic neoplasia and feline hepatic lipidosis, cytological examination of a liver aspirate can be very helpful but ultrasound-guided aspiration is preferred. Indications for hepatic biopsy include:

- persistently increased liver enzymes (extrahepatic disease must be excluded where possible)
- persistently abnormal function indicators (extrahepatic disease must be excluded where possible)
- altered hepatic size.

ASSESSMENT OF RENAL FUNCTION

The kidney plays a major role in the regulation of many body systems including water conservation, waste disposal and maintenance of blood pressure. Therefore, there are many blood parameters that may be affected in renal disease. Those commonly used for the diagnosis of disease can be divided into tests which assess glomerular function, and those which assess tubular function.

Assessing glomerular function

Urea

Urea is synthesised in the liver from intestinally derived ammonia (produced by the effect of bacteria on dietary protein). The urea formed in the hepatocytes is excreted via the kidney tubules. There is some correlation between the severity of renal disease and the plasma urea concentration. However, the urea concentration may also be increased by factors other than glomerular filtration rate (GFR) (Table 5.26). The blood urea is therefore not a reliable estimate of the GFR since both pre-renal factors, e.g. hypovolaemia, and post-renal factors may cause a rise in concentration.

Creatinine

Creatinine is formed from creatine in the muscles and is freely filtered at the renal glomerulus. It is considered a better estimate of GFR than the blood urea concentration. However, the function of approximately 75% of nephrons must be lost

Table 5.26 Factors that may affect plasma urea concentration	
Pathological process	Comment
Renal failure	Associated with reduced glomerular filtration rate
Dietary protein concentration	Ingestion of a high-protein diet can produce raised urea. 12-hour fast is recommended before sampling
Intestinal haemorrhage	
Reduced renal blood flow	Hypovolaemia, cardiac disease
Post-renal disease	Urethral obstruction, ruptured bladder

before significant increase is noted. In acute renal failure, serial monitoring of creatinine can be useful since the parameter often rises over a few days. In chronic renal disease the creatinine concentration is relatively stable.

Azotaemia is an increase in plasma urea and creatinine concentrations.

Assessing tubular function

Normal renal tubular function is required for water conservation, sodium balance and maintenance of a normal plasma and body water composition.

Urine SG and water conservation

The SG of the unaltered glomerular filtrate is 1.008–1.015. A concentration above or below this level requires tubular function.

The specific terminology used to describe the urine SG (USG) is:

- isosthenuria   USG 1.008–1.015
- hyposthenuria   USG <1.008
- hypersthenuria   USG >1.015.

Adequate concentration of urine is assumed at USG > 1.030 in the dog and USG > 1.035 in the cat. Loss of concentrating ability can be an early sign of renal disease. Measurement of USG can help to differentiate between renal disease and a pre-renal azotaemia (Fig. 5.23). The presence of a concentrated urine sample (urine SG >1.030 in dogs, >1.035 in cats) supports a pre-renal azotaemia, while azotaemia in the presence of poorly concentrated urine could reflect renal insufficiency.

Assessment of renal function is best achieved by simultaneous measurement of the blood urea and creatinine, and urine SG. Serial monitoring of the renal parameters during fluid therapy is a helpful means of establishing the reversibility of the azotaemia. Other tests which provide information regarding renal function include:

- phosphorus
- sodium
- potassium

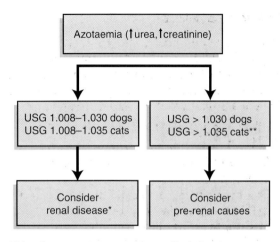

*Other disease processes can present with similar urine concentrations and should also be considered, e.g. hypercalcaemia, hypoadrenocorticism, hypokalaemia, liver disease
**In the cat, the urine concentrating ability may be maintained at this level despite early renal damage.

Figure 5.23   Differentiation between pre-renal azotaemia and renal disease.

- chloride
- total protein
- albumin
- urinalysis.

ELECTROLYTES

The water content of the body is distributed between two compartments, the extracellular fluid (ECF) and the intracellular fluid (ICF). Water passes freely between these compartments but the electrolyte composition of each is very different (Fig. 5.24). The measurement of electrolytes is indicated where intestinal disease, renal disease and hypoadrenocorticism are suspected and in seizuring and dehydrated patients. However, many other diseases produce electrolyte abnormalities (Box 5.16) which may contribute significantly to the clinical signs and in these cases, a timely correction of the electrolyte abnormalities may help the patient's recovery.

Sodium

The volume of fluid in the vascular space (circulating volume) is related to the volume of the

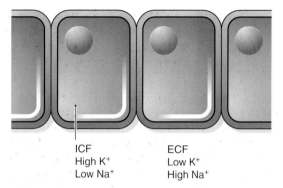

ICF
High K$^+$
Low Na$^+$

ECF
Low K$^+$
High Na$^+$

Figure 5.24 Distribution of electrolytes in the intracellular (ICF) and extracellular fluids (ECF).

Box 5.17 Diseases associated with abnormal serum sodium concentrations

Hyponatraemia	Hypernatraemia
Gastrointestinal loss	Diabetes insipidus
Hypoadrenocorticism	Heat stroke
Congestive cardiac disease	Inadequate access to water
Peritonitis	Adipsia (absence of thirst)
Pancreatitis	Diuretic therapy
Uroabdomen, e.g. ruptured bladder	
Diabetes mellitus	

Box 5.16 Diseases that may produce electrolyte abnormalities

Hypoadrenocorticism (Addison's disease)
Gastrointestinal disease with vomiting and diarrhoea
Renal disease
Diabetes mellitus
Cardiac disease
Diuretic therapy
Urethral obstruction
Ruptured bladder
Diabetes insipidus
Peritonitis

Box 5.18 Diseases associated with abnormal serum potassium concentrations

Hypokalaemia	Hyperkalaemia
Gastrointestinal loss (vomiting, diarrhoea)	Ethylenediaminetetraacetic acid (EDTA) contamination of sample
Chronic renal failure (especially cats)	Hypoadrenocorticism (Addison's disease)
Insulin therapy in diabetic patients	Urethral obstruction
Diuretic therapy	Ruptured bladder
Decreased intake	Tumour lysis syndrome (after chemotherapy)

ECF, which, in turn, varies with the total body sodium content. Maintenance of the body sodium content and total body water volume involves many hormones and mechanisms including the renin–angiotensin system, aldosterone and antidiuretic hormone. Significant hyponatraemia is most commonly associated with vomiting, hypoadrenocorticism and congestive cardiac failure (Box 5.17). Significant hypernatraemia is uncommon but is most marked in association with diabetes insipidus, where the patient is not allowed free access to fluids.

Potassium

Potassium is the major cation of the ICF. Potassium is filtered freely by the glomeruli and then reabsorbed. The excretion of the electrolyte is increased by aldosterone (with associated retention of sodium). The intracellular electrolyte plays a role in the contraction of muscle and maintenance of a normal transmembrane electrical potential. Measurement of potassium is essential in patients with bradycardia and supraventricular arrhythmias and where hypokalaemic myopathy is a differential. Hypokalaemia may be associated with muscle weakness, while concentrations >7.5 mmol/l can produce severe cardiac conduction disturbances. Hypokalaemia may be more common than currently recognised, especially in association with increased renal loss in cats (Box 5.18). Correction of hypokalaemia in such patients may require intravenous or oral supplementation.

Hyperkalaemia can be associated with hypoadrenocorticism, but pre-analytic error, associated with EDTA contamination of the sample, should always be excluded prior to further testing. This may arise by touching the hub of the needle on the inside of the EDTA tube while ejecting the sample. The potassium EDTA is then transferred to the serum tube, producing spurious hyperkalaemia and hypocalcaemia.

Chloride

Changes in relative water content usually produce parallel changes in sodium and chloride.

Magnesium

Magnesium is found in highest concentrations in bone and muscle. Unfortunately, the plasma concentration does not accurately reflect the whole body magnesium stores. Magnesium deficiency may cause abnormalities of heart rhythm or muscle weakness.

Calcium

Calcium plays an essential role in the regulation of enzymatic reactions, selective membrane permeability, muscle function and neural activity. The total blood calcium concentration is the most frequently used measurement, and is composed of the protein-bound fraction (40%), calcium complexes (citrate and phosphate) and ionised calcium (50%). The serum calcium concentration can therefore be affected by the plasma protein concentration, and in particular, the albumin concentration. In the dog, but not the cat, it is possible to calculate the corrected calcium concentration, which takes some account of the serum albumin concentration.

$$\text{Corrected Ca} = [\{\text{measured Ca(mmol/l)} \times 4\} \\ \text{(mmol/l)} \quad - \{\text{albumin (g/l)} \div 10\} + 3.5] \\ \times 0.25$$

In the future it may be possible to measure ionised calcium routinely, giving a more accurate assessment of calcium homeostasis. The ionised calcium is biologically active and is regulated predominantly by the following hormones:

- parathyroid hormone (PTH)
- calcitonin
- vitamin D.

Significant hypocalcaemia (<1.75 mmol/l) may cause nervousness, seizures, hind leg cramping or pain, muscle tremors and intense facial pruritus. It is associated with a number of diseases (Box 5.19).

The clinical signs associated with hypercalcaemia are often noted at concentrations >3 mmol/l and include polydipsia, polyuria, lethargy and weakness. Non-parathyroid neoplasia, especially lymphoma and neoplasia of the anal sac, is the most common cause of significant hypercalcaemia (Box 5.19). The investigation of hypercalcaemia, therefore, often includes survey radiography, biopsy of enlarged lymph nodes and measurement of PTH:

- calculate corrected calcium
- recheck on a fresh sample
- rectal examination for anal gland neoplasia
- survey radiography for lymphadenopathy
- haematology profile
- fine needle aspirate/biopsy of any enlarged nodes
- measurement of PTH
- bone marrow aspirate if necessary.

PLASMA PROTEINS

The plasma proteins are synthesised predominantly in the liver although plasma cells also contribute to their production. Quantitatively, the single most important protein is albumin. The other proteins are collectively known as globulins.

Box 5.19 Diseases associated with abnormal serum calcium concentrations	
Hypocalcaemia	**Hypercalcaemia**
Primary hypoparathyroidism	Immature animal
Eclampsia	Dehydration
Renal failure	Malignant neoplasm,
Ethylene glycol toxicity	e.g. lymphoma
Hypoalbuminaemia	Hypoadrenocorticism
Acute pancreatitis	Primary
Intestinal disease	hyperparathyroidism
Bilateral thyroidectomy	Renal failure
	Hypervitaminosis D

Albumin

Marked hypoalbuminaemia (<15 g/l) is associated with the development of ascites and tissue oedema. Common causes include protein-losing enteropathy, e.g. inflammatory bowel disease, and liver disease (Box 5.20). Hyperalbuminaemia is a consequence of dehydration.

Globulins

The serum concentration of globulins is calculated by subtracting the albumin concentration from the total protein concentration or is measured by SPE. Hypoglobulinaemia is most commonly caused by haemorrhage and protein-losing enteropathies. Hyperglobulinaemia is a common consequence of inflammation, feline infectious peritonitis and, less commonly, neoplasia, i.e. multiple myeloma and lymphoma.

CARBOHYDRATE METABOLISM

Glucose

Glucose is the principal source of energy for mammalian tissues. The blood concentration is controlled by hormones, which regulate its entry into, and removal from the circulation (insulin, glucagon, adrenaline (epinephrine), cortisol). In the kidney of the dog and cat, glucose entering the glomerular ultrafiltrate is reabsorbed by the renal tubules. However, the renal reabsorption of glucose is overwhelmed in the presence of blood glucose concentrations greater than 10–12 mmol/l, resulting in glucosuria.

Hyperglycaemia in the dog is commonly noted with diabetes mellitus (Box 5.21). Such cases do not present with clinical signs, i.e. polyuria and polydipsia, until the renal threshold for glucose is exceeded, resulting in osmotic diuresis. In the cat, the adrenaline (epinephrine)-induced stress response may produce a moderate or marked increase in glucose concentration. In this species, the diagnosis of diabetes mellitus is often difficult, and confirmation requires documentation of persistent hyperglycaemia with compatible clinical signs. Urinalysis (evidence of persistent glucosuria and possible ketonuria) and measure-

---

> **Box 5.20** Causes of hypoalbuminaemia
>
> Haemorrhage
> Intestinal disease
> Renal disease
> Hepatic disease
> Pregnancy
> Extensive burns

> **Box 5.21** Causes of hypoglycaemia and hyperglycaemia
>
> | **Hypoglycaemia** | **Hyperglycaemia** |
> |---|---|
> | Laboratory error | Adrenaline |
> | Insulinoma | (epinephrine) stress |
> | (insulin-secreting tumour) | response (esp. cats) |
> | Other neoplasms, e.g. | Postprandial |
> | hepatic carcinoma | Diabetes mellitus |
> | Hypoadrenocorticism | Hyperadrenocorticism |
> | Liver disease | Acromegaly |
> | Neonatal hypoglycaemia | Acute pancreatitis |
> | Hunting dog | |
> | hypoglycaemia | |
> | Sepsis | |

---

ment of serum fructosamine can also help to confirm the diagnosis in this species.

Hypoglycaemia results from excessive utilisation of glucose by normal or neoplastic cells (Box 5.21). In addition, a delay in the analysis of heparin plasma or serum can also produce spurious hypoglycaemia due to continued utilisation of glucose by the erythrocytes. If a delay in analysis is expected, e.g. referral to an external laboratory, then the blood should be collected into a sample tube containing fluoride oxalate. An insulinoma is a functioning tumour of the pancreatic islet cells, which produces biologically active insulin. Diagnosis relies upon the measurement of insulin at a time when the patient has a low blood glucose concentration. A tentative diagnosis of inappropriate insulin secretion can be made on the basis of a normal or increased insulin concentration in the face of hypoglycaemia.

Fructosamine

Fructosamine is formed by an irreversible reaction between blood glucose and plasma proteins.

The fructosamine concentration is related to the average blood glucose concentration during the preceding 1–3 weeks. It can be used as an aid in the diagnosis of feline diabetes mellitus and in evaluation of the success of insulin therapy in both the cat and the dog. However, fructosamine may be affected by other diseases, e.g. hyperthyroidism and hypoalbuminaemia.

LIPID METABOLISM

Cholesterol

High cholesterol concentrations in the dog and cat rarely have the same important health implications, e.g. coronary heart disease, as in humans. However, an abnormal serum cholesterol concentration directs the clinician towards specific disease conditions (Box 5.22), and the test is often included in general health profiles where endocrine disease is a clinical concern.

Triglyceride

Storage of triglycerides in adipose tissue provides an essential reserve of chemical energy for tissue requirements. Fasting hypertriglyceridaemia in the dog and cat is a pathological finding (Box 5.23). The triglycerides impart turbidity to the plasma or serum (lipaemia). The serum concentration should therefore be measured in all fasting blood samples which appear lipaemic. Clinical manifestations of hypertriglyceridaemia include recurrent abdominal pain, alimentary signs and ocular abnormalities.

INVESTIGATION OF INTESTINAL AND PANCREATIC DISEASE

Pancreatitis

The pancreas is situated next to the intestinal tract and produces enzymes, which are released into the gut, where they help to break down food for digestion. Pancreatitis causes leakage of the enzymes into the blood in increased quantities.

Box 5.22 Causes of abnormal cholesterol concentrations

Increased cholesterol	Decreased cholesterol
Hypothyroidism (dog)	Liver disease
Hyperadrenocorticism	Intestinal disease
Diabetes mellitus	
Liver disease (with impaired bile flow)	
Renal disease (conditions causing proteinuria)	

Box 5.23 Causes of hypertriglyceridaemia in the dog and cat

Non-fasted sample
Diabetes mellitus
Hypothyroidism
Hyperadrenocorticism
Glomerulonephritis
Acute pancreatitis
Idiopathic hyperchylomicronaemia of the Miniature Schnauzer
Familial hyperchylomicronaemia in the cat
Idiopathic hypertriglyceridaemia

Amylase and lipase are two enzymes which are commonly measured for the confirmation of canine pancreatitis. Unfortunately, mild increases in the enzyme activities (<2–3 times greater than the upper limit of the reference range) may be noted with renal, gastric or intestinal disease. In the case of lipase, administration of dexamethasone is also reported to cause a mild increase in the serum activity. In addition, normal activities of these two serum enzymes do not exclude the possibility of pancreatitis. Research into other indicators for pancreatitis has highlighted the use of ultrasound examination and biopsy for diagnosis. Measurement of canine pancreatic lipase immunoreactivity is a test which is currently being validated and may prove to be very useful.

The diagnosis of feline pancreatitis is also very difficult. The measurement of serum amylase and lipase is generally unhelpful and further investigations include feline trypsin-like immunoreactivity (fTLI), pancreatic ultrasound and biopsy of the gland.

Intestinal disease

The tests used in the investigation of intestinal disease depend on the clinical presentation and the differential diagnosis list. The following are commonly included in investigations:

- Faecal analysis. For parasitic examination (including *Giardia*) and culture. Two (ideally, three) faecal samples (not a swab) should be collected at 48 hour intervals to maximise identification of a pathogen. Faecal culture is indicated where there is bloody diarrhoea or pyrexia, and in young animals.
- Faecal parvoviral antigen. The faeces may be positive for viral antigen early in the course of the disease.
- Haematology/biochemistry. A range of abnormalities may be noted with intestinal disease (Table 5.27).
- FeLV and feline immunodeficiency virus (FIV).
- Trypsin-like immunoreactivity (TLI) is the test of choice for pancreatic insufficiency in the dog and cat.
- Serum vitamins, i.e. folate and cobalamin. Abnormalities of these vitamins may help to identify intestinal disease, including small intestinal bacterial overgrowth (SIBO).
- Intestinal biopsies are often required in the investigation of intestinal disease but do not always provide a definitive diagnosis. Samples may be collected at laparotomy or via endoscopy but irrespective of the method selected, multiple samples must be submitted to the pathologist to ensure the best chance of identifying the disease process.

BLOOD GAS ANALYSIS

Blood gas analysis is used in severely ill patients to identify acid–base disturbances and in the assessment of pulmonary gaseous exchange. Recent advances have reduced the cost of this equipment and its use may become more widespread in general practice. A careful sample collection technique and rapid analysis are required. Measurements include pH, carbon dioxide tension ($P\text{CO}_2$) and oxygen tension ($P\text{O}_2$).

Table 5.27 Haematological and biochemical abnormalities, which may be noted with intestinal disease

Abnormality	Common diseases
Anaemia: mild non-regenerative	Any chronic or inflammatory disease
Anaemia: iron deficiency	Chronic intestinal haemorrhage, e.g. neoplasm, ulceration
Leucopenia	Viral disease, e.g. parvovirus, feline infectious enteritis
Lymphopenia	Viral disease, e.g. distemper virus
Degenerative left shift	Sepsis, peritonitis
Hypoproteinaemia	Inflammatory bowel disease, neoplasia, lymphangiectasia
Increased liver enzymes (usually mild)	Any intestinal disease
Increased bile acids (usually mild)	Any intestinal disease
Hypocalcaemia	May be secondary to hypoalbuminaemia

Interpretation of blood gas results is complex and the reader is referred to Willard et al (1994) for a comprehensive review.

ENDOCRINE TESTING

Thyroid gland

In the dog and cat, the thyroid gland is a bilobed structure, which produces thyroxine (T_4) and triiodothyronine (T_3). T_3 is the biologically active hormone which regulates the basal metabolic rate and influences growth and tissue maturation.

Canine hypothyroidism

Hypothyroidism is a deficiency of the thyroid hormones T_3 and T_4. It is the most common endocrine disease of the dog and produces a wide range of pathological effects with a variable clinical presentation. It is most commonly a consequence of destruction of the thyroid gland. A range of laboratory abnormalities can be associated with hypothyroidism (Box 5.24) but definitive diagnosis is currently difficult. In many cases, a diagnosis of hypothyroidism can be made by the following in combination:

Box 5.24 Laboratory changes in canine hypothyroidism

Mild normocytic, normochromic (non-regenerative) anaemia
Von Willebrand's factor is not affected by hypothyroidism
Hypercholesterolaemia in approximately two thirds of cases
Hypertriglyceridaemia (which causes lipaemia) in some cases
Increased serum creatinine kinase (CK) activity
Low total thyroxine (TT_4)
Low free thyroxine (FT_4) by equilibrium dialysis
Raised canine thyroid-stimulating hormone (cTSH)

Box 5.25 Diseases and drugs which may affect the total thyroxine (TT_4) concentration

Diseases which affect basal T_4	Drugs which affect basal TT_4
Hyperadrenocorticism	Sulphonamides
Diabetes mellitus	Glucocorticoids
Liver disease	Anticonvulsants
Cardiac disease	
Renal failure	

Box 5.26 Laboratory changes associated with feline hyperthyroidism

Erythrocytosis
Heinz body production
Stress leucogram
Increased liver enzymes
Azotaemia
Mild hyperglycaemia
Urine specific gravity variable
Increased total thyroxine concentration

- clinical signs
- history
- laboratory screening tests
- serum total T_4 (TT_4) and canine thyroid-stimulating hormone (cTSH).

However, other disease processes and drug therapies may affect the TT_4 and cTSH concentrations (Box 5.25). In addition, the TT_4 concentration in some normal dogs is below the reference range, making confirmation of the diagnosis on the basis of TT_4 concentrations difficult. In patients where concurrent disease cannot be corrected, or treatment cannot be withdrawn, then further testing is often required for the diagnosis of hypothyroidism. These tests include:

- Free T_4 by equilibrium dialysis.
- TRH stimulation test. TT_4 is measured before and after injection of thyrotropin releasing hormone (TRH).
- Measurement of autoantibodies, including anti-thyroglobulin antibodies.
- A combination of these tests, taken with the clinical findings and therapeutic trial, may be required for the diagnosis of canine hypothyroidism.

Treatment of hypothyroidism requires administration of thyroid hormone supplements. For dogs on the same drug dosage there may be a large variation in serum TT_4 concentration, therefore adequacy of dosing should be based on serum measurements. The TT_4 allows the clinician to assess whether the supplementation has been given and if the dosage/absorption of the last tablet is sufficient. Some clinicians also measure cTSH, if the cTSH was increased at initial diagnosis. Successful therapy is associated with a decrease in the cTSH concentration.

Feline hyperthyroidism

Hyperthyroidism is characterised by increased concentrations of serum T_3 and T_4 as a result of benign adenomatous hyperplasia of the thyroid (commonly bilateral). A range of laboratory abnormalities has been described with feline hyperthyroidism. Many occur infrequently and the most common changes are increased liver enzymes (Box 5.26). Increases in ALT, ALP or AST (or a combination) are apparent in 90% of hyperthyroid cats. The liver enzymes tend to 'normalise' in parallel with a reducing TT_4 concentration and therefore marked, or persistent increases in liver enzymes in the face of marginally or mildly increased TT_4 concentration should be treated with suspicion for concurrent hepatic disease. Azotaemia, when noted, may reflect co-existing renal disease. On treatment of the hyperthyroidism, the GFR is reduced and the azotaemia may become more marked. Increased TT_4 concentrations are noted in most cats with hyperthyroidism but there may be difficulty in differentiating normal from hyperthyroid patients since some normal cats have values outside the reference range and some affected cats have values inside the range. Values in the high normal range may reflect early disease, fluctuations in TT_4, or the effect of non-thyroidal illness (which depresses TT_4). Hyperthyroidism should be suspected in a cat with known non-thyroidal illness and a TT_4 concentration at the high end of the reference range. Re-testing in 4–6 weeks, or after treatment of the non-thyroidal illness, may provide a diagnosis. Other tests which have been used in these cases include:

- T_3 suppression test (Mooney 1998)
- TRH stimulation test (Mooney 1998).

The treatment options for hyperthyroidism commonly used in the United Kingdom are medical treatment with carbimazole and thyroidectomy (uni- or bilateral). Medical therapy is advisable for all cases initially, allowing stabilisation of the hyperthyroid state and evaluation of the patient for any deterioration in renal function. The measurement of TT_4 is used to assess the return to euthyroidism. In addition, renal function should be monitored before and after the introduction of therapy. TT_4 below the reference range is not infrequently noted although cats rarely show signs of hypothyroidism. Adverse reactions to carbimazole are rare but could include leucopenia and thrombocytopenia.

Close post-surgical monitoring is essential for those patients who then proceed to thyroidectomy. Hypocalcaemia is a consequence of surgery in which the parathyroid glands have been removed or damaged. The low calcium usually develops 1–5 days post-surgery.

Adrenal gland

The adrenals are paired glands applied to the cranial pole of the kidneys. The glands contain two functionally different tissues: the cortex and medulla. The adrenal cortex produces mineralo-corticoids (mainly aldosterone), glucocorticoids and sex hormones, while the adrenal medulla secretes adrenaline (epinephrine) and noradrenaline (norepinephrine). Glucocorticoids are secreted from the cortex under the influence of adrenocorticotrophic hormone (ACTH) from the pituitary gland.

Canine hyperadrenocorticism

Two forms of hyperadrenocorticism are recognised:

- Pituitary-dependent hyperadrenocorticism is characterised by an overproduction of ACTH by the pituitary as a consequence of a microadenoma or macroadenoma. The increased production of ACTH produces hypertrophy of the adrenal glands with production of excess cortisol.
- Adrenal-dependent hyperadrenocorticism is a consequence of overproduction of cortisol by a neoplasm of the adrenal gland.

A number of laboratory changes including a stress leucogram and raised liver enzymes are noted in dogs with hyperadrenocorticism (Box 5.27). However, the absence of these changes does not exclude the diagnosis. Where hyperadrenocorticism is suspected on the basis of clinical signs there are four further tests, which may be used to screen for the disease. However, false-positive results are noted in all of these tests in dogs with diseases other than hyperadrenocorticism, and care should be taken in interpretation of the results. The tests are described below:

1. ACTH stimulation test. This is a relatively quick test, which is based on the stimulation of cortisol secretion by the adrenal gland after administration of synthetic ACTH.

Box 5.27 Laboratory changes associated with canine hyperadrenocorticism

Stress leucogram
Erythrocytosis
Increased alkaline phosphatase (can be marked)
Increased alanine aminotransferase (usually mild)
Hyperglycaemia
Low urea

Cortisol is measured before and one hour after administration of 0.25 mg synthetic ACTH (Torrance and Mooney 1998).

2. Low-dose dexamethasone suppression test. This test identifies a greater number of cases than the ACTH stimulation test, including all cases of adrenal neoplasia and 95% of cases of pituitary-dependent disease. The test takes 8 hours to perform. False-positive results can cause difficulty in interpretation. Cortisol is measured before and at 3 and 8 hours after the intravenous administration of 0.01–0.015 mg/kg dexamethasone (Torrance and Mooney 1998).

3. Measurement of 17-OH progesterone. 17-OH is a precursor of cortisol and is measured by several diagnostic laboratories in the UK. Measurement of 17-OH-progesterone after administration of ACTH is proving useful in the diagnosis of canine hyperadrenocorticism, although only a small number of cases have been assessed to date.

4. Urinary cortisol:creatinine ratio. This is a simple test, which can be performed on a morning urine sample. If the cortisol:creatinine ratio is normal then hyperadrenocorticism is unlikely. However, increased ratios are noted in many diseases and the test cannot be used to confirm the presence of hyperadrenocorticism.

Further investigation is often required to differentiate between pituitary-dependent hyperadrenocorticism and adrenal-dependent disease. The tests which may allow this differentiation are:

1. Plasma ACTH. Samples for ACTH measurement must be handled according to strict guidelines and it is essential that clinicians contact the diagnostic laboratory for instructions before sample collection. This test cannot be used as an initial screening test for hyperadrenocorticism and is only used where a diagnosis is already established.

2. High-dose dexamethasone suppression test. The protocol is the same as for the low-dose dexamethasone suppression test but 0.1 mg/kg dexamethasone is administered intravenously.

The ACTH stimulation test is used to monitor the effectiveness of mitotane or trilostane therapy. Iatrogenic hypoadrenocorticism is a potential consequence of treatment for hyperadrenocorticism, and an ACTH stimulation test and measurement of electrolytes should be performed if there is development of weakness, anorexia or profound depression during therapy.

Canine hypoadrenocorticism

Hypoadrenocorticism, or Addison's disease, is further classified as primary or secondary:

- **Primary hypoadrenocorticism.** Destruction of the adrenal cortices results in a combined deficiency of all hormones, with clinical signs relating to mineralocorticoid and glucocorticoid deficiencies.
- **Secondary hypoadrenocorticism** is a consequence of reduced ACTH secretion by the pituitary gland.

Characteristic electrolyte changes and a pre-renal azotaemia are noted in the majority of cases (Box 5.28). Diagnosis is made on the basis of results of an ACTH stimulation test. In a small number of patients the electrolytes are normal and diagnosis relies solely upon the combination of clinical signs and an abnormal ACTH stimulation test.

The basis of therapy in cases of hypoadrenocorticism is replacement of mineralocorticoids and glucocorticoids. The serum electrolyte concentrations should be checked 5–7 days after the initiation of mineralocorticoid therapy. The dosage can then be further tailored if necessary.

Box 5.28 Haematology and biochemistry changes associated with hypoadrenocorticism

Anaemia (only evident after rehydration)
Lymphocytosis
Eosinophilia
Increased urea
Increased creatinine
Hyperkalaemia
Hyponatraemia
Hypercalcaemia
Hypochloraemia
Hypoglycaemia
Abnormal adrenocorticotrophic hormone stimulation test

CANINE DIABETES MELLITUS

Diabetes mellitus is characterised by a deficiency of insulin (relative or absolute), and hyperglycaemia. Without the inhibitory effect of insulin the action of glucagon is unchecked with a consequent hyperglycaemia. The hyperglycaemia and insulin deficiency affect many tissues and metabolic pathways. When the blood glucose rises above the renal threshold there is glucosuria with ensuing osmotic diuresis. A secondary polydipsia follows. Given the insulin deficiency, the peripheral tissues cannot utilise the glucose available in the blood. Fat stores are then broken down to form an alternative energy source (ketone production). Metabolic acidosis results when the production of ketones exceeds the buffering capacity of the body. Diabetes mellitus disease is characterised by hyperglycaemia (usually >14 mmol/l) and glucosuria, but other laboratory changes are common (Box 5.29).

Monitoring insulin therapy in uncomplicated cases

Diabetic dogs are generally insulin-dependent. After introduction of insulin therapy, the blood or urinary glucose is monitored (Box 5.30) and

---

> **Box 5.29** Laboratory changes associated with canine diabetes mellitus
>
> Stress leucogram
> Inflammatory leucogram (concurrent inflammatory disease is common)
> Hyperglycaemia
> Hypercholesterolaemia
> Hypertriglyceridaemia
> Increased liver enzymes (alkaline phosphatase, alanine aminotransferase)
> Increased ketones (with ketoacidosis)
> Increased pancreatic enzymes (if concurrent pancreatitis)

> **Box 5.30** Methods for monitoring insulin therapy
>
> Nadir blood glucose
> Serial blood glucose curve
> Urine glucose (2 or 3 times daily)
> Fructosamine
> Glycated haemoglobin

---

dosage adjustments made at 3–4 day intervals. The following methods of monitoring the effectiveness of insulin therapy are used in veterinary practice:

1. Blood glucose may be measured in the practice by portable glucose meters or point-of-care analysers. The sample is collected at the point of lowest blood glucose (nadir) in order to determine the effectiveness of insulin treatment. Initially it is acceptable to use mean data for the time of peak insulin action and duration to decide on the timing of this sample, e.g. lente insulin is reported to have a peak time of action of 6–8 hours and a sample taken 6–8 hours after insulin therapy can be used in the initial stabilisation period. However, at some point during the initial stabilisation period it is advisable to perform a serial blood glucose curve to determine the actual time of the nadir for that patient. Blood glucose should not be allowed to fall below 4.5 mmol/l (Holm 1997).

2. Serial blood glucose curve. After stabilisation or partial stabilisation it is useful to perform a serial blood glucose curve to check the duration of action of insulin, to tailor the feeding times and to confirm the lowest blood glucose concentration (Holm 1997).

3. Urine glucose. Many texts describe the use of urinary glucose measurements in a sample collected prior to administration of insulin. However, many patients on once-daily treatment are adequately controlled during the morning and afternoon (assuming morning injection) but have moderate to marked hyperglycaemia overnight. The morning urinary glucose shows significant glucosuria in these patients, confirming the overnight hyperglycaemia, but gives no clue as to the effectiveness of insulin treatment at the nadir. Collection of additional urine samples in the afternoon and evening would allow a better assessment (Graham 1998).

4. Fructosamine and glycated haemoglobin are used in the long-term monitoring of diabetic patients. The fructosamine concentration is related to mean blood glucose during the

preceding 1–3 weeks while glycated haemoglobin reflects the mean blood glucose over a longer period (6–8 weeks). The fructosamine concentration can be affected by other diseases, and it is essential to measure the serum protein and albumin concentrations prior to interpretation.

Monitoring patients with ketoacidosis

Treatment of patients with ketoacidosis requires:

- Insulin therapy, by intravenous or intramuscular routes.
- Slow correction of fluid deficits.
- Intensive monitoring of blood glucose and electrolytes. Many cases undergoing intensive insulin therapy for the correction of ketoacidosis develop hypokalaemia, which requires oral or intravenous supplementation. In addition, patients may occasionally develop hypophosphataemia.
- Monitor ketone production. Urinary ketones may be measured by strip tests (which are more sensitive to acetoacetate). A quantitative method for β-hydroxybutyrate is also available at many referral laboratories. Early in the treatment of ketoacidotic patients there may be a rise in ketones measured by the strip method. This is likely to reflect a shift in production of ketones towards acetoacetate and need not reflect deterioration of the condition.

Poorly responsive cases

The treatment of diabetes mellitus is not always easy: some animals may appear to have marked fluctuations in insulin requirements, some may have very high requirements and others may have reducing requirements. The underlying problems may be associated with poor insulin activity and administration, poor technique or the presence of concurrent disease (Box 5.31).

FELINE DIABETES MELLITUS

Diabetes mellitus in the cat presents some specific problems, which are not noted in the dog. In the

---

Box 5.31 Factors affecting stabilisation in diabetes mellitus

Insulin activity and administration:
- Temperature extremes, especially heating?
- Vigorous shaking
- Injection technique
- Incorrect syringes (40 versus 100 IU/ml)
- Poor absorption: protamine zinc insulin (PZI) may be poorly absorbed in some patients)
- Short duration of action (confirm on serial glucose curve)
- Somogyi overswing (period of rebound hyperglycaemia associated with a relative overdose of insulin: confirm on serial glucose curve)

Management or monitoring failure:
- Dietary mismanagement: over-feeding or semi-moist diets (keep diary)
- Inconsistent routine with regard to feeding and exercise (keep diary)
- Rapid changes in insulin dosage (leave 3–4 days between dose adjustment)
- Large changes in insulin dosage (>20% per change)
- Inappropriate monitoring (monitor once daily lente therapy at the nadir, not prior to insulin injection)

Concurrent disease or drug therapy:
- Metoestrus: bitches diagnosed in metoestrus may undergo spontaneous remission
- 'Honeymoon': insulin requirements may be reduced or disappear in the early stages of stabilisation. The signs frequently recur at a later date
- Hyperadrenocorticism
- Thyroid disease
- Azotaemia
- Pancreatitis (may be present in newly diagnosed dogs or occurs later in the course of disease. Confirmation is difficult)
- Sepsis

---

cat, a form of diabetes (Type II) is recognised which is characterised initially by insulin resistance. Classification into three types has been proposed on theoretical grounds but may not be possible on practical grounds (Peterson 1998).

Type I

Caused by insulin deficiency. Affected cats are often thin and are predisposed to ketoacidosis. In one study, many cats with Type I disease had concurrent disease (Bruskiewicz et al 1997). Feline diabetic ketoacidosis is a clinical presentation with potentially grave consequences and it is useful to consider the possibility of concurrent disease in these cases.

Type II

Caused by insulin resistance, which is usually a consequence of loss of receptors or insulin affinity. Initially there is an increased insulin concentration but in the face of chronic hyper-glycaemia the pancreatic islet cells decrease insulin secretion/production. Cats are normal weight or obese and are not ketoacidotic but can progress to becoming insulin-dependent. These cats may respond to oral hypoglycaemic agents initially. Insulin concentration may occasionally help in differentiating between insulin-dependent and non-insulin-dependent disease but the differentiation is usually difficult.

Type III

Secondary to hyperadrenocorticism, acromegaly etc. These cases often require large daily insulin dosages. Correction of underlying disorder usually reduces (but does not often abolish) insulin requirement.

Feline diabetes mellitus is associated with many of the abnormalities described for canine disease. However, in the cat it can be difficult to differentiate between a stress hyperglycaemia and diabetes mellitus. An increased fructosamine concentration often helps to differentiate between these two possibilities but may not be helpful in cats with concurrent poorly controlled hyperthyroidism.

Transient diabetes mellitus

Some cats may recover after a few days, weeks or months. This is transient diabetes mellitus, the incidence of which is unknown. Cats with Type II are most likely to have the transient form. In these cats, the requirements for insulin therapy decline with time, leaving the patients at risk of developing hypoglycaemia (assuming that the insulin dosage has remained static). Cats particularly at risk of transient diabetes mellitus and potentially hypoglycaemia, are those obese cats in which weight loss is successful, or in cats previously treated with diabetogenic agents

(glucocorticoids, progestogens). Diabetes mellitus may recur at a later stage in some cats.

REPRODUCTIVE ENDOCRINOLOGY

Management of mating

Measurement of plasma progesterone provides a guide to the timing of ovulation and is used to optimise the timing of mating. Samples are usually collected at 48-hour intervals from around day 11. It may be advisable to start testing earlier than this in bitches who have previously proved difficult to mate, since some bitches ovulate as early as day 5 after the onset of pro-oestrus.

Pregnancy diagnosis

Measurement of circulating relaxin concentration is currently used for pregnancy diagnosis. Testing is performed at 28 days post-mating.

Ovarian remnant syndrome

A hormone challenge test performed during behavioural oestrus may allow identification of retained functioning ovarian tissue. One protocol suggests the measurement of progesterone in a sample collected 1–3 weeks after administration of human chorionic gonadotrophin hormone or gonadotrophin-releasing hormone (Wallace 1992). Practices should contact the referral laboratory prior to sample collection.

Rig testing

A stimulation test, based on a protocol for equine use, has been used in the dog. Practices should contact the referral laboratory prior to sample collection.

SEROLOGICAL TESTING

Serology is detection and measurement of anti-gens or antibodies. It is used commonly in the identification of infectious disease and immune-mediated disease (Table 5.28). The tests may detect antigens or antibodies specific to a disease process.

Table 5.28 Serological tests used in veterinary practice

Test	Comment
Acetylcholine receptor antibodies	Detected in some dogs with myasthenia gravis
Allergen-specific immunoglobulin E (Ig-E)	Where clinical signs and history suggest atopy. This test may be used to select allergens for hyposensitisation
Antinuclear antibodies	Identifies antibodies to nuclear components (DNA/RNA). Used in the investigation of systemic lupus erythematosus (SLE) but other diseases may cause increases
Antiplatelet antibodies	For confirmation of antibodies directed against platelets in immune-mediated thrombocytopenia
Aspergillus	Used to support diagnosis where clinical signs and radiographic features are suggestive
Babesia canis	Babesiosis is a tick borne disease, which may cause fever and haemolysis
Bladder tumour antigen (V-BTA)	Latex agglutination test for antigen associated with transitional cell carcinoma. False-positives associated with pyuria
Canine infectious hepatitis	Paired samples (2–3 weeks apart) may be required
Coombs test	Detection of antibody or complement attached to erythrocytes in haemolytic anaemia
Distemper	For detection of antibodies. Prior vaccination makes interpretation of results difficult
Encephalitozoon cuniculi	Can cause central nervous system and renal signs in rabbits. Serological testing may be helpful in rabbits with compatible signs
Ehrlichia canis	Antibodies to *Ehrlichia* species identified
Feline coronavirus	For detection of antibodies to coronavirus. Does not provide a definitive diagnosis of feline infectious peritonitis
Feline immunodeficiency virus (FIV)	For detection of antibodies to FIV
Feline leukaemia virus (FeLV)	For detection of FeLV antigen
Feline infectious enteritis	Serological testing may be helpful in non-vaccinated animals with compatible clinical signs
Heartworm	For the detection of *Dirofilaria immitis* antigen. Small numbers of parasites may cause a false-negative result
Leishmania	Antibody detection by IFA. Peak antibody titre noted 45–80 days post-infection
Leptospira	Diagnosis by serological methods. A high titre, or rising titre, supports the clinical suspicion
Lyme disease	Detection of antibodies to *Borrelia burgdorferi*
Masticatory muscle myositis	Antibodies to Type II muscle fibres detected
Neospora caninum	Associated with encephalomyelitis and hind limb ataxia in puppies
Parvovirus	Detection of antigen in faeces early in disease. Detection of antibodies in serum, but prior vaccination may interfere with interpretation
Rheumatoid factor	Non-specific factor, which may be identified in dogs with rheumatoid arthritis
Progesterone	For the timing of mating in dogs
Psittacine beak and feather disease	Birds often present as feather pluckers but leucopenia may be noted in young birds
Rabies	Serological testing required as part of the Pet Travel Scheme
Sarcoptes serology	Used in addition to standard investigation (including skin scrapes)
Toxoplasma gondii	Measurement of IgG and IgM is preferred for confirmation of active infection. Can also be measured in cerebrospinal fluid
Von Willebrand's factor antigen	

Test methods

- Enzyme-linked immunosorbent assay (ELISA test) (Fig. 5.25): commonly used and forms the basis of many in-clinic tests including FeLV, FIV, canine parvovirus, canine progesterone and canine heartworm.
- Immunofluorescence techniques: used to identify and detect microbial antigen in blood smears, scrapings and tissue aspirates. These tests are used in referral laboratories.
- Microscopic agglutination test. These tests are used in referral laboratories.
- Polymerase chain reaction (PCR). This is not a serological test but is a method of amplifying DNA (e.g. from the infectious agent). Small amounts of DNA are amplified allowing detection by other methods.

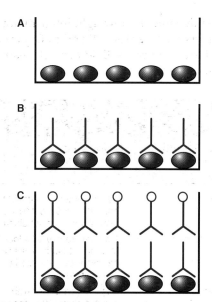

Figure 5.25 Diagrammatic representation of enzyme-linked immunosorbent assay (ELISA) testing. Antigen is bound to the test well. Patient serum contains antibody, which binds to the antigen. Antibodies directed against immunoglobulin are added, which bind to the first antibody and produce a colour change.

URINE TESTING

Urinalysis is performed where clinical signs suggest urinary tract disease, e.g. dysuria, haematuria or where there is polydipsia/polyuria.

Visual appraisal

Normal urine is yellow but the colour intensity may vary depending on concentration. The colour can be affected by drugs or dietary pigments. Normal urine is clear. Turbid urine is abnormal and is likely to contain cells, crystals or casts.

Urine specific gravity

The SG of the urine is its density or weight, compared to an equal volume of distilled water. SG should be measured using a refractometer, rather than dipstick tests. The range of SG noted in the dog (1.001–1.065) and cat (1.001–1.080) reflects the hydration status and may be affected by many disease processes. USG >1.030 in the dog, and USG >1.035 in the cat suggest adequate urinary concentration.

Urine chemistries

Urine pH

- Acidic (pH <7.0) urine may be due to fever, starvation, metabolic disease, muscle breakdown and some diets.
- Alkaline urine (pH >7.0) may be noted with urinary retention, urinary tract infection and vegetarian diets.

Blood

The test detects red blood cells, haemoglobin and myoglobin. Microscopic examination of the urine is essential to confirm the presence of intact red cells.

- Haematuria: associated with cystitis, crystalluria, neoplasia and acute nephritis.
- Haemoglobinuria: caused by intravascular haemolysis, e.g. haemolytic anaemia. Confirm by examination of a blood film and haematology profile.
- Myoglobinuria: caused by excess muscle breakdown.

Protein

Only traces of protein are usually detected. Increased protein (especially where the urine is dilute) may warrant further quantification (urinary protein:creatinine ratio) by a referral laboratory.

Glucose

Strip test reagents are usually specific to glucose; while tablet reagents may detect other sugars. Glucosuria is associated with diabetes mellitus but does not provide a definitive diagnosis. Renal tubular defects may also cause glucosuria and therefore confirmation of hyperglycaemia is essential for a diagnosis of diabetes mellitus. Monitoring urinary glucose is one of the approaches to stabilising and monitoring the diabetic patient.

Ketones

Ketonuria in small animals is most commonly associated with diabetes mellitus (diabetic ketoacidosis) but is occasionally noted with other metabolic diseases.

Bilirubin

A trace of bilirubin may be identified in normal canine urine (especially in a concentrated sample). However, greater quantities and any bilirubinuria in the cat are pathological findings. Causes include primary liver degree and biliary obstruction, e.g. associated with pancreatic neoplasia.

Sediment examination

Sediment examination is an essential part of the urinalysis. Ideally the sample should be analysed within 30 minutes of collection. If a delay cannot be avoided then refrigeration prior to analysis is recommended but the sample should be allowed to come back to room temperature before examination since there is increased crystal formation at lower temperatures. Method:

- Spin sample at 1500 rpm for 5 minutes.
- Decant supernatant leaving a small amount in which to re-suspend the cells.
- Re-suspend sediment by gently flicking bottom of tube.
- Place a drop on a microscope slide and cover with a cover slip (stained material, e.g. Sedistain, may be preferred).

- Examine under a low light intensity for cells and crystals (Tables 5.29 and 5.30). Artefacts include air bubbles, lipid droplets, hair and plant spores.

Table 5.29 The components of a urinary sediment examination

Cells and structures identified on sediment examination	Significance
Red cells	Haematuria which could be associated with cystitis, neoplasia, crystalluria or renal disease
White cells	Inflammation: further localisation to urinary tract is possible if the sample was collected by cystocentesis
Epithelial cells	May be associated with contamination from the external genitalia, traumatic catheterisation, chronic inflammation or neoplasia. Referral of sample for cytological examination indicated
Casts: hyaline, cellular or granular	Associated with tubular disease
Crystals (Table 5.30)	May be associated with urolithiasis and cystitis
Organisms	May be contaminants. A sample collected by catheterisation or cystocentesis is preferred for culture. Boric acid usually required as a urinary preservative

Table 5.30 Crystals found on examination of a urinary sediment

Crystals	Appearance	Comment
Triple phosphate	Coffin lids, 8-sided prisms with tapering ends and slides	Alkaline to slightly acidic urine
Amorphous phosphate	Granular precipitate	Common in alkaline urine. Look like amorphous urates so check the urine pH
Calcium carbonate	Dumb-bell or round with radiating lines	Common in horses
Amorphous urates	Granular precipitate	Common in acidic urine, look like amorphous phosphate so check the urine pH
Ammonium biurate	Brown, round with fine radiating lines. May also have spicules	Liver disease Dalmations
Calcium oxalate dihydrate	Squares, containing a central X	Acidic and neutral urine. Often in small numbers in canine urine
Calcium oxalate monohydrate	Small, dumb-bell	Large numbers associated with ethylene glycol (antifreeze) toxicity

Urolithiasis

Calculi are composed of precipitated minerals and determining their chemical composition helps to select appropriate therapy. The composition is usually determined at a referral laboratory either by chemical analysis or crystallography. The latter is more expensive but provides accurate quantitative results.

MICROBIOLOGICAL TESTING: SKIN EXAMINATIONS

Examination of material from the skin and hair may include:

- impression smears
- examination of coat for flea dirt using damp cotton wool or blotting paper
- hair plucks and brushings
- skin scrapes.

Microscopic examination of skin samples

For microscopic examination the material is either mounted directly in a drop of liquid paraffin or may be processed with a clearing agent, e.g. 10% or 20% potassium hydroxide. The ectoparasites that may be identified in small animal practice are listed in Box 5.32. The characteristic features of these parasites and the clinical presentations have been reviewed elsewhere (Fisher 1999, Duncan 2000).

Box 5.32 Ectoparasites of small animals

Cheyletiella blakei (cat)
Cheyletiella parasitovorax (rabbit)
Cheyletiella yasguri (dog)
Ctenocephalides felis (dog and cat)
Demodex canis (dog)
Demodex cati (cat)
Demodex criceti (hamster)
Felicola subrostrata (cat)
Leporacarus gibbus (rabbit)
Linognathus setosus (dog)
Neotrombicula autumnalis (dog and cat)
Notoedres cati (cat)
Otodectes cynotis (cat and dog)
Psoroptes cuniculi (rabbit)
Pulex irritans (dog and cat)
Sarcoptes scabiei (dog)
Trichodectes canis (dog)
Trixacarus caviae (guinea pig)

REFERENCES

Bloxham PA 1999 Clinical pathology and laboratory diagnostic aids. In: Lane DR, Cooper B (eds) Veterinary nursing, 2nd edn. Oxford, Butterworth Heinemann, pp 337–362

Bruskiewicz KA, Nelson RW, Feldman EC, Griffey SM 1997 Diabetic ketoacidosis in cats: 42 cases (1980–1995). J Am Vet Med Assoc 211: 188–192

Butcher 1999 Occupational hazards. In: Lane DR, Cooper B (eds) Veterinary nursing, 2nd edn. Butterworth Heinemann, Oxford, pp 97–103

Chandler S 1999 General nursing. In: Lane DR, Cooper B (eds) Veterinary nursing 2nd edn. Butterworth Heinemann, Oxford, pp 397–419

Duncan WG 2000 Mite infestations in small animals (Part 2). Vet Pract Nurse 12: 27–30

Duncan J, Broadley S 1999 Lab tests: collecting quality samples. Vet Nurs 14: 172–179

Feldman BF 1992 Diagnostic approach to coagulation and fibrinolytic disorders. Semin Vet Med Surg (Small Animal) 7: 315–322

Fisher M 1999 Elementary mycology and parasitology. In: Lane DR, Cooper B (eds) Veterinary nursing, 2nd edn. Butterworth Heinemann, Oxford, pp 376–396

Graham PA 1998 Canine diabetes mellitus. In: Torrance AG, Mooney CT (eds) Manual of small animal endocrinology, 2nd edn. BSAVA, Cheltenham, pp 83–96

Holm B 1997 Diabetes mellitus in the dog (part II). Eur J Companion Animal Pract VII: 68–77

Knottenbelt CM, Day MJ, Cripps PJ, Mackin AJ 1999 Measurement of titres of naturally occurring alloantibodies against feline blood groups in the UK. J Small Animal Pract 40: 365–370

Lumsden JH 1998 Laboratory data interpretation. In: Davidson MG, Else RW, Lumsden JH (eds) Manual of small animal clinical pathology. BSAVA, Cheltenham, pp 27–32

Master J, Bowden C (eds) 2001 Pre-veterinary nursing textbook. Butterworth-Heinemann in association with BVNA, Oxford, pp 33, 224

Mooney CT 1998 Feline hyperthyroidism. In: Torrance AG, Mooney CT (eds) Manual of small animal endocrinology, 2nd edn. BSAVA, Cheltenham, pp 115–128

Peterson ME 1998 Feline diabetes mellitus. In: Torrance AG, Mooney CT (eds) Manual of small animal endocrinology, 2nd edn. BSAVA, Cheltenham, pp 97–102

Reagan WJ, Sanders T, DeNicola DB 1998 Veterinary haematology. Atlas of common domestic species. Manson Publishing, London

Thrall MA 1997. Haematology. In: Pratt PW (ed) Laboratory procedures for veterinary technicians, 3rd edn. Mosby, St Louis, pp 33–84

Torrance AG, Mooney CT (eds) 1998 Manual of small animal endocrinology, 2nd edn. BSAVA, Cheltenham

Villiers E, Dunn JK 1998 Basic haematology. In: Davidson MG, Else RW, Lumsden JH (eds) Manual of small animal clinical pathology. BSAVA, Cheltenham, pp 33–60

Wallace M 1992 Ovarian remnant syndrome. In: Kirk RW, Bonagura JD (eds) Kirk's current veterinary therapy XI. WB Saunders, Philadelphia, pp 966–968

Willard MD, Tvedten H, Turnwald GH (eds) 1994 Small animal clinical diagnosis by laboratory methods. WB Saunders, Philadelphia

FURTHER READING

Davidson MG, Else RW, Lumsden JH (eds) 1998 Manual of small animal clinical pathology. BSAVA, Cheltenham

Eibert M, Lewis DC 1997 Evaluation of the feline erythron in health and disease. Compend Contin Edu Practis Vet 19: 335–346

Griot-Wenk ME, Giger U 1995 Feline transfusion medicine. Vet Clin North Am 25: 1305–1322

Harrell K, Parrow J, Kristensen A 1997 Canine transfusion reactions. Part I. Causes and consequences. Compend Contin Edu Pract Vet 19: 181–189

Harrell K, Parrow J, Kristensen A 1997 Canine transfusion reactions. Part II. Prevention and treatment. Compend Contin Edu Pract Vet 19: 193–200

Pratt PW (ed) 1997 Laboratory procedures for veterinary technicians, 3rd edn. Mosby, St Louis

Reagan WJ, Sanders T, De Nicola DP 1998 Veterinary haematology. Atlas of common domestic species. Manson Publishing, London

Reyers F 1994 Haemogram patterns in disease. In: Proceedings of the WSAVA XIX World Congress. Durban, pp 109–122

Multiple choice questions and answers

FLUID MANAGEMENT

1. The total body water content of a 12-year-old, obese Golden Retriever weighing 32 kg can be estimated as:
   a. 17.6 litres
   b. 19.2 litres
   c. 22.4 litres
   d. 25.6 litres

2. The ionic composition of ECF consists primarily of:
   a. bicarbonate, chloride and potassium
   b. bicarbonate, chloride and sodium
   c. chloride, magnesium and sodium
   d. sodium, magnesium and phosphate

3. The normal range of pH of the ECF is:
   a. 6.80–6.90
   b. 7.20–7.30
   c. 7.35–7.45
   d. 7.65–7.75

4. Two intravenous fluid therapy products that contain lactate as a precursor of bicarbonate are:
   a. Darrow's and Hartmann's solutions
   b. Darrow's and Ringer's solutions
   c. Dextran and Hartmann's solution
   d. Hartmann's and Ringer's solutions

5. The approximate volume of pre-existing fluid deficit in a 12 kg dog presented with a mild to moderate decrease in skin turgor, dry oral mucous membranes, slight tachycardia but normal pulse character is:
   a. 600 ml
   b. 840 ml

c. 1200 ml
d. 1800 ml

6. The total blood volume of a 25 kg German Shepherd can be calculated as approximately:
   a. 1500 ml
   b. 1950 ml
   c. 2250 ml
   d. 2500 ml

7. Hypocalcaemia following blood transfusion is most likely to occur:
   a. with rates of transfusion of 22 ml/kg per 24 hours or less
   b. in animals with acute renal failure
   c. in hypothermic animals
   d. when EDTA is used as the anticoagulant

8. Fatal immunologic blood transfusion reactions in cats are most commonly seen when:
   a. type A cats receive type B blood
   b. type B cats receive type A blood
   c. type B cats receive type AB blood
   d. both (b) and (c)

9. A major cross-match is necessary prior to the administration of:
   a. packed red cells
   b. plasma
   c. whole blood
   d. both (a) and (c)

10. The complication of exsanguination in fluid therapy patients is specifically prevented by:
    a. immobilising the limb that contains the catheter with a splint
    b. leaving catheters in situ for a maximum of 48 hours
    c. reinforcing giving set attachments with tape
    d. using the largest size intravenous catheter

INFECTIOUS DISEASES

11. A non-infectious disease may be defined as one that:
    a. is caused by a micro-organism and can be passed on to another susceptible animal
    b. can be spread by direct or indirect contact
    c. is caused by an upset within the various systems of the body

d. causes a rise in the number of cases in a particular area

12. The unit used to measure the size of bacteria is the:
    a. metre
    b. millimetre
    c. nanometre
    d. micrometre

13. Which of the following statements is false?
    a. Gram stain is one of the methods used to differentiate between species of bacteria
    b. *Staphylococcus, Escherichia* and *Bacillus* are all species of protozoa
    c. Viruses are obligate intracellular parasites
    d. *Rickettsia* and *Chlamydia* share characteristics with both bacteria and viruses

14. An inanimate object which may be responsible for the spread of disease is known as a:
    a. fomite
    b. vector
    c. pathogen
    d. paratenic host

15. Which of the following disinfectants is not suitable for use in cat kennels?
    a. Trigene
    b. Virkon
    c. Domestos
    d. Jeyes fluid

16. Disinfection may be defined as a process by which:
    a. bacterial growth is prevented
    b. all micro-organisms are killed with the exception of bacterial spores
    c. all micro-organisms are killed including bacterial spores
    d. growth of micro-organisms is reduced

17. The incubation period of canine distemper is:
    a. 1–6 months
    b. 3–4 weeks
    c. 7–10 days
    d. 1–2 days

18. Immunisation by antibodies derived from the dam is classified as:
    a. passive natural
    b. active natural
    c. passive artificial
    d. active artificial

19. Viral haemorrhagic disease seen in the rabbit is caused by a:
    a. poxvirus
    b. spirochaete
    c. lyssavirus
    d. calicivirus
20. Which of the following statements is true?
    a. Feline infectious anaemia is spread between cats by fomites such as feeding bowls and litter trays
    b. Cats that have recovered from feline infectious enteritis can become carriers of the virus
    c. Myxomatosis in rabbits causes a dry hacking cough and infection of the larynx and trachea
    d. Vaccination with live CAV 1 antigen protects against kennel cough and infectious canine hepatitis

COMMON MEDICAL DISEASES

21. The most appropriate method of assessment of renal function is:
    a. plain radiography and blood samples
    b. dipstick urinalysis
    c. blood sample analysis and urine analysis (dipstick and specific gravity)
    d. any of the above
22. The most appropriate diet for an underweight dog with diabetes is:
    a. high-fibre, low-fat, medium-protein diet
    b. convalescent diet (high-calorie), high-fat, high-carbohydrate
    c. meat-only (high protein)
    d. high-carbohydrate, low-fat, medium-protein diet
23. A dog with immune-mediated haemolytic anaemia is admitted to hospital for treatment. The dog is initially mildly jaundiced but you notice over the next few days that the dog is becoming more yellow although its PCV remains constant and it seems bright. What would you conclude from this finding?
    a. the doses of treatment should be increased because haemolysis is still occurring

b. the dose of treatment should be reduced because the dog is reacting to the therapy
    c. this may be normal but the dog should be closely monitored for signs of clinical deterioration
    d. the products of RBC destruction have caused liver damage
24. Pruritic skin disease is not a typical clinical sign associated with:
    a. bacterial skin disease
    b. atopy
    c. sarcoptic mange
    d. endocrine disease
25. Induction of emesis should be avoided in the management of poisoning when:
    a. the ingestion occurred more than 2 hours previously
    b. the patient has a reduced gag reflex
    c. caustic substances have been ingested
    d. all the above
26. The safest radiographic position for examination of a sedated dyspnoeic patient is:
    a. ventrodorsal view
    b. dorsoventral view
    c. lateral view
    d. none – dyspnoeic patients should not be sedated
27. Dyspnoea due to pulmonary oedema as a result of acute heart failure is best managed by:
    a. intravenous diuretics
    b. cage rest
    c. a combination of cage rest and intravenous diuretics
    d. oxygen supplementation by mask
28. Which one of the following procedures should be avoided in the pregnant bitch?
    a. physical examination
    b. routine vaccination
    c. ultrasonography
    d. treatment for worms
29. You are presented with a dog in status epilepticus – the most appropriate first line of action is:
    a. leave it in a quiet dark kennel to recover
    b. administer long-acting barbiturates to induce anaesthesia

c. attempt to control seizures with short-acting anticonvulsant, e.g. diazepam per rectum or intravenously

d. collect samples for analysis and wait for results before initiating any therapy

30. Which one of these ophthalmic conditions does not require to be seen urgently by a vet?
    a. corneal ulcer
    b. pannus
    c. glaucoma
    d. 'red eye' of unknown cause

31. Which of these drugs is *not* commonly used in the management of early canine degenerative joint disease?
    a. glycosaminoglycans
    b. carprofen
    c. phenylbutazone
    d. prednisolone

32. The most common nutritional bone disease seen in small animal patients is:
    a. metaphyseal osteopathy
    b. nutritional secondary hyperparathyroidism
    c. hypertrophic osteopathy
    d. craniomandibular osteopathy

33. What will the results of synovial fluid analysis be in a patient with septic arthritis?
    a. turbid, decreased viscosity, increased volume, increased numbers of neutrophils
    b. turbid, increased viscosity, increased volume, increased numbers of neutrophils
    c. turbid, increased viscosity, decreased volume, increased numbers of neutrophils
    d. turbid, decreased viscosity, increased volume, increased numbers of monocytes

34. Which of the following disorders tends to show erosive changes on radiography?
    a. systemic lupus erythematosus
    b. idiopathic polyarthritis
    c. haemophilic arthritis
    d. rheumatoid arthritis

35. Which of the following terms accurately describes all ligament injuries?
    a. sprain
    b. strain
    c. rupture
    d. avulsion

MEDICAL DIAGNOSTICS

36. The menace response is a test of cranial nerves
    a. II (optic) and III (oculomotor)
    b. III (oculomotor) and IV (trochlear)
    c. II (optic) and VII (facial)
    d. II (optic) and V (trigeminal)

37. All of the following statements about hind-limb spinal reflexes are true *except*:
    a. they depend on the presence of an intact reflex arc
    b. they are a good test of pain sensation in animals with traumatic spinal cord damage, particularly the withdrawal reflex
    c. reflexes are usually reduced to absent with lower motor neurone disease
    d. reflexes are usually normal to increased in upper motor neurone disease

38. All of the following statements about the total T_4 assay are correct *except*:
    a. Total T_4 is cheap and widely available
    b. it is generally preferred over the use of T_3 assay for diagnosis of both canine hypothyroidism and feline hyperthyroidism
    c. it may be combined with endogenous TSH for greater specificity in the diagnosis of canine hypothyroidism
    d. it is unaffected by concurrent drug therapy

39. All of the following statements about the diagnosis of hyperadrenocorticism (Cushing's disease) are true *except*:
    a. the ACTH stimulation test may be used to monitor efficacy of treatment in dogs on Mitotane therapy
    b. the low-dose dexamethasone suppression test requires care in accurately drawing up the dexamethasone as only very small quantities are used
    c. the urine cortisol:creatinine ratio can be used as a sole diagnostic test for positively identifying Cushing's disease
    d. samples for endogenous ACTH measurement require special handling and immediate freezing

40. Of the following statements about canine pancreatic disease which is true?
    a. amylase and lipase are invariably raised in the presence of pancreatitis
    b. the TLI test is the most reliable diagnostic test for exocrine pancreatic insufficiency (EPI)
    c. serum lipase levels are unaffected by any concurrent medications
    d. amylase and lipase are unaffected by the presence of renal disease

41. Which of the following statements is false?
    a. a raised serum total bilirubin may be due to haemolysis
    b. a raised serum total bilirubin may be due to hepatocellular damage
    c. a raised serum total bilirubin may be due to post-hepatic obstruction
    d. analysis of the ratio of conjugated: unconjugated bilirubin is a useful test to discriminate between these

42. Which of the following should *not* be performed prior to collecting cerebrospinal fluid (CSF) for diagnostic purposes?
    a. administration of corticosteroids
    b. a neurological examination
    c. an ophthalmic examination
    d. assessment for the possibility of a cervical fracture

43. Which of the following statements concerning urine collection by cystocentesis are false?
    a. cystocentesis is rapidly and easily performed and is well tolerated by most conscious patients
    b. there is considerable risk in performing cystocentesis on an overly distended bladder
    c. urine samples collected by cystocentesis should be allowed to stand and be refrigerated prior to analysis
    d. urine collected by cystocentesis is preferred over other methods for culture

44. Which of the following statements about bone marrow aspiration is false?
    a. it is a painful procedure and should be pre-empted with appropriate analgesia or general anaesthesia
    b. sterile technique is essential, particularly in neutropenic patients
    c. it is indicated in many cases of non-regenerative anaemias
    d. there is significant risk of haemorrhage in thrombocytopenic animals

45. Which of the following statements concerning pericardiocentesis is false?
    a. an enlarged heart due to dilated cardiomyopathy should always be differentiated from pericardial effusion before drainage is attempted
    b. blood drained from the heart should clot if left to stand and this should always be performed soon after drainage is commenced
    c. the character of the drained fluid is usually diagnostic of the underlying disease
    d. ultrasonography is invaluable in assessing the heart for tumours that may cause effusion

46. Which of the following instruments would be most useful for rhinoscopy?
    a. arthroscope
    b. gastroscope
    c. bronchoscope
    d. proctoscope

47. The diameter of each glass fibre in a fibre-optic endoscope is approximately:
    a. 1 µm
    b. 10 µm
    c. 100 µm
    d. 10 mm

48. Which of the following statements is true?
    a. video-endoscopes are cheaper than fibre-optic endoscopes
    b. video-endoscopes have an eyepiece
    c. Xenon light sources are brighter than tungsten–halogen bulbs
    d. the insertion tube is the part inserted into the light source

49. Which of the following is a contraindication for endoscopy?
    a. heart murmur
    b. coughing
    c. vomiting
    d. bleeding disorder

50. The correct positioning for gastroscopy is:
    a. left lateral recumbency
    b. dorsal recumbency
    c. right lateral recumbency
    d. sternal recumbency
51. The correct positioning for percutaneous endoscopic placement of a gastrostomy tube is:
    a. left lateral recumbency
    b. dorsal recumbency
    c. right lateral recumbency
    d. sternal recumbency
52. Nitrous oxide should not be used during gastroscopy because:
    a. it is explosive
    b. it damages the gastric mucosa
    c. it causes over-distension
    d. it damages the endoscope
53. The correct order in which to clean an endoscope is:
    a. external cleaning – brushing – flushing – drying
    b. brushing – external cleaning – flushing – drying
    c. external cleaning – brushing – drying – flushing
    d. flushing – external cleaning – brushing – drying
54. A flexible endoscope can be sterilised with all except one of the following:
    a. ethylene oxide
    b. ethyl alcohol
    c. gluteraldehyde
    d. steam
55. The electrocardiograph is:
    a. the machine that detects and records the electrical activity of the heart
    b. the recording of the electrical activity of the heart
    c. the study of the electrical activity of the heart
    d. the recording of the physical activity of the heart
56. The ECG trace indicates:
    a. the contraction of the heart
    b. the pulse rate
    c. the electrical activity of the heart
    d. the cardiac output
57. Which of the following does not reduce the quality of the ECG trace?
    a. patient movement
    b. poor electrode contact
    c. electrical fields generated by other equipment
    d. use of electroconductive gel
58. Which of the following may produce a 50 Hz fluctuation in the ECG trace?
    a. patient movement
    b. fluorescent lighting
    c. sinus arrhythmia
    d. good electrode contact
59. The P wave is a result of:
    a. atrial repolarisation
    b. ventricular depolarisation
    c. ventricular repolarisation
    d. atrial depolarisation
60. Which of these is not a feature of atrial fibrillation?
    a. absence of P waves in all leads
    b. irregular R-R intervals
    c. bradycardia
    d. associated with atrial enlargement
61. In the context of the ECG, the term 'lead' is most appropriately used to indicate:
    a. the supply cord of the machine
    b. the cable between each electrode and the machine
    c. the electrical connection between two points on the patient's body surface
    d. the connection of the electrode to the patient
62. Electrical interference artefact can *not* be reduced by:
    a. patient positioning
    b. turning off unnecessary equipment
    c. avoiding tangling the ECG cables
    d. ensuring good contact between the patient skin and electrode
63. Which dysrhythmia is often associated with splenic disease?
    a. sinus arrhythmia
    b. ventricular premature complexes
    c. third-degree AV block
    d. atrial fibrillation
64. The standard position of the dog for a diagnostic ECG is:

a. standing
b. sternal recumbency
c. left lateral recumbency
d. Right lateral recumbency

LABORATORY DIAGNOSTICS

65. Which one of the following statements is false?
    a. food should not be consumed in a laboratory
    b. latex gloves are recommended when working with blood
    c. smoking should not be permitted in the laboratory
    d. mouth pipetting is an acceptable technique

66. Which of the following are potential sources of error in laboratory testing?
    a. collection of a non-fasted sample, resulting in lipaemia
    b. failure to label the sample with the owner's name and time of collection
    c. improper use of pipettes
    d. all of the above

67. Samples which are required for a routine haematology profile are:
    a. lithium heparin + blood smear
    b. EDTA + blood smear
    c. sodium citrate + blood smear
    d. EDTA

68. A reticulocyte count helps to differentiate between:
    a. regenerative and non-regenerative anaemia
    b. haemolytic anaemia and haemorrhage
    c. inflammation and a corticosteroid-mediated leucocytosis
    d. inflammation and an adrenaline (epinephrine)-mediated leucocytosis

69. Döhle bodies are associated with:
    a. viral disease
    b. neoplasia
    c. haemorrhage
    d. bacterial infection

70. Which of the following tests is used in the confirmation of vitamin K antagonism, e.g. in rodenticide toxicity?

a. platelet count
b. buccal mucosal bleeding time
c. one-stage prothrombin time
d. Von Willebrand's factor

71. Which one of the following tests is not a hepatic function indicator:
    a. albumin
    b. bilirubin
    c. bile acids
    d. GGT

72. Which of the following could affect the liver enzymes:
    a. glucocorticoid therapy
    b. cardiac disease
    c. intestinal disease
    d. all of the above

73. Hypercalcaemia is commonly associated with:
    a. hyperadrenocorticism
    b. diabetes mellitus
    c. hypothyroidism
    d. neoplasia

74. Which of the following is not used in the investigation of hyperadrenocorticism?
    a. low-dose dexamethasone suppression test
    b. urinary cortisol:creatinine ratio
    c. high-dose dexamethasone suppression test
    d. urinary protein:creatinine ratio

MULTIPLE CHOICE ANSWERS

1 a
2 b
3 c
4 a
5 b
6 c
7 c
8 d
9 d
10 c
11 c
12 d
13 b
14 a
15 d
16 b

17	c		46	a
18	a		47	b
19	d		48	c
20	b		49	d
21	c		50	a
22	d		51	c
23	c		52	c
24	d		53	a
25	d		54	d
26	b		55	a
27	c		56	c
28	b		57	d
29	c		58	b
30	b		59	d
31	d		60	c
32	b		61	c
33	a		62	a
34	d		63	b
35	a		64	d
36	c		65	d
37	b		66	d
38	d		67	b
39	c		68	a
40	b		69	d
41	d		70	c
42	a		71	d
43	c		72	d
44	d		73	d
45	c		74	d

Index